CRASH COURSE

Third Editio

Neurology

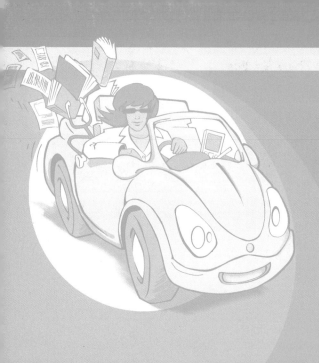

First edition authors:

Anish Bahra and Katia Cikurel

CRASH COURSE

Third Edition

Neurology

Series editor
Daniel Horton-Szar
BSc (Hons), MBBS (Hons), MRCGP
Northgate Medical Practice
Canterbury
Kent, UK

Faculty advisor
Jeremy Gibbs
MD, FRCP
Consultant Neurologist and Honorary
Senior Lecturer
Department of Neuroscience
Royal Free Hospital
London, UK

Christopher Turner
BSc, MBChB, MRCP

Consultant Neurologist
National Hospital for Neurology and
Neurosurgery Hospital
London, UK

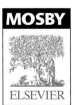

MOSBY
ELSEVIER

Edinburgh • London • New York • Oxford • Philadelphia • St Louis • Sydney • Toronto 2009

MOSBY
ELSEVIER

Commissioning Editor: Alison Taylor
Development Editor: Clive Hewat
Project Manager: Christine Johnston
Page Design: Sarah Russell
Icon Illustrations: Geo Parkin
Cover Design: Stewart Larking
Illustration Management: Merlyn Harvey

First edition 1999
Second edition 2006
Third edition 2009

ISBN: 978-0-7234-3469-6

British Library Cataloguing in Publication Data
A catalogue record for this book is available from the British Library

Library of Congress Cataloging in Publication Data
A catalog record for this book is available from the Library of Congress

Note
Knowledge and best practice in this field are constantly changing. As new research and experience broaden our knowledge, changes in practice, treatment and drug therapy may become necessary or appropriate. Readers are advised to check the most current information provided (i) on procedures featured or (ii) by the manufacturer of each product to be administered, to verify the recommended dose or formula, the method and duration of administration, and contraindications. It is the responsibility of the practitioner, relying on their own experience and knowledge of the patient, to make diagnoses, to determine dosages and the best treatment for each individual patient, and to take all appropriate safety precautions. To the fullest extent of the law, neither the Publisher nor the Authors assumes any liability for any injury and/or damage to persons or property arising out of or related to any use of the material contained in this book.

The Publisher

Working together to grow
libraries in developing countries

www.elsevier.com | www.bookaid.org | www.sabre.org

ELSEVIER   **BOOK AID**   Sabre Foundation
                International

ELSEVIER   **your source for books,**
              journals and multimedia
              in the health sciences
www.elsevierhealth.com

The
publisher's
policy is to use
**paper manufactured
from sustainable forests**

Printed in China

Preface

Neurology often appears a daunting subject for most medical students and junior doctors. This book aims to provide a logical and simple approach to understanding the fundamental concepts that underlie most common neurological diseases. Illustrations and diagrams have been used as much as possible to emphasize these concepts. In the third edition comprehension boxes have been added, to focus the reader on the essential topics, and communication boxes which highlight dealing with common but difficult, clinical scenarios. There has been a move towards removing unnecessary and over-detailed material and replace it with more in depth discussions of important concepts.

Crash Course Neurology will provide a solid foundation not only for medical students preparing for exams and postgraduates working towards MRCP but also an excellent reference book for those working in hospital medicine and general practice.

Chris Turner

All medical students and doctors need to acquire and maintain some basic skills in neurology. Neurological symptoms account for a high proportion of consultations in general practice, 20% of acute medical admissions and many complications of trauma, critical illness, anaesthesia, and surgery. Diagnosis is primarily clinical, based on a careful history and physical examination, and any number of subsequent investigations can only supplement and never replace the process of clinical assessment.

Crash Course Neurology is a concise text presenting a lucid and systematic approach to neurological diagnosis and management. Part I of the book deals with the analysis and differential diagnosis of common presenting symptoms such as headache, dizziness, speech disturbance and limb weakness. In Parts II and III the clinical features, investigation and management of specific neurological disorders are discussed in more detail. The self-assessment questions and patient management problems at the end provide a useful check on the learning process and additional stimulus to effective reading.

The book is clearly written and logically set out, with numerous diagrams, lists and tables to facilitate learning and revision. It is primarily designed as an introduction to neurology for students, and a revision text for both finals and MRCP, but the general approach and much of the material could be usefully revisited by fully qualified doctors who encounter neurological problems during the course of their work.

Jeremy Gibbs
Faculty Advisor

More than a decade has now passed since work began on the first editions of the Crash Course series, and over four years since the publication of the second editions. Medicine never stands still, and the work of keeping this series relevant for today's students is an ongoing process. These third editions build upon the success of the preceding books and incorporate a great deal of new and revised material, keeping the series up to date with the latest medical research and developments in pharmacology and current best practice.

As always, we listen to feedback from the thousands of students who use Crash Course and have made further improvements to the layout and structure of the books. Each chapter now starts with a set of learning objectives, and the self-assessment sections have been enhanced and brought up to date with modern exam formats. We have also worked to integrate material on communication skills and gems of clinical wisdom from practising doctors. This will not only add to the interest of the text but will reinforce the principles being described.

Despite fully revising the books, we hold fast to the principles on which we first developed the series: Crash Course will always bring you all the information you need to revise in compact, manageable volumes that integrate pathology and therapeutics with best clinical practice. The books still maintain the balance between clarity and conciseness, and providing sufficient depth for those aiming at distinction. The authors are junior doctors who have recent experience of the exams you are now facing, and the accuracy of the material is checked by senior clinicians and faculty members from across the UK.

I wish you all the best for your future careers!

Dr Dan Horton-Szar
Series Editor

Acknowledgements

My gratitude goes to Jeremy Gibbs for providing a constant source of questioning, guidance and feedback.

Chris Turner

Dedication

To my loving wife, Emma, for her love and patience

To my special little girl, Sophie Olivia, for all the happiness she brings

To my parents for their unwavering belief in truth and honesty

To my brother for his incentive and inspiration.

Contents

Contents

Glossary

A

acalculia difficulty in performing simple mental arithmetic.

ageusia loss of taste sensation.

agnosia deficit of higher sensory processing caused by impaired recognition.

agraphaesthesia loss of the ability to recognize numbers or letters traced on the skin.

akathisia feeling of inner restlessness associated with repetitive movements of a purposeless nature.

akinesia inability to initiate a voluntary movement.

amyotrophy wasting of muscle.

anarthria inability to articulate.

anisocoria unequal pupil size.

anosognosia patients unawareness of their illness.

apraxia inability to perform a motor sequence with preserved motor, sensory and coordination functions.

astereognosis inability to recognize an object placed in the hand with eyes closed and intact peripheral sensation.

athetosis involuntary movements characterized by slow writhing purposeless movements.

aura a neurological phenomenon occurring seconds to minutes before a migraine headache or epileptic seizure.

B

ballismus wild flailing movements of the limbs.

Broca's aphasia non-fluent, slow, laboured effortful speech, but patient can recognize errors in own speech. Comprehension often preserved for simple material. Repetition, reading, writing and naming impaired, but naming may be helped by contextual cues.

C

cataplexy sudden loss of lower limb tone leading to falls without loss of consciousness.

chorea involuntary hyperkinetic movement disorder associated with jerky, restlessness, purposeless movements which move from one part of the body to another in an unpredictable way.

coma a state of unresponsiveness to verbal or mechanical stimuli.

D

déjà vu an inappropriate feeling of overfamiliarization with the environment.

delirium a neurobehavioural syndrome associated with problems with attention.

dementia loss of intellectual functions leading to impaired function or behaviour.

dissociated sensory loss impairment of some but not all sensory modalities.

dysdiadochokinesia difficulty in performing rapid alternating movements.

dyskinesia excessive involuntary movements, e.g. chorea, athetosis.

dysmetria abnormal control of range of movement.

dysphagia difficulty swallowing.

dysphonia disorder of volume, pitch or quality of voice due to dysfunction of the larynx.

dystonia sustained involuntary muscle contraction.

E

encephalopathy general term for diffuse disturbance of brain function.

F

fasciculation rapid, flickering movements within a muscle associated with spontaneous activity of a motor unit. Sometimes described as 'worms under the skin'.

fibrillation spontaneous contraction of single muscle fibres. These cannot be seen by eye and are detected electrophysiologically.

frontal release signs a group of reflexes which are usually absent in healthy adults but may be found following a wide range of disorders of the CNS. Their anatomical localization is vague even though they are still referred to as the 'frontal release signs' and 'primitive reflexes' may be a more appropriate term as it suggests that these are reflexes which are inhibited as the brain develops.

G

gait apraxia the inability/impairment to walk in spite of preserved motor sensory and coordination functions. It usually occurs with lesions of the frontal lobes and its white matter connections.

Gower's sign a typical movement made by a patient with proximal lower limb weakness where the arms are used to climb up the legs in order to stand from lying on the floor.

'glove and sock' sensory/motor loss the loss of sensation and power in a polyneuropathy is typically worse distally then proximally. This is often referred to as 'glove and stocking' but the loss rarely extends up to the mid-thigh and usually stops mid-calf.

glabellar tap reflex tap on the forehead produces blinking which habituates in most people. If this fails to habituate then it used to be felt that it was a useful diagnostic sign of idiopathic Parkinson's disease. Unfortunately, it is often positive in normal aged individuals and in other extra-pyramidal disorders and is therefore usually not clinically useful.

H

hemianopia a defect of one half of the visual field.

Horner's syndrome partial ptosis, meiosis and anhydrosis associated with dysfunction in the sympathetic supply to the eye.

hypomimia reduction of voluntary facial expression.

I

internuclear ophthalmoplegia failure or slowing of adduction during horizontal conjugate gaze with or without gaze-evoked nystagmus in the abducting eye secondary to a lesion in the medial longitudinal fasciculus.

J

Jacksonian march sequential spread of a simple partial usually motor seizure, e.g. hand, elbow then shoulder which may terminate spontaneously or with a secondary generalized seizure.

K

Kayser–Fleischer rings green/brown deposits of copper in Descemet's membrane which can usually only be seen with slit lamp examination and highly suggestive of Wilson's disease.

Kernig's sign pain in the lower back and neck and resistance to passive extension of the knee when the thigh is flexed secondary to meningitis.

L

Lhermitte's sign electric shock-like sensation down the arms and legs following flexion of the neck due to a lesion within the cervical cord.

locked-in syndrome severe damage to the ventral pons causing loss of the ascending and descending tracts to the spinal cord, pons and medulla so that the patient can only move the eyes, often vertically, and blink. It is usually caused by basilar artery thrombosis.

M

marche à petit pas small stepped, often wide based, shuffling gait without a flexed posture or festination of idiopathic Parkinson's disease caused by bilateral frontal cortical or white matter damage usually secondary to small vessel disease.

Marcus Gunn pupil delay or failure of constriction of a pupil to direct light due to a lesion in the optic nerve.

micrographia small handwriting. This is often seen in idiopathic Parkinson's disease and starts normally but fatigues and becomes small.

myelopathy a disorder of the spinal cord which is usually associated with a sensory level near the level of the lesion, upper motor neuron weakness below the lesion, sometimes lower motor neuron signs at the level of the lesion and sphincter disturbance.

myoclonus involuntary 'shock-like' contraction resulting in a jerking movement usually of the limbs, trunk or neck.

myotonia inability to relax a muscle following contraction.

N

neglect inability to respond to or attend to a sensory stimulus.

nystagmus involuntary oscillation of the eyes which can be pathological or physiological.

O

oculocephalic response (Doll's eye movements) the eyes remain fixated on an object when the head is passively moved and is a sign of an intact pontine brainstem reflex.

optokinetic nystagmus a physiological involuntary conjugate pursuit eye movement in response to a moving object with a return saccade when the object disappears out of vision, e.g. looking out of a moving train.

P

papilloedema swelling of the optic disc head secondary to raised intracranial pressure.

paraplegia severe/total weakness of both legs.

parkinsonism a constellation of signs associated with some or all of the features of bradykinesia, rigidity, tremor and postural instability.

pes cavus high arched feet due to imbalance in the muscular contractions acting on the feet usually associated with genetic neuropathies, e.g. Charcot–Marie–Tooth or due to an early neurological insult, e.g. cerebral palsy.

Phalen's sign tingling in the distribution of the median nerve when the wrist is forced flexed at 90° and is associated with carpal tunnel syndrome.

phonophobia dislike or fear of loud noises.

photophobia dislike or fear of bright lights.

pseudobulbar palsy impairment of bilateral corticobulbar fibres associated with dysphagia, dysarthria, brisk jaw jerk slow and spastic tongue and exaggerated gag reflex.

pseudodementia global impairment of cognitive functions due to affective disorders (anxiety/ depression) which mimics dementia caused by organic pathology, e.g. Alzheimer's disease.

ptosis drooping of the eylid.

pyramidal synonymous with corticospinal and upper motor neuron.

Q

quadrantanopia loss of a quarter of the visual field.

quadriplegia total or severe loss of power in all four limbs.

R

radiculopathy disorder of the nerve roots causing sensory loss in the corresponding dermatome, motor loss in the corresponding myotome, reflex loss and pain in a radicular distribution.

rigidity increased resistance to passive movement that is equal throughout the range of movement and is associated with extra-pyramidal disease.

Romberg's sign increase in unsteadiness when a standing patient closes their eyes and is associated with proprioceptive loss to the feet.

S

saccades rapid movements of the eyes which move the focus from one point to another.

scotoma a localized area of impaired vision.

spasticity increased resistance to passive movement at a joint which varies with amplitude and velocity and is associated with a lesion in the upper motor neuron.

supranuclear gaze palsy impairment of the supranuclear connections to the nuclei of the nerves supplying the extraocular muscles leading to preservation of reflex, but loss of voluntary, eye movements.

T

tandem gait the ability to walk in a straight line with one foot in front of the other. This is impaired in midline cerebellar disorders.

Tinel's sign parasthaesia following tapping of a trapped or regenerating peripheral nerve.

Todd's paresis transient localized weakness following a seizure usually lasting seconds or minutes.

U

Uhthoff's phenomenon worsening of visual acuity with exercise or other causes of increased body temperature in optic neuritis related to temperature sensitivity of demyelinated axons.

upper motor neuron the cell in the primary motor cortex which projects its axon down through the internal capsule and spinal cord to synapse with the lower motor neuron.

V

vegetative state clinical syndrome associated with extensive loss of cognitive function but preserved vegetative function, e.g. respiration and autonomic. It has a very poor prognosis.

W

Wernicke's aphasia fluent aphasia with phonemic and semantic paraphrasias, impaired comprehension, impaired repetition, severely impaired naming, reading and writing.

THE PATIENT PRESENTS WITH

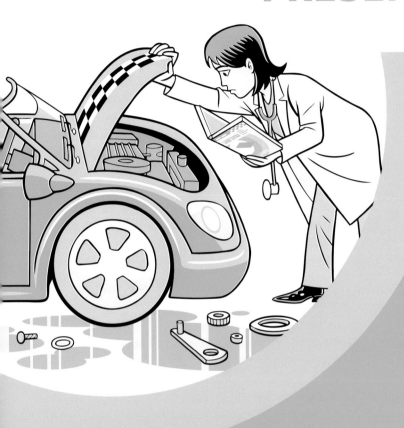

Disorders of higher cerebral function

The term 'cognition' refers to our ability to perform complex intellectual behaviours such as speaking and writing, navigating our way around our environment, recognizing other people, and comprehending time.

Dementia is a syndrome in which several aspects of cognitive function are impaired; it is often associated with diffuse disease of the cerebral cortices. Disease of structures encased by the cerebral cortices or 'subcortical structures', such as the basal ganglia, also has a role in cognition and these structures are affected in many dementias (e.g. Huntington's disease).

Alzheimer's disease and generalized vascular disease are the most common causes of dementia. Localized cortical lesions cause more well-defined cognitive dysfunction, such as isolated aphasia or agnosia, and are called 'focal deficits'.

The left and right cerebral hemispheres each contain a frontal, parietal, temporal, and occipital lobe (Fig. 1.1). Each lobe has distinct cognitive functions. The side of the brain that controls writing and speech is called the 'dominant' hemisphere and the other side is the 'non-dominant' hemisphere.

The left hemisphere is dominant in over 90% of right-handed people and in about 60% of left-handed people.

FRONTAL LOBE

Normal functions

- Primary motor cortex: this is located in the precentral gyrus and is concerned with motor function of the opposite side of the body. The upper motor neuron cell bodies are topographically organized in the primary motor cortex in a 'homunculus' (Fig. 1.2). These neurons project axons in the corticospinal and corticobulbar tracts. The axons travel in the internal capsule to reach the brainstem and spinal cord to synapse with lower motor neuron cell bodies.
- Supplementary motor and premotor cortices: these areas are concerned with coordinating and planning complex movements.
- Frontal eye field: this is involved in making eye movements to the contralateral side.
- Broca's area (dominant hemisphere only): the motor or 'expressive' centre for the production of speech.
- Prefrontal cortex: the anterior and orbital parts of the frontal cortex govern personality, emotional expression, initiative, and the ability to plan.
- The cortical micturition centre: this region lies in the paracentral lobule and is involved in the cortical inhibition of voiding of the bladder and bowel.

The blood supply to the frontal lobe is from the anterior cerebral artery (ACA) and middle cerebral artery (MCA). The ACA supplies the medial surface of the primary motor cortex, which controls the leg; the MCA supplies the lateral surface of the primary motor cortex, which controls the face and arm (see Chapter 26).

Symptoms from lesions of the frontal lobe

- Precentral gyrus: contralateral mono- or hemiparesis and facial weakness in an upper motor neuron pattern.

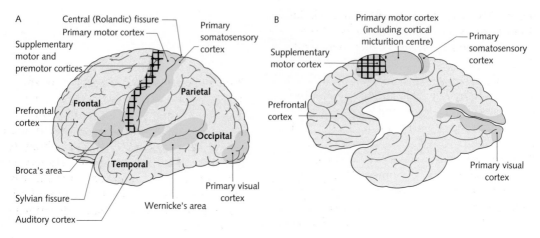

Fig. 1.1 Functional regions of the cerebral cortex. (A) Lateral left hemisphere. (B) Medial right hemisphere.

Fig. 1.2 Topographical distribution of the sensorimotor cortices or 'homunculus'.

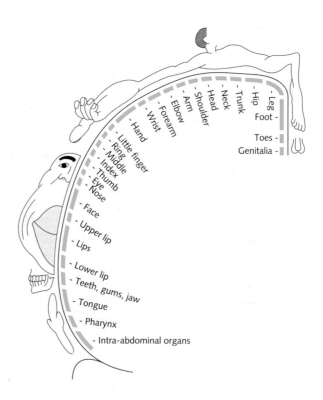

- Supplementary motor and premotor cortices: disorders of complex motor planning.
- Frontal eye field: impairment of eye movements to the contralateral side (gaze paresis). This is most commonly seen in a large middle cerebral artery stroke and carries a worse prognosis.
- Broca's area: expressive dysphasia. This comprises non-fluent, hesitant speech with intact comprehension. The patient knows what he or she

wants to say but has difficulty finding the correct words, often producing the wrong word. The ability to repeat words is better than spontaneous speech. Handwriting is also often poor.
- Prefrontal cortex: this causes altered behaviour including social disinhibition, loss of initiative and interest, inability to solve problems with loss of abstract thought, and impaired concentration and attention without intellectual or memory

decline. This usually occurs with bilateral lesions resulting from head injury, small vessel disease, frontal degenerations (e.g. the frontotemporal dementias) and acute hydrocephalus. Severe bilateral pathology, especially of the orbital surfaces, can result in akinetic mutism, in which the patient appears awake and is able to move the eyes but does not spontaneously move and is incontinent.

- Elicitation of primitive (grasping, sucking, pouting, rooting and palmomental) reflexes: these reflexes may originate from the parietal cortex and are usually inhibited by the prefrontal cortex, although the exact anatomical substrate is uncertain. They are essential as a baby but are subsequently suppressed as the child grows.
- Apraxia of gait: this is the inability to walk normally in spite of preservation of normal power, coordination, and sensory function. The gait is slow and shuffling but upright and wide based, distinct from the flexed posture and narrow base of the Parkinsonian gait (see Chapter 14).
- Incontinence of urine and/or faeces: this results from loss of cortical inhibition. There is no desire to micturate. Milder symptoms are frequency and urgency of micturition.

Focal seizures arising from the frontal cortex give rise to clonic movements of the contralateral lower face, arm, and leg, and conjugate deviation of the head and eyes towards the convulsing side (i.e. away from the side of the lesion).

Lesions of the inferior or 'orbital' frontal lobes can be accompanied by disturbances of the olfactory pathway and optic nerves as a result of the close proximity of these pathways to the orbital surfaces of the lobes.

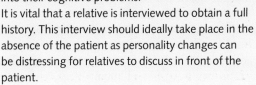

Patients with frontal lobe disease often have poor insight into their cognitive problems. It is vital that a relative is interviewed to obtain a full history. This interview should ideally take place in the absence of the patient as personality changes can be distressing for relatives to discuss in front of the patient.

PARIETAL LOBE

Function

- Primary somatosensory cortex (dominant and non-dominant): this is located in the postcentral gyrus and is concerned with perceiving complex somatosensory stimuli from the contralateral side of the face and body. It receives afferent (incoming) projections via the thalamus from the somatosensory pathways. The fibres are represented topographically, in a homunculus, similar to that of the primary motor cortex.
- Language (dominant hemisphere): pathways within the arcuate fasciculus connecting Broca's area (frontal) with Wernicke's area (posterior temporal) pass through the inferior parietal region.
- Use of numbers, e.g. calculation (dominant hemisphere).
- Integration of somatosensory, visual, and auditory information (mainly non-dominant): this allows awareness of the body and its surroundings, appropriate movement of the body, and constructional ability.
- Visual pathways (dominant and non-dominant): the upper part of the optic radiation (subserving the lower quadrant of the contralateral visual field) passes deep within the parietal lobe and might be affected in lesions of the deep white matter.

The blood supply to the parietal lobe is from the MCA.

Symptoms from lesions of the parietal lobe

- Discriminative sensory impairment of the opposite side of the face and limbs (dominant and non-dominant): there is impairment of joint position sense and two-point discrimination, and inability to recognize objects by form and texture (astereognosis) or figures drawn on the hand (agraphaesthesia). Pain, temperature, touch, and vibration are intact, although their localization when applied to the body might be impaired.
- Visual disturbances. If the deeper fibres of the parietal lobe are involved, a contralateral homonymous inferior quadrantanopia can arise.

Syndromes of the dominant parietal lobe

- Wernicke's receptive 'fluent' dysphasia: this arises from inferior parietal and superior temporal lesions (Wernicke's area and dorsally). There is impaired comprehension of speech and written language. The speech is fluent but words are replaced with partly correct words and an incorrect word related to the word intended (paraphasia) or newly created meaningless words (neologisms). The speech does not make sense and the patient has poor insight into the problem.
- Gerstmann's syndrome: this consists of the inability to differentiate the right and left sides of the body, inability to distinguish the fingers of the hands (finger agnosia), and impairment of calculation (dyscalculia) and writing (dysgraphia). Difficulty with reading (dyslexia) may also occur; this is a function of the dominant parieto-occipital cortex.
- Bilateral ideomotor and ideational apraxia: this is the inability to carry out a sequence of tasks when there is normal comprehension and intact motor and sensory function. Ideomotor apraxia occurs when a patient fails to copy an action, and ideational or 'conceptual' apraxia is more profound, e.g. the patient fails to understand use of tools and objects at a basic level.

Syndromes of the non-dominant parietal lobe

- Constructional apraxia (visuospatial dysfunction): there is difficulty in drawing simple objects (e.g. a house) and with construction (e.g. using building blocks). This also occurs to a lesser extent with dominant lesions.
- Dressing apraxia: there is difficulty with putting on clothes.
- Topographical disorientation: the patient cannot find his or her way around normally familiar spaces, e.g. home.
- Contralateral sensory inattention: there is neglect of the opposite side of the body; this can be motor, sensory, or visual. For example, a hemiplegic patient may ignore the paralysed side or there may be denial of the hemiplegia (anosognosia). Sensory and visual neglect are discussed in Chapter 13.

Focal seizures of the parietal cortex manifest as sensory symptoms on the contralateral side of the body.

Descriptions on various sensations may be given (e.g. 'pins and needles', tingling) and the symptoms often 'march' from the lips and extremities to adjacent areas of the body.

TEMPORAL LOBE

Function

- Wernicke's area (dominant hemisphere): this area, in the posterior part of the superior temporal gyrus, is concerned with comprehension of written and spoken language.
- The auditory and vestibular cortices: the primary auditory cortex receives fibres arranged in order of frequency of tone. The auditory pathways from each ear project to both auditory cortices. The dominant temporal lobe is important for the comprehension of spoken words, and the non-dominant for the appreciation of sounds and music. Vestibular fibres terminate just posterior to the auditory cortex.
- The limbic system: the olfactory and gustatory cortices lie in the medial temporal lobe. The limbic system is important in memory, learning, and emotion.
- Visual pathways: the fibres of the lower part of the optic radiation (subserving the upper quadrant of the contralateral visual field) pass deep through the white matter of the temporal lobe.

The blood supply to the temporal lobe is from the posterior cerebral (medial part of the lobe) and middle cerebral (lateral part) arteries.

Symptoms from lesions of the temporal lobe

- Wernicke's area: receptive dysphasia (temporoparietal region). This is associated with fluent speech.
- Auditory agnosia: this is the inability to recognize sounds, e.g. ringing of a bell, whistling of a kettle, a melody. It occurs in lesions of the non-dominant hemisphere.
- Cortical deafness: this will occur only with bilateral lesions of the primary auditory cortices and is uncommon. The patient might be unaware of the deficit. Auditory hallucinations can occur in temporal lobe epilepsy.

Hearing is normal in auditory agnosia and Wernicke's receptive dysphasia, but the interpretation of sounds and speech are abnormal.

- Vestibular dysfunction: vestibular dysfunction from a lesion of the vestibular cortex is uncommon, but vertigo might occur as part of the aura of temporal or parietal lobe seizures.
- Olfactory and gustatory hallucinations: olfactory hallucinations and, less commonly, gustatory hallucinations can arise from lesions within the medial temporal lobe, particularly during seizures.
- Learning difficulties: difficulties with learning auditory information occur in dominant hemisphere lesions; difficulties with learning visual information occur in non-dominant hemisphere lesions.
- Memory impairment: this occurs with lesions of the medial temporal lobe involving the hippocampus and parahippocampal gyrus. Bilateral damage results in marked impairment of retention of new information.
- Emotional disturbances: emotional disturbances from damage to the limbic system can include aggression, rage, apathy, hyperorality and hypersexuality.
- Visual disturbances: a lesion involving the deeper fibres within the temporal lobe will cause a contralateral superior homonymous quadrantanopia. Complex visual hallucinations can occur in temporal lobe seizures.

Temporal lobe seizures begin with a prodrome of auditory, olfactory, gustatory, or visual hallucinations, a sensation of anxiety or fear, and often a rising epigastric sensation. There may be disturbances of memory, with feelings of familiarity (*déjà vu*) or unfamiliarity (*jamais vu*). Behavioural changes can occur. Aggression and hypersexuality are reported but are uncommon.

Dysphasia

Dysphasia is a disorder of spoken and written language; it occurs with damage of the frontal, parietal, or temporal cortices. Broca's expressive and Wernicke's receptive dysphasias occur with damage of the dominant hemisphere and are discussed

above (see pp. 4 and 6). The cortical areas subserving these functions are linked by the arcuate fasciculus, which runs in the subcortical white matter. This enables the comprehension of language with subsequent production of speech. There are other types of dysphasia associated with more isolated focal lesions:

- Conduction dysphasia: occurs with damage to the arcuate fasciculus in the dominant parietal lobe. The speech is fluent but 'jargon' and nonsensical, with paraphrasia and neologisms as in Wernicke's dysphasia. However, comprehension of language is intact, the patient is aware of the problem, and repetition is markedly impaired.
- Global dysphasia: occurs with lesions of both Broca's and Wernicke's areas. There is a combination of non-fluent speech and impaired comprehension of language. This is the most common type of dysphasia and is usually caused by a stroke affecting the left MCA territory.
- Nominal dysphasia: is an inability to name objects and arises from a lesion of the dominant parietotemporal cortex. It may occur during recovery from other dysphasias.

OCCIPITAL LOBE

Function

The function of the occipital cortex (Fig. 1.3) is the perception of vision and recognition of whatever is visualized. The blood supply is from the posterior cerebral artery but the occipital poles, subserving macular vision, have additional supply from a branch of the MCA.

Symptoms from lesions of the occipital lobe

- Contralateral homonymous hemianopic field defect: if this arises from a lesion of the posterior cerebral artery, there will be sparing of the macular area leaving central vision intact with loss of peripheral vision (see Fig. 1.3).
- Cortical blindness: bilateral occipital lesions render the patient blind, with retention of the pupillary reflexes. The patient might deny the blindness (Anton's syndrome).
- Visual agnosia: lesions of the visual association cortices cause impairment of recognition of faces and objects.

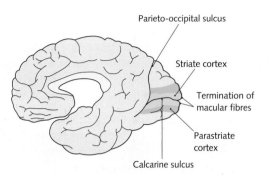

Fig. 1.3 The occipital lobe. The striate (primary visual) and parastriate (visual association) cortices are shown, and termination of the macular fibres at the poles.

- Visual illusions: objects might appear larger (macropsia) or smaller (micropsia); there might be disturbances of shape, colour, and number. This is more common with lesions of the non-dominant hemisphere.

Visual hallucinations in seizures of the primary visual cortex are unformed (flashes of light and geometric shapes); those due to seizure activity from the visual association cortex or its connections with the temporal cortex are formed (objects, people).

DIFFUSE VERSUS FOCAL CORTICAL DYSFUNCTION

Focal damage to the cerebral hemispheres usually results from vascular events (infarction or haemorrhage), tumours, trauma, or localized inflammatory/infective lesions (e.g. abscess, tuberculoma). Generalized or multifocal cerebral dysfunction results from degenerative diseases (Alzeimer's disease, dementia with Lewy bodies), multiple infarcts, demyelination, or diffuse infections (encephalitis, meningitis).

A summary of the localization of symptoms arising from focal syndromes is shown in Fig. 1.4.

Frontal lobe

Contralateral mono-/hemiparesis, facial weakness
Broca's dysphasia: Motor, expressive dysphasia (dominant)
Behavioural change: Social disinhibition, loss of abstract thought, apathy, mutism
Primitive reflexes: Grasp and sucking
Apraxic gait
Urinary incontinence
Contralateral horizontal gaze paresis

Parietal lobe

Contralateral discriminatory sensory impairment
Wernicke's dysphasia: Sensory, receptive dysphasia (dominant)
Visual field deficit: Contralateral lower homonymous quadrantanopia
Dominant syndromes: Gerstmann's syndrome, bilateral ideomotor and ideational apraxia
Non-dominant syndromes: Constructional apraxia, dressing apraxia, contralateral sensory inattention

Temporal lobe

Wernicke's dysphasia: Sensory receptive dysphasia (dominant)
Auditory agnosia: Inability to recognize sounds (non-dominant)
Visual field deficit: contralateral upper homonymous quadrantanopia
Learning difficulties: Auditory (dominant) and visual (non-dominant) information
Memory impairment
Emotional disturbances: Aggression, rage, hypersexuality, olfactory and gustatory hallucinations

Occipital lobe

Visual field deficit: Contralateral homonymous hemianopia
lesions of posterior cerebral artery – spare the macula
lesions of the middle cerebral artery/occipital pole – contralateral macular homonymous hemianopic field defect
Visual agnosia: Impaired recognition of faces and objects
Visual illusions: Disturbance of size, shape, colour and number of objects
Visual hallucinations: Unformed and formed

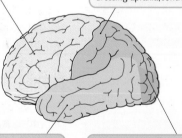

Fig. 1.4 Summary of localization of symptoms arising from focal lesions of the cerebral hemispheres.

Objectives

- Describe the common causes of transient and persistent loss or change in consciousness
- What are the clinical differences between the presentation of syncope and epilepsy?
- How would you assess a patient in a coma? What is the Glasgow Coma Scale? What are the factors that predict prognosis?
- Define the terms persistent vegetative state, non-convulsive status epilepticus, catatonia, akinetic mutism, and locked-in syndrome

When consciousness is disturbed, patients usually exhibit a loss of awareness of their external environment. The neuroanatomical and neurophysiological bases of consciousness are uncertain. The cerebral cortex is important in integrating and responding to external stimuli. The reticular system, within the brainstem, which is also modulated by external stimuli, is probably important in maintaining an 'active' or conscious cerebral cortex.

These two anatomical sites form a useful and practical way of approaching impairment of consciousness clinically, which can range from either complete loss of awareness or 'unconsciousness' through varying degrees of impairment. The duration of impaired consciousness is also important in formulating a differential diagnosis. Impairment of consciousness can be transient or short-lived with a return to normal function between attacks or ongoing, prolonged unconsciousness otherwise called 'coma'.

TRANSIENT LOSS OF CONSCIOUSNESS

Transient loss or disturbance of consciousness is a very common presenting problem. The patient usually has no ongoing symptoms or physical signs when seen, and subsequent investigations are often unhelpful in ascertaining the cause. The diagnosis depends on taking a careful history from the patient and from any available witness. Recurrent loss or disturbance of consciousness is usually due to hypotensive syncope, epilepsy, or migraine.

Hypotensive syncope

Syncope is the transient loss of consciousness and posture that results from a global reduction in blood flow to the brain. There are five common causes:

1. Vasovagal syncope

Vasovagal syncope, or 'fainting', is caused by a sudden drop in blood pressure resulting from peripheral vasodilatation. There is a subsequent reduction in cardiac output, which is followed by vagal stimulation and therefore bradycardia. Typical precipitating situations are strong emotion, sudden intense pain, and prolonged standing in hot oppressive circumstances such as a crowded train.

The patient is usually upright at the onset of syncope. Prodromal symptoms include feeling lightheaded, gradual dimming of vision, ringing in the ears, salivation, sweating, nausea, and sometimes vomiting. These symptoms can last from several seconds to a few minutes. The attack can be aborted if the patient lies flat but a patient who remains standing will lose consciousness and fall. The patient is usually pale and clammy, the pulse is low volume and slow, and the systolic blood pressure drops to approximately 60 mmHg. If this state persists for a sufficient time to cause cerebral hypoxia, the eyes may roll upward and there may be brief myoclonic movements, which can be mistaken for a seizure. This typically occurs if the patient is kept standing by unwitting onlookers and prevents a return of blood flow to the brain. Sphincter control is usually maintained and a typical postictal state is not seen, although malaise may persist.

2. Micturition and cough syncope

Micturition syncope usually occurs in men who get up during the night to pass urine. It results from a combination of vasodilatation (which occurs with emptying of the bladder), a degree of postural hypotension on standing, and bradycardia. The loss of consciousness is sudden with a rapid recovery.

Sustained coughing can elevate the intrathoracic pressure sufficiently to impair the venous return to the heart. Increase of the cerebrospinal fluid pressure, reduction in pCO_2, and resultant vasoconstriction may also be contributory. Unconsciousness may be associated with the Valsalva manoeuvre (exhalation against a closed glottis) and is seen in syncope following breath-holding attacks in children and strenuous activity (e.g. heavy lifting or laughing). The mechanism here is probably similar to cough syncope.

3. Postural hypotension

In a number of clinical conditions, the upright posture is accompanied by an uncompensated fall in blood pressure and therefore also cerebral blood flow. Postural hypotension can occur in:

- Normal individuals, especially adolescents.
- Debilitating illness with prolonged recumbency.
- Autonomic neuropathy, e.g. diabetes, Guillain–Barré syndrome, amyloidosis.
- Hypovolaemia, e.g. loss of blood, diuretic therapy, Addison's disease.
- Neurodegenerative diseases, e.g. Parkinson's disease, multisystem atrophy.
- Drugs, e.g. antihypertensives.

4. Carotid sinus disease

The carotid sinus responds to stretch by sending signals via a branch of the glossopharyngeal nerve to the medullary cardiac centre. This produces a reflex bradycardia or a reduction in arterial pressure without the bradycardia. A syncopal attack may ensue in patients in whom the carotid sinus is hypersensitive (probably due to atheromatous disease or ageing of the receptor). If the patient turns the head rapidly when wearing a tight collar or scarf, or if the carotid sinuses are massaged, then the patient can become hypotensive and lose consciousness. Carotid sinus massage should therefore only be performed with cardiac monitoring and atropine present.

5. Syncope due to primary cardiac dysfunction

Syncope of cardiac origin is usually abrupt and without prodrome. The upright position is not a prerequisite. Loss of consciousness is brief and classically accompanied by marked pallor with a rapid return of colour as cardiac output is restored (pallor is prolonged after vasovagal syncope). Brief tonic or clonic movements might occur but recovery is usually rapid. The history, examination and further investigations including a 24-hour electrocardiogram (ECG) monitoring and an echocardiogram will further support a cardiac cause. These include:

- Cardiac arrhythmias (usually profound bradycardia or pulseless ventricular tachycardia).
- Left ventricular outflow obstruction: aortic stenosis, hypertrophic obstructive cardiomyopathy (HOCM).
- Right ventricular outflow obstruction: pulmonary stenosis, pulmonary hypertension, pulmonary embolism.
- Ventricular failure, e.g. acute anterior myocardial infarction.

Seizures

The most common diagnostic problem is distinguishing a syncopal attack from a seizure. Certain clinical features aid the differentiation of these common problems:

- A seizure can occur in any position. Syncopal attacks tend to occur in the upright position, although this is less so with those of cardiac origin, particularly Stokes–Adams attacks.
- The onset of a seizure is more sudden. There may be preceding aura symptoms but these usually last only seconds, shorter than the characteristic prodrome of syncope. The notable exception is the abrupt onset of a Stokes–Adams attack.
- Urinary and faecal incontinence often accompany a seizure, although urinary incontinence can occur with syncope.
- During a seizure, patients may bite their tongue, especially the lateral edge.
- Following recovery from a seizure, the patient may be confused, drowsy, with a headache, associated with some of the features of migraine, and aching muscles. This is called the 'postictal' state. The patient recovers consciousness and

orientation more rapidly from a syncopal attack, but there may be prolonged malaise.

- Injury is more common during a seizure.

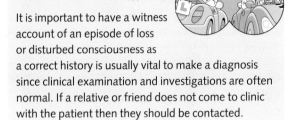

It is important to have a witness account of an episode of loss or disturbed consciousness as a correct history is usually vital to make a diagnosis since clinical examination and investigations are often normal. If a relative or friend does not come to clinic with the patient then they should be contacted.

The different types of seizure are dealt with in more detail in Chapter 16.

As well as syncope and epilepsy, further differential diagnoses might be considered (Fig. 2.1):

- Vertebrobasilar ischaemia causing transient ischaemic attacks (TIAs).
- Vertebrobasilar migraine.
- Hypoglycaemia.
- Psychogenic or 'non-epileptic' attacks.
- Drop attacks.
- Narcolepsy/cataplexy.
- Hyperventilation.

Vertebrobasilar ischaemia

The reticular formation is supplied by the vertebrobasilar system and, if this is compromised, LOC might occur. If this is due to a TIA then LOC may be transient but if there is prolonged loss of vertebrobasilar flow then infarction and death can occur. Symptoms of brainstem origin, such as vertigo and diplopia, are often associated. Thrombi from the aortic arch or left atrium are the most common causes of vertebrobasilar transient ischaemia but rarer causes, such as subclavian steal syndrome or Takayasu's arteritis, may occur. Similar symptoms may occur in vertebrobasilar migraine.

Hypoglycaemia

Hypoglycaemia is accompanied by a surge in catecholamine secretion. The patient begins to feel hungry, tremulous, and sweaty, has palpitations, is confused, and ultimately loses consciousness. Seizures can occur as a secondary phenomenon following prolonged hypoglycaemia.

Hyperventilation

Over-breathing results in a reduction of pCO_2, cerebral vasoconstriction, a metabolic alkalosis, and a reduction in ionized calcium. Characteristic features are:

- Breathlessness and air hunger with rapid respiration.
- Light-headedness.
- Perioral and digital paraesthesia.
- Carpopedal spasm.
- Variable submammary or axillary chest pain.
- Anxiety and fatigue.

The attacks may occur in particular situations due to phobic anxiety, commonly in crowds, or sometimes after physical exertion. Hyperventilation rarely causes complete LOC.

Loss of consciousness due to a TIA is extremely rare and is usually associated with focal symptoms of brainstem ischaemia. This should therefore be a diagnosis of exclusion. Seizures are relatively common in the elderly and are often associated with small-vessel disease. Elderly patients with temporal lobe complex partial seizures can often be misdiagnosed and a history specifically looking for its features should be taken, e.g. oro-lingual and hand automatisms.

Investigating transient loss of consciousness

In patients presenting with episodes of transient loss of consciousness (LOC), the first step is to establish whether the attacks might have been syncopal or a seizure. The history is most important in determining this. If a seizure is suspected, electroencephalography (EEG) may give information about the presence of abnormal activity but it is not a diagnostic test. Twenty percent of non-epileptic patients will have non-specific EEG abnormalities and the EEG is often normal in patients with seizures. The diagnosis is made primarily from the history, and an eyewitness account of the event is essential. Any structural

Fig. 2.1 Differential diagnosis of transient loss of consciousness

Seizure	Can occur in any position and time of day Preceding aura symptoms Sudden onset Urinary or faecal incontinence Tongue biting Postictal confusion, drowsiness, and headache	
Syncope	Upright position usually Prodrome – light headed, nausea, ringing in ears, dimming of vision, pallor, sweating Hypotension and bradycardia Relatively rapid recovery	*Situational* Emotion or pain Micturition Coughing Postural
		Cardiovascular Left or right ventricular outflow obstruction Arrhythmia Acute left ventricular failure Carotid sinus disease
Vertebrobasilar ischaemia	Additional brainstem symptoms, e.g. vertigo, diplopia Cerebrovascular risk factors, e.g. hypertension, diabetes, ischaemic heart disease Check peripheral upper limb pulses to look for evidence of subclavian steal syndrome	
Hyperventilation	Anxiety or situational, e.g. crowded rooms Perioral and/or digital tingling, carpopedal spasm, chest pain High respiratory rate, low pCO_2, metabolic alkalosis	
Narcolepsy/cataplexy	Inappropriate desire to sleep Falls with emotional situations, e.g. laughing Family history and presence of HLA-DR2	
Hypoglycaemia	Diabetic on treatment or relative of such a patient Hepatic failure Hypopituitarism, Addison's disease Insulinoma Glycogen storage disease Excess alcohol Ideal diagnosis is the documentation of a low blood glucose whilst symptomatic	
Vertebrobasilar migraine	Look for a history of migrainous headache and other brainstem symptoms	
Psychogenic attacks	Diagnosis based on exclusion of other causes and positive features of a psychological illness	

Note: If a patient presents with episodes of transient loss of conciousness, the first step is to establish whether the attacks are syncopal or due to a seizure. The history is most important in determining this. Thereafter further differential diagnoses may be investigated as shown above.

abnormality that may or may not be suggested by EEG can be visualized with computed tomography (CT) or magnetic resonance imaging (MRI).

If the history and examination are more suggestive of syncope, then a 12-lead ECG, 24-hour ECG monitoring and echocardiogram need to be considered. If the attacks have a postural component then tilt table testing should also be considered. Twenty-four-hour ECG monitoring may detect arrhythmias if they occur every day. For less frequent attacks, a REVEAL device may need to be inserted to detect infrequent, but clinically important, arrhythmias.

COMA

Coma is a state of impaired consciousness in which the patient is not roused by external stimuli. Inattention, confusion, stupor, and coma are terms describing progressive states of impaired consciousness. However, they are not clearly defined and therefore interobserver interpretation is highly variable. The Glasgow Coma Scale (Fig. 2.2) provides a more objective and reproducible method by which conscious level can be assessed and documented.

Fig. 2.2 Glasgow Coma Scale

Eye opening
1   None
2   In response to pain
3   In response to speech
4   Spontaneous

Verbal responses
1   None
2   Incomprehensible sounds
3   Inappropriate words
4   Disorientated speech
5   Orientated speech

Motor responses
1   None
2   Extensor response to pain
3   Flexor response to pain
4   Withdrawal to pain
5   Localization of painful stimulus
6   Obeys commands

It is based on eye opening and verbal and motor responses. A patient with a normal conscious state will score a total of 15.

Differential diagnosis of coma

Certain conditions may resemble coma:

Akinetic mutism

Patients with akinetic mutism are able to comprehend what is occurring around them and appear alert, but are silent and do not move spontaneously or respond to external stimuli. This arises from bilateral frontal lobe damage involving the corticoreticular pathways but sparing the motor and sensory pathways.

Locked-in syndrome

Locked-in syndrome results from an extensive lesion of the ventral pons which interrupts the corticobulbar and corticospinal pathways, with sparing of the reticular pathways and therefore sparing of consciousness. Patients are alert but unable to speak or move their face or limbs. The pathways for eye movement are relatively spared, so patients can communicate with vertical eye movements and blinking. This carries a grave prognosis and requires ventilatory support.

Persistent vegetative state

A persistent vegetative state, which can follow coma, refers to a state in which individuals have lost cognitive neurological function and awareness of the environment but retain non-cognitive function and a preserved sleep–wake cycle. The individual loses the higher cerebral powers of the brain but the functions of the brainstem, such as respiration and circulation, remain relatively intact. Spontaneous movements may occur and the eyes may open in response to external stimuli, but the patient does not speak or obey commands. Patients may occasionally grimace, cry, or laugh. This condition usually follows diffuse damage to the cerebral cortex.

Catatonia

A catatonic patient is silent and there is no volitional motor or emotional response to external stimuli. The patient may resist an examiner's attempt to move, for example, a limb, and if the limb is moved, the patient may keep it fixed in this position for some time. This may be seen in catatonic depressive and schizophrenic states.

Non-convulsive status epilepticus

Non-convulsive status epilepticus should be suspected in patients who do not regain consciousness after convulsive status epilepticus. It can also occur spontaneously and should be suspected in any patient with ongoing confusion/disturbance of consciousness. An EEG usually confirms ongoing non-convulsive epileptic activity.

Causes of persistent disturbance of consciousness

The causes of persistent loss or disturbance of consciousness may be cerebral and extracerebral (Figs 2.3 and 2.4).

Clinical approach to the comatose patient

The first step is to ascertain:

- Airway: establish and clear the airway.
- Breathing: ensure the patient is adequately ventilated with oxygen.
- Circulation: ensure there is cardiac output, otherwise begin external cardiac massage.

If there is respiratory or circulatory failure, this must be corrected and the potential causes investigated. Once a stable cardiorespiratory status has been established, a history should be taken from a relative,

Fig. 2.3 Cerebral causes of persistent loss (coma) or disturbance of consciousness

Intracranial cause	Clinical features	Investigations
Epilepsy	Status epliepticus Convulsive movements Incontinence Tongue biting	EEG CT or MRI
Trauma Extradural haemorrhage	Evidence of head injury – laceration, bruising, blood or CSF from nose or ear	Fracture on skull X-ray CT or MRI of head
Subdural haemorrhage	Past history of head injury several weeks previously; the elderly and alcoholics are prone to falls and tearing of penetrating veins	CT or MRI of head
Vascular Subarachnoid haemorrhage	History of explosive-onset headache Collapse Subhyaloid haemorrhage Pyrexia Neck stiffness, +ve Kernig's sign Focal neurological signs if there is intracerebral extension of the blood	CT of head – should be performed within 48 hours to avoid false negative results Lumbar puncture (LP) – if CT is normal, an LP should be done between 12 hours and 1 week after the initial event – xanthochromic CSF
Intracerebral haemorrhage	Collapse, seizures, focal signs	CT or MRI of head
Hypertensive encephalopathy	Hypertension, retinopathy, seizures, nephropathy	Investigation of secondary hypertension
Vertebrobasilar thromboembolism	History of TIAs or stroke, valvular or ischaemic heart disease, predisposition to thromboembolism	MRI head MRA vertebrobasilar system
Infective Meningitis	Headache Pyrexia Neck stiffness, +ve Kernig's sign	If there is no evidence of raised intracranial pressure, an LP should be done; otherwise CT should be performed first
Encephalitis	Clouding of consciousness, confusion, behaviour and memory disturbance, headache, pyrexia, seizures, focal signs	CT or MRI – focal or diffuse cerebral oedema EEG LP
Cerebral abscess	Subacute onset Headache Usually focal symptoms and signs Often seizures Source of infection elsewhere – ears, sinuses, lungs, valvular heart disease	CT or MRI of head Blood cultures Microbiology from potential source of infection

friend, or eyewitness, and a clinical examination and initial investigations must be performed to ascertain the cause of coma.

Examination of the comatose patient

Examine the patient for:

- Signs of head injury.
- Neck stiffness (if no evidence of cervical spine injury).
- Respiratory pattern.
- Pupil responses.
- Ocular movements.
- Fundoscopic abnormalities.
- Limb posture and spontaneous movements.
- Reflexes and plantar responses.
- Assess Glasgow Coma Scale.

Signs of head injury

Lacerations and bruising may be present and occur over an underlying fracture. A basal skull fracture may

Fig. 2.4 Extracerebral causes of persistent loss (coma) or disturbance of consciousness

Extracranial cause	Clinical features	Investigations
Circulatory collapse Cardiac, e.g. arrhythmia, myocardial infarction	Hypotension, tachycardia, rhythm disturbance, cardiac failure	ECG, cardiac enzymes, echocardiogram
Septicaemic shock	Rigors, pyrexia, vomiting, peripheral vasodilatation	Cultures – blood, sputum, urine, throat, stool
Hypovolaemia, e.g. blood loss, profuse diarrhoea	Melaena, haemetemesis, abdominal pain (ruptured aortic aneurysm)	
Hypotensive drugs		
Metabolic Hypo- or hypernatraemia	**Subacute onset** Muscle twitches, dehydration	
Hypo- or hypercalcaemia	Carpopedal spasm Polyuria and/or polydipsia, abdominal pain, vomiting	Biochemical confirmation
Hypo- or hyperglycaemia	Hemiplegia (reversible), seizures Dehydration, hyperventilation, ketotic fetor	
Hypo- or hyperthermia	Bradycardia, hypotension, hypoventilation, rigidity, cardiac arrest	Rectal temperature
Uraemia	Sallow skin, uraemic fetor, pale conjunctivae, hypertension	Raised creatinine, acidosis, anaemia
Hepatic failure	Jaundice, signs of portal hypertension, GI bleed, sedative drugs, sepsis	Abnormal LFTs, raised ammonia, electrolyte imbalance
Hypoxia	Following respiratory failure, cardiorespiratory arrest; brain damage occurs after 4 minutes of anoxia	
Hypercapnia	Bounding pulse, papilloedema, asterixis	Elevated pCO_2
Endocrine Adrenal crisis	Hypotension, abdominal pain, buccal and flexure pigmentation	Low Na^+, Ca^{2+}, glucose Raised K^+, urea, Synacthen test
Hypopituitarism	Pallor, hypogonadism, bitemporal hemianopia	Low pituitary and target hormones, CT/MRI of head
Myxoedema	Dry and coarse facies, hypotension, bradycardia, hypothermia	Clinical diagnosis confirmed by thyroid function tests; pituitary failure
Hypo- or hyperparathyroidism	As for hypo- and hyperthyroidism	$\downarrow/\uparrow Ca^{2+}$, $\downarrow/\uparrow$ parathyroid hormone
Toxins Alcohol	Ethanolic fetor Wernicke's encephalopathy	Raised blood alcohol level Low thiamine
Carbon monoxide	Pink skin colour	Elevated carboxyhaemoglobin
Drugs Opiates	Slow respiratory rate, pin-point pupils	Reversible with naloxone +ve blood and urine toxicology
Sedatives	Barbiturates – hypotension and hypothermia	+ve toxicology
Tricyclic antidepressants	Dilated pupils with sluggish responses, hypothermia	
Psychiatric Catatonia	As described above (p. 13)	
Psychogenic coma	Eyelids resist opening; normal reflexes and plantar responses; corneal reflex cannot be suppressed; normal optokinetic and caloric responses	

present with a normal skull X-ray. It is important to look for evidence of an anterior fossa fracture such as rhinorrhoea, bilateral periorbital haematoma, and subconjunctival haemorrhage. A fracture of the petrous bone may produce cerebrospinal fluid (CSF) or blood otorrhoea and be associated with Battle's sign (swelling and bruising over the mastoid process).

Respiratory pattern

- Cheyne–Stokes respiration: alternate hyper- and hypoventilation; seen in metabolic and iatrogenic (opiate) disturbances, and bilateral deep hemisphere lesions (thalamus or internal capsule).
- Central neurogenic hyperventilation: metabolic disturbances, e.g. diabetic and salicylate acidosis, and lesions of the reticular formation.
- Ataxic respiration: irregular respiratory pattern seen in lesions of the medulla.
- Apneustic respiration: pauses of 2–3 seconds occur after inspiration; seen in pontine lesions.

Pupil responses

- Pin-point pupils: pontine lesions, opiates, parasympathomimetics.
- Bilateral fixed mid-position: midbrain lesion.
- Unilateral or bilateral fixed and dilated: supratentorial mass with uncal herniation, or overdose of anticholinergics or sympathomimetics.
- Enlarged, slowly reactive pupils: metabolic or toxic.

Ocular movements

- Oculocephalic reflex: seen in patients with an intact brainstem. On rotating the head to the left and right, the eyes will maintain their position by conjugate movement in the opposite direction. This is called the 'doll's eye' reflex.
- Oculovestibular reflex: pouring cold water into the ear, or 'caloric stimulation', causes deviation of the eyes towards the side irrigated.
- Lesions of the midbrain or pons may result in dysconjugate movements of the eyes.

Fundoscopic abnormalities

Look for papilloedema, raised intracranial pressure and subhyaloid haemorrhage associated with subarachnoid haemorrhage.

Limb posture and movement

- Decerebrate posturing: neck extension, extension, abduction and/or pronation of arms, extension of legs and plantar flexed feet.
- Decorticate posturing: flexion and/or adduction of arms, extension of legs.

These reflexes have no localizing value in humans but decorticate posturing often carries a better prognosis than decerebrate posturing.

Investigations in the comatose patient

Immediate investigations include:

- Temperature.
- Blood glucose.
- Electrolytes, calcium, urea, and creatinine.
- Full blood count and coagulation screen.
- Arterial blood gases.
- Blood culture and toxicology.
- ECG and chest X-ray.

Neurological investigations in selected cases include:

- Brain imaging (CT or MRI).
- CSF examination.
- EEG.
- Angiography.

Prognosis of coma

In patients where a drug overdose or a reversible metabolic cause has caused coma and there has not been a prolonged period of unsupported cardiorespiratory failure, then the prognosis can be excellent with appropriate critical care. Unfortunately, other causes have a poorer prognosis. In patients with a Glasgow Coma Scale score of 3 for more than 6 hours there is a mortality of over 50% and, of the remainder, only a small minority will return to independent existence.

Two common causes of coma are post-anoxic brain injury following partially successful cardiopulmonary resuscitation and head injury. Post-anoxic brain injury carries a grave prognosis whereas prognosis after head injury should be more guarded and open.

BRAINSTEM DEATH

If the cardiorespiratory centre in the brainstem is damaged then spontaneous breathing can be impaired. In many cases, it is not entirely clear whether brainstem function will return. Guidelines have been drawn up to diagnose brainstem death. Certain preconditions need to exist before testing can take place:

- The patient requires ventilatory support in the absence of drugs.
- There is a known cause for the coma, capable of resulting in brainstem death.
- The patient's core temperature and any metabolic abnormality or effects of drugs must be normalized.
- The effects of any neuromuscular drugs must have worn off.

It should be noted that the tendon reflexes might be intact because these occur at spinal level. There might also be limb posturing to painful stimuli in some cases. The examination should be repeated within 24 hours by a second experienced clinician to confirm that irreversible brainstem death has occurred. Electroencephalography is not a diagnostic investigation. It might show slight residual activity in some brain-dead subjects and, exceptionally, might be flat in reversible coma resulting from hypothermia, drug intoxication, or recent cardiac arrest.

Examination of brainstem reflexes used in the diagnosis of brain death are listed in Fig. 2.5.

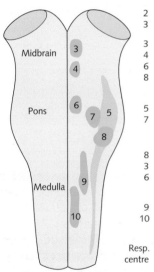

2 3	Absent pupillary responses to light
3 4 6 8	Absent oculocephalic ('doll's eye') reflexes The eyes move passively in the direction of horizontal or vertical head movements, rather than maintaining their position of gaze while the head is being moved by the examiner
5 7	Absent corneal reflexes No blink with corneal stimulation No grimace in response to facial pain (firm supraorbital pressure)
8 3 6	Absent caloric reflexes (vestibulo-ocular responses) An intact reflex consists of transient tonic deviation of the eyes towards the stimulated side when 20–50 mL of ice-cold water is instilled into the ear
9 10	Absent gag reflex No cough in response to pharyngeal or tracheal stimulation and suction
Resp. centre	Absence of any respiratory effort, even after fully oxygenating the patient and then allowing the pCO_2 to rise to 50–60 mmHg (apnoea test)

Fig. 2.5 Brainstem reflexes used in the diagnosis of brain death.

- Describe the structures that are pain-sensitive in the head and neck.
- What are the main four clinical presentations of headache and what are the common causes?
- Which features in the history and examination would suggest a secondary cause for headache?

Most patients with headaches have tension-type or migraine headache. The diagnosis in these cases is made entirely from the history because there are usually no physical signs. However, headache can also be secondary to other disorders affecting the head and neck, and it is sometimes the predominant symptom of serious intracranial disease such as tumour, CNS infections or subarachnoid haemorrhage.

Pain in the head and neck may be referred from the ears, eyes, nasal passages, teeth, sinuses, facial bones, and cervical spine. It is conveyed predominantly by the trigeminal nerve (fifth cranial nerve), and also by the seventh, ninth, and tenth cranial nerves, and the upper three cervical roots. Structures of the anterior and middle cranial fossa generally refer pain to the anterior two-thirds of the head via the branches of the trigeminal nerve and structures of the posterior fossa refer pain to the back of the head and neck via the upper cervical roots (Fig. 3.1).

Do not forget that the brain parenchyma is insensitive to pain. This enables patients to have surgical procedures performed on their brain whilst conscious. Headache arises from the structures encasing and within the brain such as meninges and blood vessels. Primary headaches, such as migraine, are probably a result of neuronal activity which secondarily causes changes in cranial pain-sensitive structures leading to cranial pain and other symptoms.

The approach to assessing a patient with headache should be based on the temporal pattern of symptoms, especially the mode of onset and subsequent course. This may be:

- Recurrent and episodic with acute or subacute onset.
- Chronic and daily with fluctuations in severity over months or years.
- Subacute onset and progressive over days to weeks.
- Acute onset and progressive over hours.

Recurrent episodic headache

Recurrent episodic headache is usually benign and is very rarely due to sinister pathology. Common causes and their clinical features are listed in Fig. 3.2.

Chronic daily headache

Chronic daily headache is most often diffuse tension-type headache or chronic migraine and is rarely due to serious intracranial disease (Fig. 3.3).

Subacute-onset and progressive headache

The category of subacute-onset headache includes most of the serious causes of headache. Worrying features include a progression of the headache, persisting focal symptoms or signs, deterioration of conscious level, seizures, and associated fever (Fig. 3.4).

Acute-onset headache

Instantaneous onset should always raise the suspicion of intracranial haemorrhage or arterial dissection. There are also benign causes such as recurrent coital or exertional headache and thunderclap-type migraine, as listed in Fig. 3.5.

Headache

Fig. 3.1 The pain-sensitive structures in the head and neck, and disorders that may give rise to secondary headache.

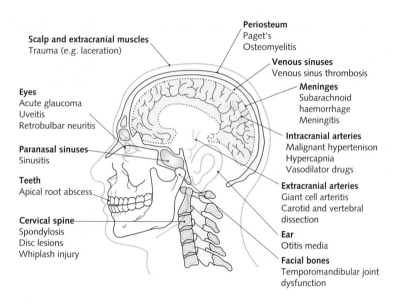

Scalp and extracranial muscles
Trauma (e.g. laceration)

Eyes
Acute glaucoma
Uveitis
Retrobulbar neuritis

Paranasal sinuses
Sinusitis

Teeth
Apical root abscess

Cervical spine
Spondylosis
Disc lesions
Whiplash injury

Periosteum
Paget's
Osteomyelitis

Venous sinuses
Venous sinus thrombosis

Meninges
Subarachnoid
haemorrhage
Meningitis

Intracranial arteries
Malignant hypertenison
Hypercapnia
Vasodilator drugs

Extracranial arteries
Giant cell arteritis
Carotid and vertebral
dissection

Ear
Otitis media

Facial bones
Temporomandibular joint
dysfunction

Fig. 3.2 Differential diagnosis of recurrent episodic headache

Cause	Clinical features
Migraine	Unilateral throbbing headache exacerbated by movement Accompanied by nausea, vomiting, photo-, phono- and osmophobia ± aura symptoms
Cluster headache	Severe unilateral retro-orbital ± temporal pain Ipsilateral conjunctival injection, lacrimation, partial Horner's syndrome, nasal blockage, rhinorrhoea Attacks last 15–180 minutes and occur several times a day for about 2–3 months at a time
Benign coital, exertional and cough headache	Headaches precipitated by exertion, coughing, straining and sexual activity; may be benign, but this diagnosis is one of exclusion
Intermittent hydrocephalus (rare)	Intermittent severe headaches accompanied by drop attacks, weakness of the legs and unsteady gait, e.g. intermittent obstruction of the third ventricle by a colloid cyst
Paroxysmal hypertension (rare)	This may occur in patients with a phaeochromocytoma

Fig. 3.3 Differential diagnosis of chronic daily headache

Cause	Clinical features
Tension-type headache ± analgesic overuse	Bilateral featureless headache; usually fluctuating severity
Chronic migraine ± analgesic overuse	Daily, mild, bilateral, usually featureless headache with superimposed episodes of characteristic migraine headaches
Post-traumatic headache	Post-traumatic headache syndromes include: • Post-concussion headache • Episodic headaches which may be migrainous • Generalized featureless daily headache • Tenderness or pain located to the site of the injury • Occipital and/or neck pain from upper cervical spine injury
Low pressure headache	This occurs following lumbar puncture or spontaneous or traumatic chronic leakage of CSF

Fig. 3.4 Differential diagnosis of subacute-onset headache

Cause	Clinical features
Intracranial tumour	Headache exacerbated by coughing, sneezing, or straining may occur with obstruction of the CSF pathways Focal neurological signs, seizures
Meningitis/encephalitis	± history of recent respiratory tract infection Fever, neck stiffness, +ve Kernig's sign, inflammatory CSF: Bacterial, viral, Tuberculosis (note ethnic origin and HIV status), cryptococcal (HIV), malignant, syphilitic, sarcoid
Venous sinus thrombosis	Drowsiness, vomiting, seizures, focal signs
Subdural haematoma	History of head injury (elderly and alcoholics in particular), fluctuating level of consciousness, confusion, focal neurological signs (usually a hemiparesis)
Intracranial abscess	Direct extension from local disease (e.g. frontal sinusitis) or metastatic spread (e.g. lung abscess) Fever, systemically unwell, focal neurological signs
Giant-cell arteritis	Patients usually over 50 years of age; female preponderance Visual disturbance-ischaemic papillopathy Associated polymyalgia rheumatica Elevated ESR Tender thickened superficial temporal artery; giant-cell arteritis on biopsy Urgent steroid therapy often prior to biopsy
Benign intracranial hypertension	Young, overweight females Papilloedema, raised CSF pressure, sixth nerve palsies. CT or MRI usually normal, although the lateral ventricles often appear small
Acute hydrocephalus	Nausea, vomiting, diplopia (6th nerve palsy-false localizing sign) ± papilloedema, ataxia of gait diagnosis confirmed on CT head scan
Hypertensive crisis	Very high blood pressure There may be papilloedema There may be other features of phaeochromocytoma
Acute glaucoma	Pain typically frontal, orbital or ocular, accompanied by persisting visual impairment, fixed oval pupil and conjunctival injection. This is an ophthalmological emergency

Fig. 3.5 Differential diagnosis of acute-onset headache

Cause	Clinical features
Subarachnoid haemorrhage	Explosive-onset 'thunderclap headache' Neck stiffness, photophobia, +ve Kernig's sign ± focal neurological signs if there has been intracerebral extension of blood CT head scan—subarachnoid blood (within 48 hours) CSF—xanthochromia (12 hours to 1 week)
Intracerebral haemorrhage	Note history of hypertension, anticoagulation Focal neurological signs depending on site of bleed CT head scan – intracerebral blood
Arterial Disection	This presents with head and neck pain sometimes following rapid deceleration or twisting injuries.
First episode of migraine/cluster headache	Migraine can present with an explosive 'thunderclap' onset; the diagnosis of a migrainous aetiology is then one of exclusion, unless recurrent stereotyped episodes have occurred over several years.
Coital/excertional headache	Can occur with an explosive onset before or during orgasm

HISTORY

A good history is essential to differentiate the type of headache. Determine:

- Mode of onset: acute, subacute, chronic, or recurrent and episodic.
- Subsequent course: episodic, progressive, or chronic.
- Site: unilateral or bilateral; frontal, temporal, or occipital; radiation to neck, arm, or shoulder.
- Character of pain: constant, throbbing, stabbing, or dull/pressure-like.
- Frequency and duration.
- Accompanying features: additional neurological symptoms, neck stiffness, autonomic symptoms.
- Exacerbating factors: movement, light, noise, smell (e.g. migraine), coughing, sneezing, bending (e.g. raised intracranial pressure).

- Precipitating factors: alcohol (cluster headache and migraine), menstruation (migraine), stress (most headaches are worse with stress), postural change (high or low intracranial pressure headache), head injury (subdural haemorrhage or post-traumatic headache).
- Particular time of onset: mornings (migraine, raised intracranial pressure), awoken at night (cluster headache).
- Past history of headache.
- Family history: migraine, intracranial haemorrhage.
- General health: systemic ill health, existing medical conditions.
- Drug history: analgesic abuse, recreational drugs, vasodilators, e.g. nitrates, nifedipine.

EXAMINATION

When examining a patient with headache, look for:

- Level of consciousness including GCS.
- Focal neurological signs.
- Signs of local disease of the ears, eyes, or sinuses; restriction of neck movements and pain; temporomandibular joint dysfunction; thickening of the superficial temporal arteries.
- Signs of systemic disease.
- Abnormal blood pressure.

The clinical examination is often entirely normal in patients with headache. The history is therfore vital, especially with regard to migrainous symptoms and overuse of analgesics, particularly codeine.

SUMMARY

Headache might be:

- Primary, e.g. migraine, tension-type headache, cluster headache.
- Secondary, e.g. subarachnoid haemorrhage, meningitis, raised intracranial pressure.

The temporal pattern of symptoms should be established (i.e. the mode of onset and subsequent course – recurrent and episodic, chronic, subacute, or acute). A list of differential diagnoses based on the established temporal pattern of symptoms should be drawn up.

The examination may demonstrate focal neurological signs, e.g. papilloedema, which suggests a secondary headache.

Features that should alert the clinician to the presence of a secondary headache and prompt further investigation are:

- Recent onset/short history (particularly in middle or old age with no previous history of headache).
- Acute onset or progressive course.
- Recent change in established pattern or character of headache.
- Increasing severity with resistance to appropriate and adequately tried treatment.
- Associated features – neurological signs, seizures, personality change, fever, systemic illness.

Disorders of smell and taste

4

Objectives

- Understand the major anatomy of the olfactory system
- Describe the common causes of disturbances of smell
- Be aware of the serious pathologies which may rarely present with loss of smell

Alteration of the sense of smell is not a common presenting symptom, and impairment of olfaction as a physical sign is not often important in making a neurological diagnosis. Consequently, smell is not always tested during a routine clinical examination. However, anosmia is a significant problem after some head injuries and, rarely, it can be the only physical sign of a serious structural lesion involving the frontal lobes.

Odours enter the nose and sinuses where they stimulate olfactory receptors on cells of the nasal mucosa. These cells are bipolar neurons that have peripheral and central processes. The peripheral processes contain many cilia, which carry the olfactory receptors. The unmyelinated central processes enter into the cranial cavity through the cribriform plate of the ethmoid bone to synapse with dendrites of the mitral cells in the olfactory bulb. The central processes of the bipolar neurons constitute the first (olfactory) nerve. Axons from mitral cells, in the olfactory bulb, form the olfactory tract. This runs in the olfactory groove of the cribriform plate beneath the frontal lobes and above the optic nerve and chiasm. Some of these axons synapse within the anterior perforated substance but most continue into the brain and ultimately terminate in the primary olfactory cortex (in the anterior aspect of the parahippocampal gyrus and the uncus of the temporal lobe) and nuclei of the amygdaloid complex (Fig. 4.1).

DIFFERENTIAL DIAGNOSIS

Anosmia and hyposmia

Anosmia is loss of the sense of smell. Hyposmia is impairment of the sense of smell. Anosmia or hyposmia may be due to:

- Inability of odours to reach the olfactory receptors (hypertrophy or oedema of the nasal mucosa).
- Destruction of the receptor cells and their central connections.
- Central lesions.

The anosmia or hyposmia may be temporary or permanent. The patient will not notice unilaterally impaired olfaction. Olfaction tends to deteriorate with age.

The following causes should be considered:

- Upper respiratory tract infection: chronic rhinitis, sinusitis (allergic, vasomotor, or infective).
- Heavy smoking causing metaplastic changes in the nasal epithelium.
- Viral infections, e.g. influenza, herpes simplex (may cause permanent destruction of the receptor cells).
- Drugs, e.g. antibiotics, antihistamines, penicillamine.
- Local trauma to the olfactory epithelium.
- Head injury: unmyelinated fibres from the receptor cells are damaged along their vulnerable course through the cribriform plate, particularly if there is an associated fracture. If the dura is torn there may be cerebrospinal fluid rhinorrhoea; this can be differentiated from mucous secretion by its higher glucose concentration. This is the most common neurological cause of anosmia.
- Tumours: meningioma of the dura in the olfactory groove may extend posteriorly to involve the optic nerve. Rarely, frontal lobe gliomas and pituitary tumours.
- Aneurysm of the anterior cerebral or anterior communicating artery.
- Raised intracranial pressure: olfaction may be impaired without evidence of damage to the olfactory structures.

23

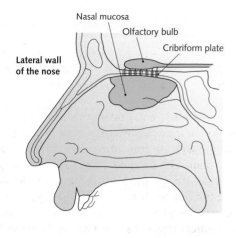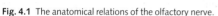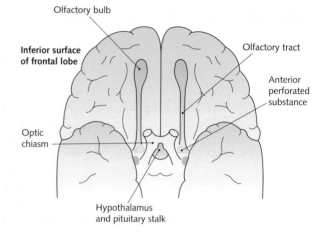

Fig. 4.1 The anatomical relations of the olfactory nerve.

- Frontal lobe abscess
- Degenerative disorders such as Alzheimer's disease and idiopathic Parkinson's disease are often associated with anosmia.

Ageusia and dysgeusia

Ageusia is the perception of loss of taste. Dysgeusia is the perception of an impaired sense of taste.

Many patients with bilateral anosmia complain of loss or impairment of taste. This is because much of our appreciation of food and drink is by olfaction rather than by elemental taste. Taste itself is normal if tested formally in anosmic subjects.

Hyperosmia

Hyperosmia is an abnormally increased sensitivity to odours and may be seen in the following conditions:

- Anxious patients may complain of hypersensitivity to various odours.
- Migraine attacks with and without aura may be accompanied by hypersensitivity to light, sound, and smell (osmophobia).

Olfactory hallucinations

- Complex partial seizures of temporal lobe origin can give rise to brief olfactory hallucinations, which are part of the aura.
- Olfactory hallucinations may occur following alcohol withdrawal.

- Olfactory hallucinations and delusions of unpleasant nature can be due to a psychotic illness, e.g. depression or schizophrenia.
- Hallucinations and delusions may also occur in patients with some forms of dementia.
- A persistent unpleasant smell may occur from local disease of the nasopharynx such as purulent sinusitis.

Disorders of smell:
- Anosmia/hyposmia is the loss/impairment of smell. The patient will notice this if the impairment is bilateral but not if it is unilateral. It is most often caused by disease of the nasopharynx and alterations of the nasal epithelium in smokers but head injury is the most common neurological cause.
- Ageusia/dysgeusia is an apparent alteration in taste perception in individuals with bilateral anosmia.
- Hyperosmia is a hypersensitivity to odours and is usually seen in anxious patients or migraine.
- Olfactory hallucinations may occur with temporal lobe seizures, following alcohol withdrawal, as a manifestation of psychosis or in patients with some dementias.

EXAMINATION

A characteristic-smelling object (e.g. peppermint, clove oil) is held under each nostril in turn while the other is occluded and the patient keeps the eyes closed. An individual with intact olfaction will be able to detect the smell and name it. The recommended special testing bottles are rarely available when needed and most clinicians perform preliminary assessment with nearby objects such as fruit, a coffee jar, or cigarette packet. When examining patients with anosmia, it is important to look carefully for frontal lobe signs and evidence of optic nerve or chiasmal damage.

Pathology in the nasal passages or sinuses is a more common cause of anosmia than any neurological condition.

In any patient complaining of loss of smell, it is important to take an accurate history for use of recreational drugs such as alcohol (head trauma) and smoking (olfactory epithelial metaplasia) as these are the commonest causes. Visual fields and frontal release signs should be accurately assessed as dysfunction in these systems may be the only other abnormal physical signs. If no obvious cause can be found then CT or MRI of the brain and sinuses is warranted. It should be noted that the sinuses are not formally assessed on a routine CT scan of the brain and appropriate views need to be requested specifically.

INVESTIGATIONS

Unexplained anosmia may require referral for more expert ear, nose, and throat (ENT) examination if there is no suspicion of a neurological cause or obvious ENT cause.

If the patient has any evidence in the history or examination of frontal lobe or visual field defects in combination with anosmia, then it is appropriate to image the brain with computed tomography or magnetic resonance imaging to look for a structural lesion such as a tumour or abscess. Established post-traumatic anosmia requires no investigation unless there are also features to suggest a cerebrospinal fluid fistula or intracranial infection. The prognosis for a return of smell in post-traumatic patients is often poor, but late recovery can occur.

Visual impairment

Objectives

- Understand the anatomical path of light stimulation from retina to visual cortex
- Be able to sketch the common visual field defects associated with abnormalities in the visual pathway
- Describe the main causes of acute transient and persistent visual loss

Disturbance of vision is often due to ocular disease and is largely dealt with by the ophthalmologist. Visual impairment presenting to the neurologist usually involves a lesion in the visual pathway from the retina to the occipital cortex.

The anatomical path of light stimulation

1. Retina to optic nerve

- The retina consists of three distinct neuronal levels: photoreceptors, bipolar and ganglion cells (Fig. 5.1).
- There are two types of photosensitive cells: 'rods' and 'cones'.
- Rods are responsible for night vision and detection of peripheral movement and are in greatest density in the periphery of the retina. They do not detect colour.
- Cones are responsible for daytime and colour vision and are concentrated at the macula.
- The macula is a region of the retina specialized for perception of detailed images and colour.
- The rods and cones convert light into electrical impulses and transmit these to bipolar cells, which in turn pass the signal to the ganglion cells.
- The ganglion cells have unmyelinated axons so that their fibres do not interfere with the path of light reaching the rods and cones.
- The unmyelinated axons converge at the optic disc and at that point become myelinated as they form the second cranial or 'optic' nerve.

2. Optic nerve to optic chiasm

- Light from an object in the right temporal field of vision will cast an image on the temporal retina

of the left eye and the nasal retina of the right eye, and vice versa (Fig. 5.2).
- Light from the upper field of vision will cast an image in the lower part of the retina, and vice versa.
- Fibres from the temporal region of each retina run in the temporal half of the optic nerve and those from the nasal region of the retina, in the nasal half of the nerve. The macular fibres run centrally.
- The optic nerve then passes through the orbit and exits at the optic foramen. It then passes on the undersurface of the frontal lobe to join the other optic nerve to form the optic chiasm.

3. Optic chiasm to lateral geniculate nucleus

- The optic chiasm lies anterior to the pituitary stalk, superior to the pituitary, and inferior to the hypothalamus (see Fig. 5.3).
- Optic nerve fibres carrying impulses from the nasal part of the retina cross in the chiasm whereas fibres subserving the temporal retina stay on the same side.
- Fibres in the inferior part of the chiasm carry information regarding the upper visual field and upper part from the lower visual field.
- The ipsilateral temporal fibres and the contralateral nasal fibres join to form the optic tract. This travels around the midbrain to the posterior thalamus where it synapses within the lateral geniculate nucleus (LGN).
- A few fibres leave the tract before the LGN and pass directly to the tectal area at the back of the upper midbrain. These fibres mediate the light and accommodation reflexes.

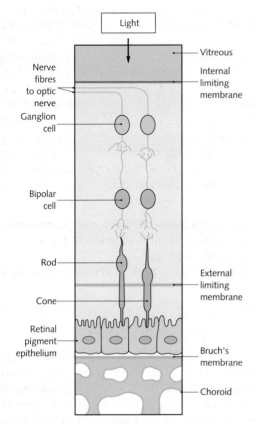

Fig. 5.1 Layers of the retina.

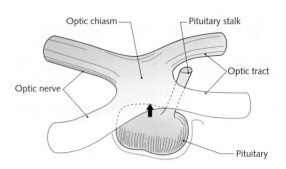

Fig. 5.3 Relation of the optic chiasm to its surrounding structures and in particular to the pituitary fossa, with which it is closely associated. The arrow indicates upward pressure on the inferior part of the chiasm by a pituitary tumour.

4. Lateral geniculate nucleus to occipital cortex

- The axons from the cell bodies in the LGN form the optic radiation, which passes in the posterior part of the internal capsule. The fibres within the optic radiation that subserve the upper part of the visual field travel around the temporal portion of the lateral ventricle. The fibres subserving the lower visual field pass around the parietal portion of the lateral ventricle (see Fig. 5.2).
- Both paths terminate in the calcarine or primary visual cortex on the medial surface of the occipital cortex.

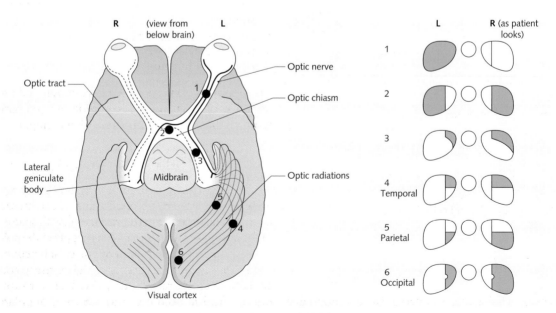

Fig. 5.2 Lesions of different parts of the visual pathway produce characteristic field defects.

Blood supply to the visual pathway

The ophthalmic artery is the first branch of the internal carotid artery and gives rise to the central retinal and posterior ciliary arteries, which supply the retina and optic nerve. The optic radiations are supplied by the middle cerebral artery. The posterior cerebral artery supplies the LGN and the occipital cortex.

Visual field defects

Lesions at different sites of the optic pathway give specific visual field defects, as shown in Fig. 5.2.

CLINICAL FEATURES TO AID LOCALIZATION OF A LESION

Optic nerve lesion (see 1, Fig. 5.2)

The patient with an optic nerve lesion complains of impaired vision in one eye. If the cause is inflammatory, then there may be pain with movement of the eye. On examination, there is reduced visual acuity, reduction of colour vision, and a central scotoma. An afferent pupillary defect may be present. If the lesion is longstanding, the vision may be completely lost in the affected eye and the optic disc becomes pale; this is the appearance of optic atrophy.

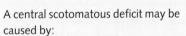

A central scotomatous deficit may be caused by:
- Retinal disease involving the macula.
- Lesions of the optic nerve.

Lesions of the optic nerve include:
- Optic neuritis, e.g. multiple sclerosis.
- Optic nerve or orbital neoplasm, e.g. meningioma or glioma.
- Nutritional deficiency, e.g. vitamin B_{12}.
- Toxins, e.g. methanol, alcohol.
- Vascular, e.g. giant cell arteritis, small vessel disease due to hypertension or diabetes.

Optic chiasm lesion (see 2, Fig. 5.2)

A chiasmal lesion causes a bitemporal hemianopia due to involvement of the decussating fibres. Pressure from

a lesion below the chiasm (e.g. pituitary tumour) will involve the inferior nasal fibres first, resulting in a bitemporal superior quadrantanopia; pressure from a lesion above the chiasm (e.g. hypothalamic craniopharyngioma) will cause a bitemporal inferior quadrantanopia. The patient often either complains of unilateral visual disturbance or does not complain of visual problems at all but may bump into objects in either temporal field.

The anatomical relations of the optic chiasm are shown in Fig. 5.3. Double vision is uncommon but can occur if the lesion extends to involve the oculomotor nerves in the cavernous sinus.

Lesions of the optic chiasm include:

- Tumours, e.g. pituitary adenoma, meningioma, craniopharyngioma, or metastatic deposits.
- Cerebral aneurysm.
- Granulomatous disease: tuberculosis, sarcoidosis.

Optic radiation and optic tract lesions (see 3, 4, 5, Fig. 5.2)

Lesions of the optic radiation cause a contralateral homonymous hemianopia or quadrantanopia. Those confined to the parietal fibres give rise to an inferior quadrantanopia and those confined to the temporal lobe fibres give rise to a superior quadrantanopia. The patient often attributes the problem only to the eye on the hemianopic side. Lesions of the optic tract and optic radiation include:

- Infarction, such as a lesion of the middle cerebral artery.
- Intracerebral haemorrhage.
- Tumours.
- Trauma.

Isolated optic tract lesions are uncommon and are usually caused by posterior extension of a pituitary tumour. They cause an incongruous hemianopia.

Occipital cortex lesions (see 6, Fig. 5.2)

Unilateral lesions of the posterior cerebral artery, e.g. embolism from the vertebrobasilar arterial tree, cause a contralateral homonymous hemianopia with sparing of the macula because of dual blood supply to the pole of the visual cortex which subserves macular function.

Bilateral occipital cortex damage gives rise to cortical blindness characterized by visual loss throughout the field in both eyes and preserved pupillary responses. If the visual association areas are involved, the patient is sometimes apparently unaware of the loss of vision: this is Anton's syndrome.

Descriptive terms for field defects

Visual field defects can confuse students initially. There are several basic principles.

- 'Monocular' deficits occur anterior to the optic chiasm in the retina or optic nerve.
- 'Binocular' deficits occur posterior to the optic chiasm.
- 'Hemianopia' means affecting half the vision in one or both sides.
- 'Quadrantanopia' means affecting a quarter of the visual field in one or both eyes.
- 'Homonymous' means affecting the same part of the visual field in both eyes.
- 'Incongruous' means the affected part of the visual field is in the same region in both eyes (i.e. homonymous) but it is asymmetrically affected, e.g. lesions of the optic tract.
- If you have difficulty understanding a visual field defect then try and follow the anatomical path it takes from the retina to the lesion.

DIFFERENTIAL DIAGNOSIS

When a patient presents with visual impairment it is important to establish the temporal pattern, including the mode of onset and subsequent course. The patient's characteristics are also important: a hypertensive diabetic male is more likely to have anterior ischaemic optic neuropathy compared to a young female who is more likely to have optic neuritis.

Patients with acute monocular

visual loss will complain of unilateral visual disturbance and seek medical attention. Patients with more posterior deficits, especially homonomous hemianopia, often do not realise they have a deficit if it is isolated, even if the cause is acute, e.g. stroke. They may present with 'bumping into objects' on the hemianopic side and car accidents are not an uncommon prequel to presentation. Patients rarely complain of binocular deficits from bilateral field deficits.

Severe papilloedema can be a cause of bilateral visual impairment, transient ('obscurations') or persistent, but most patients with papilloedema have normal or near-normal vision. Less common causes of bilateral visual impairment are cortical blindness and functional ('hysterical') blindness.

Acute visual impairment

The first step is to ascertain whether the acute visual impairment is transient or persistent.

Acute transient visual impairment

- Amaurosis fugax.
- Migraine with aura.
- Papilloedema.

Amaurosis fugax

The patient complains of sudden unilateral altitudinal visual loss, often described as a shutter coming down from the superior to inferior part of the visual field. This lasts several seconds or minutes, followed by complete recovery.

The most common cause is atheroma of the ipsilateral carotid artery, causing embolism into the central retinal artery and its distal branches.

Migraine with aura

The visual symptoms, or 'aura', that precede migraine headache can consist of unformed flashes of white or, less commonly, coloured lights (photopsia) or formations of dazzling zig-zag lines (fortification spectra or teichopsia). This visual aura can move across the visual field over several minutes leaving scotomatous defects that are bilateral and may be homonymous. Aura symptoms generally precede the headache and last less than 60 minutes, although they can occur during the migraine.

The diagnosis is made from a history of recurrent paroxysmal attacks with headache, nausea, vomiting and photophobia. Migraine aura can occur without the headache and is known as 'migraine equivalent'. Focal symptoms such as tingling in a hand or the face as well as visual loss can occur and may be difficult to differentiate from a transient ischaemic attack. The key to making the diagnosis is in the history: migraine equivalent events usually occur in patients who have a preceding history of migraine headache but, more importantly, the neurological symptoms come on gradually over minutes, unlike a transient ischaemic attack, which usually comes on over seconds. The visual symptoms in migraine often move slowly across the visual field.

Papilloedema

Papilloedema is swelling of the optic disc due to raised intracranial pressure. It is almost invariably bilateral. The optic nerve is covered with meninges and therefore surrounded by subarachnoid fluid. The surrounding dura mater eventually fuses with the periosteum of the orbit, and the pia and arachnoid mater with the sclera. Raised intracranial pressure in the optic nerve sheath impedes venous drainage and restricts axoplasmic flow in the nerve. Patients with moderate papilloedema may have no visual symptoms. In severe cases, fleeting bilateral loss of vision, lasting a few seconds, may be experienced which are called 'visual obscurations'. On examination, visual acuity is often normal but the blind spot is enlarged, with restriction of the peripheral field of vision. The disc is swollen, pink and has blurred disc margins. There is engorgement of the retinal veins, and, if severe, flame-shaped haemorrhages on or adjacent to the disc. If the condition becomes chronic, optic atrophy and visual failure ultimately occur.

Acute persistent visual impairment

- Optic neuritis.
- Retinal or optic nerve ischaemia.
- Arterial thromboembolism of the middle or posterior cerebral artery.

Differential diagnoses of tunnel vision include:
- Papilloedema.
- Glaucoma.
- Peripheral retinopathy, usually pigmentary.
- Conversion disorder (functional visual impairment).
- Migraine with aura (transient tunnel vision).

Optic neuritis

Optic neuritis is inflammation of the optic nerve. Anterior optic nerve involvement causes visible swelling of the optic nerve head or 'papillitis'. This can have a similar appearance to papilloedema. If the optic nerve is inflamed in the posterior part of the optic nerve then the optic disc will appear normal and the syndrome is 'retrobulbar neuritis'. Loss of central vision may be mild or severe. There is often a dull ache with eye movements, particularly elevation. A central scotoma, defective colour vision, and an afferent pupillary defect are often elicited. Following recovery, temporal pallor of the optic disc is common. The most common cause is demyelination either confined to the optic nerve or as a symptom of multiple sclerosis.

The swollen optic disc seen in papillitis and papilloedema can appear clinically very similar. However, papillitis is typically associated with visual symptoms (impaired acuity and colour vision, central scotoma, afferent pupillary defect) whereas patients with papilloedema typically have preserved vision.

Retinal or optic nerve ischaemia

Sudden monocular visual loss results from embolism into the central retinal artery (retinal ischaemia) or occlusion of small posterior ciliary arteries by local small-vessel disease or inflammation such as giant cell arteritis (optic nerve ischaemia).

Arterial thromboembolism of the middle or posterior cerebral artery

Arterial thromboembolic events are usually of sudden onset, although the patient might not always notice the deficit immediately. The characteristic findings described are of a homonomous hemianopia (occipital cortex) or quadrantanopia (optic radiation). The history and examination should focus on cerebrovascular risk factors, e.g. ischaemic heart disease, diabetes, hyperlipidaemia, hypertension, atrial fibrillation.

Optic atrophy

This results from damage to the nerve fibres in the visual pathway at any point between and including the ganglion cells of the retina and the lateral geniculate nucleus. Visual loss is often central but can also be peripheral. There is central disc pallor, which can also be seen with a normal large physiological cup and in the myopic eye. Optic atrophy can be distinguished by attenuation of the retinal vessels, poor colour vision, a central scotoma, atrophy in the nerve fibre layer of the retina and impaired afferent pupillary responses to light. Once established, the disc appearance will not return to normal despite relieving the cause, although vision may improve. It is rare to see persistent blindness in patients who have had optic neuritis due to MS, and vision often returns to a good functional level, even though the disc is pale.

Causes of optic atrophy include:

- Retinal disease: persistent central retinal artery occlusion, retinitis pigmentosa, toxins, e.g. quinine.
- Optic nerve: optic neuritis, chronic glaucoma, long-standing papilloedema, tumours, metabolic deficiency, e.g. vitamin B_{12} deficiency, toxic, e.g. ethyl and methyl alcohol, tobacco, hereditary, trauma.
- Chiasm and optic tract, e.g. pituitary tumours and craniopharyngioma.

Visual impairment due to ocular disease is likely to be painful. The pain is usually localized to the eye and there are accompanying signs in the eye. Headache and visual impairment are associated with:

- Giant-cell arteritis.
- Optic neuritis (pain on eye movement).
- Glaucoma.
- Migraine (if transient).
- Severely raised intracranial pressure.
- Pituitary tumour.

INVESTIGATION OF VISUAL SYMPTOMS

The investigation plan will be determined entirely by the differential diagnosis resulting from a careful clinical history and examination (Fig. 5.4).

Fig. 5.4 Investigation plan for visual impairment

Acute transient visual impairment	
Amaurosis fugax	Carotid Doppler study (cartoid artery stenosis) CT brain ECHO (mural thrombus) 24 hr tape (AF)
Migraine with aura	No investigation if the history is typical
Papilloedema	MRI/CT scan of the brain (raised intracranial pressure)
Acute persistent visual impairment	
Optic neuritis	MRI of the brain, visual evoked responses and CSF examination to look for oligoclonal bands (multiple sclerosis)
Retinal or optic nerve ischaemia	ESR, temporal artery biopsy (giant cell arteritis)
Arterial thromboembolism of the middle or posterior cerebral artery	Fasting cholesterol and glucose, blood pressure, ECG, echocardiogram (cerebrovascular risk factors)
Chronic visual impairment	
Anywhere in visual pathway and often associated with optic atrophy	MRI of the brain (tumour, multiple sclerosis), VEPs and CSF examination (multiple sclerosis), tonometry (glaucoma), vitamin B_{12} (pernicious anaemia), cerebrovascular risk factors as above

Disorders of the pupils and eye movements

Objectives

- Understand the anatomy of the sympathetic and parasympathic innervation of the eye
- Describe the major causes of unilateral and bilateral meiosis and mydriasis
- Understand the innervation and function of the extraocular muscles
- Describe the main causes of lesions affecting the third, fourth and sixth cranial nerves
- Understand the difference between jerky and pendular nystagmus and the causes of central and peripheral nystagmus

Changes of pupillary size and reactions can provide important clues not only to disorders of the eye itself, but also disorders of the second and third cranial nerves, the cervical sympathetic outflow, and the central connections of these nerves within the brainstem. Abnormalities of eye movements may also result from lesions arising in many different anatomical sites, ranging from the frontal and occipital cortex, the basal ganglia, cerebellum, brainstem, the third, fourth, sixth and eighth cranial nerves, the neuromuscular junction, to the eye muscles themselves.

PUPIL DISORDERS

The size of the pupils is determined by the balance between two groups of smooth muscle within the iris:

- Sphincter pupillae: a circular constrictor muscle innervated by the parasympathetic nervous system.
- Dilator pupillae: a radial dilator muscle innervated by the sympathetic nervous system.

Anatomical pathway of fibres controlling the pupillary muscles

Parasympathetic fibres arise in the Edinger–Westphal nucleus in the dorsal midbrain. These fibres join those of the third cranial (oculomotor) nerve and synapse in the ciliary ganglion within the orbit. The postganglionic fibres travel in the short ciliary nerves to innervate the sphincter pupillae muscle and ciliary body (Fig. 6.1).

Sympathetic fibres arise in the hypothalamus and descend uncrossed to the midbrain, pons, medulla, and lower cervical and upper thoracic spinal cord, where they synapse with the lateral or intermediate horn cells. These cells form preganglionic fibres, which exit the cord in the anterior roots of T1 and T2 spinal nerves and pass through the thorax in the sympathetic chain to synapse in the superior cervical ganglion. Postganglionic fibres course along the internal carotid artery and through the cavernous sinus to the long ciliary nerve, which innervates the dilator pupillae. Some fibres follow the external carotid artery and innervate the blood vessels and sweat glands of the face apart from fibres responsible for sweating of the medial aspect of the forehead, which follow the internal carotid artery (Fig. 6.2).

The light reflex

When light is shone into the eye, this afferent stimulus travels via the retina, optic nerve, and then both optic tracts. Before the fibres in the optic tracts synapse in the lateral geniculate nuclei in the posterior thalamus, fibres concerned with the light reflex are given off (see Fig. 6.1). These fibres synapse in the pretectal nucleus with neurons that project bilaterally to both Edinger–Westphal nuclei in the dorsal midbrain. Efferent fibres projecting from the Edinger–Westphal nuclei travel within the third cranial nerve to innervate the sphincter pupillae and ciliary body muscles within the orbit. The bilateral innervation of the Edinger–Westphal nuclei by fibres bringing light impulses from each eye enables light shone in one eye to have an effect on both pupils. The effect on the pupil, where the light has been shone into, is called the direct response and the response in the other eye is called the consensual response (see Fig. 6.1).

Fig. 6.1 Pathway for the light reflex and pupillary constriction.

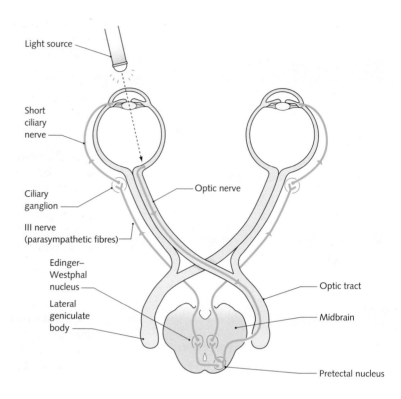

Fig. 6.2 The sympathetic pathway for pupillary dilatation.

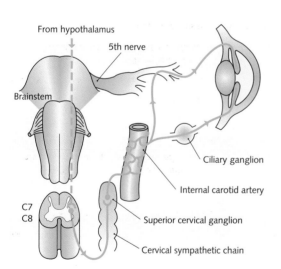

The accommodation reflex

When looking at a near object, the eyes converge and no longer have parallel axes; the pupils constrict and the ciliary body contracts to increase the thickness of the lens and therefore its refractive power. This complex reflex probably involves coordination between several anatomical regions including the parieto-occipital cortex, the Edinger–Westphal nuclei (pupillary constriction), and medial recti components of the nuclei of the third cranial nerve in the midbrain (convergence). A lesion of pupillary constrictor fibres will affect accommodation.

DIFFERENTIAL DIAGNOSIS OF PUPIL DISORDERS

Anisocoria

Anisocoria is inequality in the size of the pupils and can be a normal finding in 20% of the population. The pupillary responses to light and accommodation are unaffected. In pathological anisocoria there is interruption of the pathways of the light and/or accommodation reflexes and these reflexes will be abnormal.

Changes in pupil size and their causes are summarized in Fig. 6.3.

To identify which pupil is abnormal in a patient with anisocoria, the following should be assessed:

- Pupillary responses: the abnormal pupil will have an impaired response to light, and accommodation in most cases.
- Evidence of ptosis: if there is ptosis accompanying a small pupil, look for other signs associated with a Horner's syndrome; if the ptosis is accompanied by a large pupil, look for other signs of a third nerve palsy.
- Response to dark: place the patient in a dark environment, if a pupil fails to dilate then it is probably the pathological pupil.

Small constricted (miotic) pupil

This is caused by:

- Old age.
- Drugs (topical or systemic).

- Horner's syndrome.
- Pontine lesion.
- Argyll Robertson pupils.

Old age

Both pupils are constricted, with absent or poor dilatation in the dark.

Drugs

Both pupils are constricted and dilatation in the dark is absent or poor. Drugs include opiates and pilocarpine drops, which are used to treat chronic glaucoma.

Horner's syndrome

Interruption of the sympathetic pathway gives rise to Horner's syndrome. This is characterized by:

- Pupil constriction: the pupil reaction to light and accommodation is reduced. Dim light accentuates the anisocoria because the pupil dilates less than the normal pupil.
- Ptosis (usually partial).
- Anhidrosis of the ipsilateral side of the face (lesion proximal to the carotid bifurcation) or

Fig. 6.3 Pupil abnormalities

Unilateral (dilated)			Reaction to light (direct)	Associated signs
Third nerve palsy			None	Ptosis (partial or complete), external ophthalmoplegia
Holmes–Adie syndrome			Slow	Better response to accommodation, areflexia
Local lesion of the iris			Variable depending on extent of local damage	Irregular pupil
Unilateral (constricted)				
Horner's syndrome			Reduced dilatation to shade	Ptosis (partial), ipsilateral facial anhidrosis, 'enophthalmos'
Bilateral (dilated)				
Midbrain lesion			None	Mid-position pupils; impaired vertical gaze
Iatrogenic – atropine, tricyclic antidepressants			None or reduced	
Bilateral (constricted)				
Senile			None or reduced	
Iatrogenic – opiates, pilocarpine drops			None or reduced	
Pontine lesion			None	Pin-point pupils, coma, Cheyne–Stokes respiration
Argyll Robertson			None	Irregular pupils, normal accommodation

medial side of the forehead only (lesion distal to the bifurcation).

- 'Enophthalmos' (a sunken eye): this is apparent rather than actual; the eye appears sunken because of the narrowed palpebral fissure.

Horner's syndrome occurs from a lesion at any of the following levels (see Fig. 6.2):

- Hypothalamic lesions, e.g. craniopharyngioma.
- Brainstem, e.g. multiple sclerosis, infarction, tumour (glioma).
- Cervical cord, e.g. syringomyelia, ependymoma.
- T1 root, e.g. Pancoast tumour, cervical rib or band.
- Sympathetic chain, e.g. neoplastic infiltration or surgical damage in the neck involving the larynx, pharynx, thyroid; carotid artery lesions such as a carotid dissection or trauma from a misguided central line.

It should be noted that cervical spondylosis rarely causes Horner's syndrome because the T1 root is usually spared.

Pontine lesion

Bilateral unreactive pin-point pupils in a comatose patient suggest a large intrapontine lesion, such as haemorrhage, causing bilateral interruption of the sympathetic pathways within the brainstem. The differential includes an iatrogenic cause such as opiates, or pilocarpine unrelated to the coma.

Argyll Robertson pupils

An Argyll Robertson pupil is small and irregular. There is no response to light but there is a response to accommodation. The lesion is thought to be within the midbrain. Argyll Robertson pupils have characteristically been associated with tertiary neurosyphilis.

Pseudo-Argyll Robertson pupils can occur in midbrain lesions (e.g. pinealoma, diabetes). There is dissociation between the light reflex and that of accommodation and convergence; however, the pupils may be neither small nor irregular.

Large dilated (mydriatic) pupil

Causes:

- Lesions of the eye, e.g. damage to the iris in acute glaucoma, trauma to the sphincter muscle.
- Drugs: parasympathetic paralysis (e.g. atropine), sympathetic stimulation (e.g. adrenaline [epinephrine]).
- Third nerve lesion.

- Midbrain lesion.
- Holmes–Adie pupil.
- Afferent pupillary defect.

Disorders of the iris and iatrogenic mydriasis

Local lesions of the iris may produce a dilated, usually irregular pupil. The pupillary response will depend on the degree of damage to the muscle (e.g. adhesions anteriorly to the cornea or posteriorly to the lens following inflammation or trauma, iridectomy, or tumour infiltration).

The drug history should be noted for sympathomimetics and those causing parasympathetic paralysis.

Third nerve lesions

The pupil is dilated and both direct and consensual light responses on the affected side are absent. This is an efferent pupillary defect, so the consensual response on the unaffected side is present if light is shone onto the affected side. It is often associated with ptosis and ophthalmoplegia caused by impaired innervation of levator palpebrae muscle and the superior, inferior, and medial recti and inferior oblique muscles, which are supplied by the third nerve. Common causes of a third nerve palsy include diabetic mononeuropathy, posterior communicating artery aneurysm, and herniation of the uncus of the temporal lobe in raised intracranial pressure.

Midbrain lesions

Midbrain lesions involving the decussating fibres of the light reflex result in bilateral semi-dilated pupils without response to light. The area responsible for vertical gaze is in the midbrain, so there may also be impaired upward or downward gaze (e.g. pinealoma, infarction, demyelination, tumour deposits).

Holmes–Adie pupil

Holmes–Adie pupil is dilated and responds sluggishly, if at all, to light, but there is a better response to accommodation. It is thought to be due to degeneration of the ciliary ganglion. It usually occurs in young females and may be associated with absent tendon reflexes (Holmes–Adie syndrome). The pupils may later become smaller and unreactive to all stimuli.

Relative afferent pupillary defect

A lesion of the visual pathway anterior to the lateral geniculate body may result in an afferent pupillary defect. If a light is shone into the normal eye, the direct and consensual responses are normal; if a light is shone into the affected eye, the reaction to constrict is slow and may be incomplete. If the light is swung from one eye to the other (3–4 seconds on each eye), both pupils will constrict appropriately during illumination of the normal eye but both will then dilate as the light shines into the abnormal visual pathway (Fig. 6.4); this results from impairment of the afferent arc of the light reflex on the abnormal side, e.g. optic neuropathy caused by demyelination or tumours.

Pupil responses are normal in lesions of the optic radiation and occipital cortex.

DISORDERS OF EYE MOVEMENTS

Binocular vision allows light from an object to fall onto corresponding parts of each retina so that the brain registers a single image. If there is impaired movement of one eye, the image will be projected onto the macula in the normal eye and to one side of the macula in the affected eye and two images of the same object are then perceived by the higher centres of the brain.

The synchronous movements of the eyes is termed conjugate gaze. This maintains binocular vision. Three pairs of extraocular muscles move the eyeball:

- Superior and inferior recti (third nerve).
- Medial and lateral recti (third and sixth nerves, respectively).
- Superior and inferior oblique (contralateral fourth and ipsilateral third nerves, respectively).

All eye muscles are innervated by the third cranial nerve apart from the superior oblique (innervated by the contralateral fourth cranial nerve) and lateral rectus (innervated by the sixth cranial nerve). The function of each muscle is summarized in Fig. 6.5.

Conjugate gaze

The ipsilateral parietal cortex controls and initiates slow smooth pursuit movements and is used to maintain fixation of a moving image, e.g. following a patient walking. The contralateral frontal cortical pathway is responsible for rapid jumping or 'saccadic' movements, which enable fixation from one image to another in a distant part of the visual field (Fig. 6.6).

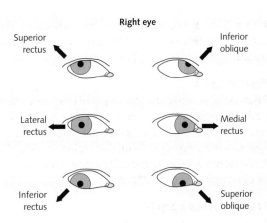

Fig. 6.5 Muscles responsible for eye movements (the right eye is shown above).

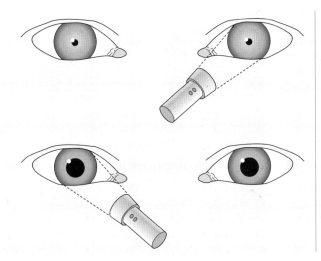

Right afferent pupillary defect
- Optic nerve lesion in right eye (e.g. MS)
- Light shone into unaffected left eye produces normal consensual pupillary constriction (intact left afferent pathway, both efferent pathways intact)
- Switching the light quickly to the abnormal right eye is followed by consensual dilation of both pupils, due to impaired afferent (optic nerve) response to the stimulus (they may then constrict again partially or slowly)

Fig. 6.4 The swinging light test – a sensitive test of optic nerve damage.

Fig. 6.6 Pathway for lateral gaze to the left, including right third nucleus and nerve, the medial longitudinal fasciculus and the left sixth nucleus and nerve. PPRF = Parapontine reticular formation. MLF = medial longitudinal fasciculus.

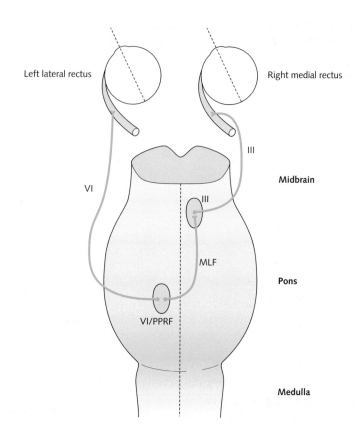

Both cortical pathways converge on the pontine centre for horizontal gaze, the parapontine reticular formation (PPRF) and on the midbrain for vertical gaze. From the PPRF there are connections to the sixth nerve nucleus, supplying the ipsilateral lateral rectus muscle, and to the contralateral third nerve nucleus, via the medial longitudinal fasciculus, supplying the contralateral medial rectus muscle. Vestibular and cerebellar influences are important for modulating eye movements.

Strabismus (squint)

A squint, or strabismus, is when the visual axes are not aligned. Light from an image falls on non-corresponding parts of the retinae. Everyone has some tendency to misalign the visual axes; however, this is overcome by mechanisms of fusion of the images. This ensures that light from an image falls onto corresponding parts of the retinae so that the brain registers a single image. In adulthood, the strabismus is accompanied by diplopia, or double vision, as the brain fails to fuse the two images and is termed a paralytic strabismus.

Binocular vision is established by the age of 6 months, so that when non-paralytic strabismus occurs

at a very young age, the brain suppresses one of the two images so that diplopia does not occur. This suppression of one image interferes with the development of normal vision in that eye at the cortical level. If this persists beyond the age of 6 years, an amblyopic or 'lazy' eye develops, which has a reduced visual acuity and poor depth perception. Non-paralytic strabismus is one cause of amblyopia. Refractive lens problems or any other disturbance of light reaching the retina (e.g. trauma to the eyeball) may cause amblyopia if it remains untreated before 6 years of age.

In both paralytic and non-paralytic strabismus, the visual axis of the abnormal eye can be away from the midline (a divergent strabismus [exotropia]) or inwards towards the midline (a convergent strabismus [esotropia]).

Non-paralytic strabismus

- Eye movements are full when each side is tested separately while covering the other eye.
- Visual acuity is reduced and cannot be corrected in the abnormal eye.
- When fixating on an object, if the normal eye is covered the squinting eye will move to take up

fixation. This is called a positive cover test. It is the basis for correction of a non-paralytic strabismus in childhood by using a patch over the normal eye to force use of the squinting eye and therefore encourage the development of normal vision in that eye.

Paralytic strabismus

Paralytic strabismus is accompanied by diplopia. The approach to assessing a patient with diplopia is discussed on p. 235.

Monocular diplopia

Monocular diplopia is double vision that occurs in one eye when the other eye is covered. It is due to a lesion of the eye itself. The most common organic causes are cataracts and corneal scarring. Some patients can present with monocular diplopia and no organic cause can be found.

Binocular diplopia

Binocular diplopia occurs when there is failure of already established binocular vision. Unlike monocular diplopia, the double vision resolves when one eye is covered. Misalignment of the visual axes may result from paralysis of the extraocular muscles or restriction of their normal movements by mechanical factors within the orbit. A paralytic strabismus from paralysis of the extraocular muscles may be evident. If the paralysis is incomplete, there may be diplopia without overt strabismus.

Causes of diplopia

- Lesions of the third, fourth, and/or sixth cranial nerves.
- Brainstem lesions affecting the nuclei of the third, fourth, and sixth nerves, or their connections.
- Lesions of the neuromuscular junction or extraocular muscles.
- Mechanical lesions impairing movement of the extraocular muscles within the orbit.

Lesions of the third (oculomotor) nucleus and nerve

The nucleus of the third cranial nerve is situated in the dorsal midbrain. It consists of a motor nucleus for the ocular muscles, and the Edinger–Westphal nucleus for pupillary constriction. The nerve emerges

from the midbrain and passes near to the posterior communicating artery to enter the cavernous sinus. It enters the orbit through the superior orbital fissure to supply part of levator palpebrae superioris; the inferior oblique; and the superior, inferior, and medial recti muscles. A parasympathetic branch is also given off to supply the pupil and ciliary body.

With compressive lesions of the third nerve (e.g. aneurysms, tumours, herniation of the temporal lobe), the superficially sited pupillary constrictor fibres are affected early. By contrast, in diabetes, there is infarction of the centre of the nerve and the more superficial fibres may be unaffected. This tends to spare the pupillary responses (Fig. 6.7).

Lesions of the fourth (trochlear) nucleus and nerve

The nucleus of the fourth cranial nerve is in the lower dorsal midbrain. The fourth nerve arises from the nucleus and decussates as the nerve emerges from

---

Fig. 6.7 3rd (oculomotor) cranial nerve lesions

3rd nerve and nucleus lesions give rise to:
Diplopia in all directions of gaze
Lateral and downward deviation of the eye
Ptosis (partial or full)
A dilated pupil unresponsive to light and accommodation

Causes

3rd nerve lesions
Posterior communicating artery aneurysm
Cavernous sinus thrombosis
Lesions of the superior orbital fissure (malignant infiltration)
Diabetes

Midbrain lesions affecting the 3rd nucleus
Infarction
Demyelination
Glioma
Metastatic deposits

In midbrain lesions, also look for:
A contralateral hemiplegia
Ipsilateral limb ataxia
Coarse red nuclear tremor (involvement of cerebellar and red nuclear fibres)

Patient looking forwards

Patient looking in the direction of the arrow

the dorsal midbrain. It has a long intracranial course as it passes ventrally and enters the cavernous sinus with the third, sixth, and ophthalmic and maxillary branches of the trigeminal (fifth) nerve. It then enters the orbit through the superior orbital fissure to supply the superior oblique muscle (Fig. 6.8).

Lesions of the sixth (abducens) nucleus and nerve

The nucleus of the sixth cranial nerve lies in the floor of the fourth ventricle in the lower pons, encircled by the emerging fibres of the seventh nerve. The sixth nerve exits the brainstem, passes over the tip of the petrous temporal bone, and enters the cavernous sinus. It enters the orbit through the superior orbital fissure to supply the lateral rectus muscle (Fig. 6.9).

Lesions of the brainstem

Pathology involving the brainstem may involve one or more of the third, fourth, and sixth ocular motor nuclei, as detailed individually (see Figs 6.7, 6.8 and 6.9). The blood supply to these nuclei is from the vertebrobasilar arterial tree, so occlusive vascular disease may cause transient or permanent diplopia due to involvement of all the ocular motor nuclei.

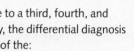

If diplopia is due to a third, fourth, and sixth nerve palsy, the differential diagnosis includes lesions of the:

- Brainstem.
- Cavernous sinus.
- Superior orbital fissure.

If examination does not reveal the diplopia to be consistent with defined weakness of one or more of the extraocular muscles (see p. 39–40), look for proptosis and a mechanical aetiology, muscle disease (e.g. thyroid eye disease, mitochondrial cytopathy), myasthenia gravis or a functional cause.

Fig. 6.8 4th (trochlear) cranial nerve lesions

4th nerve and nucleus lesions give rise to paralysis of the superior oblique muscle:
Vertical and oblique diplopia on looking down and inwards
The eye sits rotated slightly outwards and upwards (extorsion)
The patient tries to compensate by tilting the head away from the affected eye

Causes

4th nerve lesions
Isolated 4th nerve lesions are rare and usually due to diabetes (ischaemic infarction of the nerve) or trauma
Lesions of the cavernous sinus and superior orbital fissure will involve the 3rd and 6th nerves, and branches of the 5th nerve

Midbrain lesions affecting the 4th nucleus
Infarction
Demyelination
Glioma
Metastasis

Patient looking forwards

Patient looking in the direction of the arrow
The right eye fails to depress and adduct.

Note: the weakness of the superior oblique muscle is contralateral to the side of a lesion at nuclear level.

Fig. 6.9 6th (abducens) cranial nerve lesions

6th nerve and nucleus lesions give rise to paralysis of the lateral rectus muscle:
Horizontal diplopia maximal on lateral gaze to the side of the lesion

Causes

6th nerve lesions
Gradenigo's syndrome – due to infection of the petrous temporal bone
Cavernous sinus thrombosis
Fracture or malignant infiltration (nasopharyngeal carcinoma) of the skull base
Lesions of the superior orbital fissure

Pontine lesions affecting the 6th nucleus
Same as for the 3rd and 4th nucleus (see Fig. 6.7)

In pontine lesions, also look for:
A contralateral hemiplegia
Ipsilateral weakness of the upper and lower face (7th nerve fibres hooking around the 6th nucleus)

Patient looking forwards

Patient looking in the direction of the arrow

Note: in cases of raised intracranial pressure, due to its long course, the sixth nerve may become stretched as it passes over the tip of the petrous temporal bone, giving rise to a sixth nerve palsy – this is a false localizing sign.

Vascular or demyelinating disease of the medial longitudinal fasciculus gives rise to diplopia due to an internuclear ophthalmoplegia (INO) (see p. 41). An INO is common in multiple sclerosis.

Disorders of the neuromuscular junction

Diplopia and ptosis are common presenting features of myasthenia gravis and both demonstrate fatiguability on repetitive movements. Ocular involvement may be the only manifestation of myasthenia gravis initially although many of these patients eventually develop weakness elsewhere.

Disorders of muscle

Dysthyroid myopathy most frequently involves the medial and inferior recti, although soft tissue infiltration is the most common cause of proptosis and mechanical disruption of the extraocular muscles.

Oculopharyngeal muscular dystrophy causes diplopia from weakness of the extraocular muscles as well as ptosis. These patients also develop weakness of their bulbar musculature affecting speech and swallowing and eventually progress to involve the limb muscles.

Mitochondrial disease can often affect the extraocular muscles and cause severe ptosis and ophthalmoplegia. There may be no family history and the weakness may be isolated to the eyes.

Orbital lesions

- Intraorbital tumours and vascular malformations cause proptosis and diplopia.
- A 'blow-out' fracture of the orbital floor with herniation of the soft tissues into the maxillary sinus can cause tethering of the extraocular muscles. Enophthalmos (sunken eye), restricted eye movements, and loss of sensation in the area supplied by the inferior orbital nerve can be seen.

Abnormalities of conjugate gaze

Horizontal gaze palsy

The inability to move the eyes in a conjugate manner hortizontally (a 'horizontal conjugate gaze palsy') is caused by a lesion in the contralateral frontal cortex or ipsilateral pons. These structures are both anatomically close to the upper motor neurons and hemiparesis is therefore often seen in association with horizontal gaze palsy. The direction of deviation of the eye relative to the neurological deficit will aid localization of the lesion:

- Eyes deviating away from the hemiparetic side: frontal lobe lesion contralateral to the hemiparesis.
- Eyes deviating towards the hemiparetic side: pontine lesion contralateral to the hemiparesis.

During a focal seizure, the converse pattern is seen (i.e. in a frontal lobe seizure, the eyes deviate away from the side of the lesion and towards the convulsing limbs).

Internuclear ophthalmoplegia

A lesion of the medial longitudinal fasciculus results in paralysis of the medial rectus muscle on the ipsilateral side. There is failure of adduction of the eye on attempted lateral gaze away from the side of the lesion; this is can be associated with asymmetrical jerky nystagmus in the opposite abducting eye.

The most common causes are demyelination and vascular lesions. Bilateral lesions are almost pathognomonic of demyelination (Figs 6.6 and 6.10).

Nystagmus

Nystagmus is an involuntary oscillatory movement of the eyes. There are two types:

1. Jerky nystagmus is characterized by a slow pathological phase and a fast corrective phase in the opposite direction. The direction of the nystagmus is described in terms of the direction of the fast component. This type of nystagmus can be pathological or non-pathological and will be discussed in further detail below.
2. Pendular nystagmus is characterized by equal oscillations in both directions as occurs in a swinging pendulum.

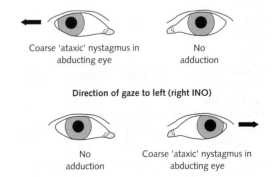

Direction of gaze to right (left INO)

Coarse 'ataxic' nystagmus in abducting eye   No adduction

Direction of gaze to left (right INO)

No adduction   Coarse 'ataxic' nystagmus in abducting eye

Fig. 6.10 Bilateral internuclear ophthalmoplegia.

Pendular nystagmus due to visual impairment

An acquired pendular nystagmus occurs in patients with marked visual impairment or loss in early life (e.g. albinism, congenital cataracts). The nystagmus is always in the horizontal plane whether the eye movements are vertical or horizontal and jerk nystagmus may be seen at the extremes of gaze.

Congenital nystagmus

Congenital nystagmus is a pendular nystagmus present in all positions of gaze, often including the resting position. The condition is present from birth and has an autosomal dominant inheritance. The patient is unaware of the movement due to synchronized oscillations of the head in the opposite direction, which steadies the image.

Jerky nystagmus

The causes of jerky nystagmus can be subdivided into central and peripheral pathways. It can be important to differentiate the side on which the fast phase nystagmus occurs because this points towards the lesion if it is central and away from the lesion if it is peripheral.

The central pathways involve:

- Vestibular nuclei in the brainstem and their connections.
- Cerebellar disease and its brainstem connections. Nystagmus from cerebellar disease is uncommon and usually involves the brainstem connections.

The peripheral pathways include the:

- Vestibulocochlear, or eighth, nerve.
- Inner ear vestibular apparatus.

It is first important to establish non-pathological from pathological nystagmus.

Non-pathological nystagmus

'Nystagmoid jerks'

Physiological nystagmus can be seen if eye movements are tested too fast or at the extremes of lateral gaze beyond the range of binocular vision.

Optokinetic nystagmus (OKN)

When we follow a moving object (e.g. trees from a moving train or vertical stripes on a rotating drum) jerky nystagmus occurs. The slow component represents normal pursuit movements to the limit of conjugate gaze and the fast component in the opposite direction represents rapid saccadic movements with subsequent fixation on a new object entering the field of view. Optokinetic nystagmus is interrupted in lesions of the ipsilateral parietal cortex and its connections to the brainstem centres involved in conjugate gaze. If a striped drum is rotated towards the side of the lesion, OKN is lost or reduced and if rotated in the opposite direction, OKN is normal. OKN is normal in disorders of the peripheral vestibular system and in non-organic blindness (i.e. hysterical blindness).

Pathological nystagmus

Central nystagmus

Lesions of the brainstem, including the vestibular nuclei, as well as the cerebellum and its connections to the brainstem usually cause horizontal nystagmus. Vertigo is not common in central nystagmus.

Asymmetrical nystagmus mainly occurs in internuclear ophthalmoplegia (see p. 41) associated with lesions of the pons.

Vertical nystagmus is less common in brainstem disease and there are two types:

1. Upbeat nystagmus is seen in lesions of the midbrain, e.g. in multiple sclerosis, vascular disorders, or tumours.
2. Downbeat nystagmus is characteristic of lesions at the foramen magnum, e.g. Arnold–Chiari malformation, foramen magnum meningioma.

Both types of vertical nystagmus are seen in Wernicke's disease following vitamin B_1 insufficiency.

'Ocular bobbing' may be seen in comatose patients with extensive pontine lesions and absent horizontal eye movements. This is fast, jerky, downward movements followed by a slow drift upwards.

Peripheral nystagmus

Vertigo is a common feature in peripheral nystagmus. Nystagmus is horizontal or rotatory and the fast phase is away from the side of the lesion in all positions of gaze. There may be unsteadiness of gait towards the side of lesion, as well as deafness and tinnitus on the affected side. Nausea and vomiting often accompany the vertigo.

Causes include:

- Labyrinthine disease (common): benign positional vertigo, Ménière's disease, infection, trauma.
- Vestibular nerve lesion (rare): acoustic neuroma (vertigo is uncommon), aminoglycoside toxicity, herpes zoster infection.

Facial sensory loss and weakness

Objectives

- Understand the basic anatomy of the fifth and seventh cranial nerves
- Describe the associated neurology with lesions along the course of the trigeminal nerve
- Understand the difference between upper and lower motor neuron facial weakness
- Describe the causes and associated differentiating features of types of facial weakness

Facial sensory disturbance may result from disorders affecting the trigeminal (fifth cranial) nerve or its central connections within the brainstem and high cervical cord, thalamus, internal capsule, and sensory cortex. The upper cervical nerves (C2, C3) supply sensation over a small part of the face, along the lower jaw, as well as the back of the head to the vertex and under the chin.

Facial weakness may result from lesions involving the seventh cranial nerve and its central connections in the brainstem, internal capsule, and motor cortex, as well as from disease of the neuromuscular junction (myasthenia) or of muscle (myopathies).

THE TRIGEMINAL NERVE

The trigeminal or fifth cranial nerve is a mixed motor and sensory nerve. It arises from the inferolateral aspect of the pons and has a large sensory root and a small motor root.

From the pons, the sensory root pierces the dura mater to join the Gasserian (trigeminal) ganglion, which contains cell bodies of the somatic sensory nerves. The ganglion lies at the apex of the petrous temporal bone and gives rise to three peripheral divisions:

1. Ophthalmic branch (V_1): this traverses the lateral wall of the cavernous sinus and enters the orbit through the superior orbital fissure. Its cutaneous distribution is shown in Fig. 7.1; it also supplies the cornea, mucosae of the nasal cavity and frontal sinuses, dura mater of the falx, and the superior surface of the tentorium.

2. Maxillary branch (V_2): this traverses the lower lateral wall of the cavernous sinus and exits the skull in the foramen rotundum. It enters the floor of the orbit via the inferior orbital fissure. In addition to supplying the skin (see Fig. 7.1), it supplies the floor of the middle cranial fossa, the upper teeth and gums, and the adjacent palate. It contributes secretomotor parasympathetic fibres to the lacrimal gland.

3. Mandibular branch (V_3): this carries the motor component of the nerve that supplies the muscles of mastication (chewing) including masseter and temporalis. It exits the skull via the foramen ovale. Its sensory supply is to the lower face (see Fig. 7.1), mucosa of the cheek, lower lip, jaw, incisor and canine teeth, floor of the mouth, lower gums and anterior two-thirds of the tongue.

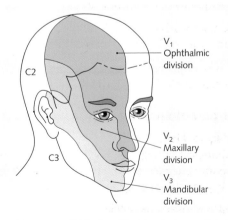

Fig. 7.1 The cutaneous distribution of the trigeminal nerve. Note that the upper cervical dermatomes (C2, C3) extend onto the face, above the angle of the jaw, and onto the back of the head to the vertex.

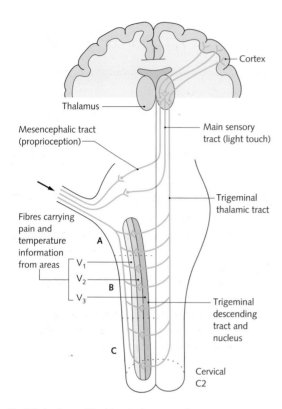

Fig. 7.2 Anatomy of the trigeminal sensory pathways.

The proximal axons of the somatic sensory Gasserian ganglion cells divide in the pons into short ascending and long descending branches. The short fibres carry light touch and deep pressure to the main sensory nucleus, and proprioception to the mesencephalic nucleus in the mid pons. The long descending fibres form the spinal trigeminal tract and carry information about pain and temperature. The nucleus of the spinal trigeminal tract extends from the junction of the pons and medulla to C2 of the spinal cord and fibres cross to the opposite side and ascend to the thalamus in the trigeminothalamic tract (Fig. 7.2).

The motor nucleus of the fifth nerve is in the mid pons. The fibres from the motor root pass below the Gasserian ganglion to join the sensory fibres in the mandibular nerve (V_3) and innervate the muscles of mastication.

DIFFERENTIAL DIAGNOSIS OF FACIAL SENSORY LOSS

The wide anatomical distribution of the fifth nerve means that complete motor and sensory lesions of the fifth

nerve are uncommon. The sensory component is mostly affected and the motor component is often spared.

On examination look for:

- Sensory deficit in the distribution of the three branches of the fifth nerve: loss of the corneal reflex is an early sign of damage to the ophthalmic branch as seen in lesions at the cerebellopontine angle, e.g. acoustic neuroma. Lesions of the lower pons, medulla, or upper cervical cord produce dissociated (i.e. sparing light touch, vibration and proprioception), sensory loss of pain, and temperature in a 'Balaclava' distribution (Fig. 7.3). As the lesion extends up the brainstem, the sensory deficit spreads towards the nose.
- Motor involvement: this may be manifested by weakness of the muscles of mastication and deviation of the jaw towards the side of the lesion because of weakness of the pterygoid muscles.
- The jaw jerk (a trigeminal pontine reflex): this is brisk in upper motor neuron lesions above the motor nucleus of the fifth nerve.

Facial sensory loss can be caused by a lesion anywhere from the cerebral cortex to the cranial nerve and its terminal branches. The site of the lesion can be determined by the associated neurological signs.

A supranuclear lesion is contralateral to the facial sensory loss because the sensory fibres cross the midline after they synapse in the brainstem. Lesions at all other sites are therefore ipsilateral to the facial sensory loss.

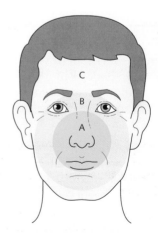

Fig. 7.3 Low pontine (A), medullary (B), and cervical lesions (C) produce an 'onion skin' distribution of pin-prick (pain) and temperature loss due to lesions in the descending trigeminal tract and nucleus (see also Fig. 7.2).

Supranuclear lesions

These include lesions to the primary sensory cortex, internal capsule and upper brainstem:

- Ipsilateral 'pyramidal' weakness.
- Ipsilateral lower facial weakness (upper motor neuron).
- Other cortical signs such as dysphasia, inattention, apraxia, hemianopia.

Causes:

- Cerebral infarction/haemorrhage.
- Demyelination, e.g. multiple sclerosis.
- Neoplasms (glioma, metastatic deposits).

Brainstem lesions

These include lesions of the pons for all sensory modalities and the medulla/upper cervical cord for pain and temperature sensation only:

- Contralateral 'pyramidal' weakness.
- Ipsilateral cranial nerve lesions in close proximity to the fifth nerve nuclei.
- Horizontal conjugate gaze palsies if the pons is involved.
- Lesions of the lower pons, medulla, or upper cervical cord can produce dissociated sensory loss due to involvement of the descending trigeminal spinal tract and/or nucleus. There is ipsilateral loss of pain and temperature in an 'onion skin' distribution with preservation of light touch, vibration, and proprioception.

Causes:

- Infarction.
- Demyelination.
- Neoplasia (glioma, metastatic disease).

Cerebellopontine angle lesions

Lesions at the cerebellopontine angle (CPA) are often associated with a disturbance in facial sensation and a reduced corneal reflex early in the disease even before facial weakness:

- Contralateral 'pyramidal' weakness.
- Damage of the ipsilateral seventh and eighth cranial nerves with late involvement of the sixth, ninth and tenth nerves.
- Ipsilateral cerebellar signs in the limbs.

Causes:

- Acoustic neuroma (vestibular schwannoma).
- Meningioma.
- Metastatic deposits.
- Trigeminal neuroma.

An acoustic neuroma often causes unilateral hearing loss which may go unrecognized by the patient and physicians as bilateral hearing loss is very common with age. A patient with unilateral sensorineural hearing loss of recent onset should be fully investigated. There may also be loss of corneal sensation which should be one of the clues that the patient with unilateral hearing loss has a lesion at the cerebellopontine angle. Facial weakness is also uncommon early in acoustic neuromas.

Cavernous sinus lesions

Patients with a lesion of the cavernous sinus may have lesions of the third, fourth, and sixth cranial nerves as well as the ophthalmic branch, and occasionally the maxillary branch, of the fifth nerve.

Causes:

- Meningioma.
- Aneurysm of the intracavernous portion of the internal carotid artery.
- Metastatic infiltration.
- Granulomatous conditions including sarcoidosis.
- Extension of a pituitary tumour.
- Thrombosis of the cavernous sinus, e.g. thrombophilia, following infections in the face.

Lesions of the trigeminal root, ganglion, and peripheral branches of the nerve

These lesions include:

- Herpes zoster: this manifests as a vesicular rash in the cutaneous distribution of the nerve.

- Skull fractures affecting the superficial branches of the trigeminal nerve (cutaneous deficit) or at the skull base (additional cranial nerve palsies).
- Neoplastic infiltration or compression: tumours of the sinuses, cholesteatoma, fifth nerve neuroma, nasopharyngeal carcinoma at the skull base, lesion of the superior orbital fissure (third, fourth and sixth nerve palsies).
- Granulomatous disease: tuberculosis, sarcoidosis.
- Connective tissue disease: Sjögren's syndrome, scleroderma and systemic lupus erythematosus.
- Trigeminal neuralgia.

FACIAL NERVE

Facial nerve anatomy

- The seventh cranial nerve is composed of motor fibres, which innervate the muscles of facial expression, and the nervus intermedius, which carries taste fibres from the anterior two-thirds of the tongue and parasympathetic fibres to the salivary glands and stapedius.
- The motor nucleus of the facial nerve lies in the lateral pons and its intrapontine fibres

hook around the nucleus of the sixth nerve (abducens) before emerging from the pons at the cerebellopontine angle.

- The facial nerve enters the internal auditory meatus with the nervus intermedius and the eighth nerve.
- The eighth nerve subsequently dives deep within the petrous bone to the middle ear and the nervus intermedius and facial nerve enter the geniculate ganglion. This contains the cell bodies of taste fibres subserving the anterior two-thirds of the tongue.
- The greater petrosal nerve comes off the geniculate ganglion and carries parasympathetic fibres to the lacrimal gland.
- The seventh nerve then courses through the facial canal in the petrous temporal bone and gives off two important branches within the canal. The first is a small branch to the stapedius muscle, which is involved in controlling the sensitivity of the ossicles to sound. If it is damaged then sounds become louder (hyperacusis). The second branch is the chorda tympani, which subserves taste to the anterior two-thirds of the tongue as well as parasympathetic fibres to the submandibular and sublingual glands.

Fig. 7.4 The anatomy of the facial nerve and its branches. The chorda tympani supplies taste sensation to the anterior two-thirds of the tongue. GPN, greater petrosal nerve to lacrimal gland.

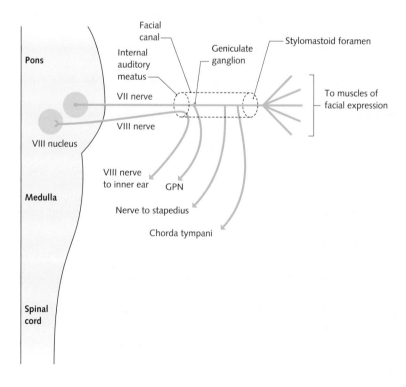

- The main facial nerve continues in the facial canal and leaves the skull through the stylomastoid foramen. It enters the parotid gland and divides into branches that supply the muscles of facial expression (Fig. 7.4).

Upper and lower motor neuron facial weakness

- The facial motor nucleus is supplied by upper motor neurons from the primary motor cortex, which travel in the corticobulbar pathway in the internal capsule to synapse on the lower motor neurons in the facial nerve nucleus in the pons.
- The lower facial muscles receive input from the contralateral hemisphere only, whereas the upper facial muscles have input from both cortices. Consequently, a supranuclear (upper motor neuron) lesion will cause contralateral weakness of only the lower facial muscles, because the upper facial muscles have an additional supply from the intact ipsilateral pathway. In contrast, a lower motor neuron lesion will cause ipsilateral weakness involving both the upper and lower facial muscles.

Differential diagnosis of facial weakness

Facial weakness arises from a lesion anywhere from the motor cortex to the seventh cranial nerve and its distal connections (including the neuromuscular junction and muscle).

To differentiate the site of the lesion, the first step is to determine whether the weakness involves the upper and lower or only the lower part of the face, and then whether it involves one side or both. Lesions of the neuromuscular junction and muscle itself cause weakness of the upper and lower face as in a lower motor neuron lesion, but it is bilateral and usually symmetrical. A summary of the differential diagnosis of facial weakness is shown in Fig. 7.5 (overleaf).

When a patient presents with unilateral lower motor neuron facial weakness it is important to ask about associated neurological symptoms such as loss of taste, perception of loud sounds and a dry eye. If these symptoms are absent then be suspicious that the lesion may be distal to the facial canal, e.g. tumour within the parotid gland.

Fig. 7.5 Differential diagnosis of facial weakness

Syndrome	Clinical features and causes
Unilateral upper motor neuron facial weakness	**Unilateral weakness of the lower face** Unilateral weakness of the lower face is due to a contralateral supranuclear (upper motor neuron) lesion. It is usually caused by a contralateral stroke or tumour
Unilateral lower motor neuron facial weakness	**Unilateral weakness of the upper and lower face** Unilateral weakness of the upper and lower face is due to disorder of the nucleus of the 7th nerve, the geniculate ganglion, or the peripheral nerve; additional clinical features aid lesion localization; lesions may occur at the following sites: • Pons – features include ipsilateral 6th nerve lesion and contralateral 'pyramidal' weakness (recall that the intrapontine fibres hook around the nucleus of the 6th nerve); e.g. infarction, demyelination, tumour deposits • Cerebellopontine angle: facial sensory loss, loss of corneal reflex, hearing loss • Facial canal – features include hyperacusis (involvement of nerve to stapedius) and loss of taste in the anterior two-thirds of the tongue (involvement of the chorda tympani); e.g. middle ear infection, Bell's palsy, tumour deposits, fracture of the skull base. Lacrimation is often spared. • Geniculate ganglion – e.g. herpes zoster infection of the ganglion; look for pain and vesicles in the auditory canal • Peripheral branches of the nerve – e.g. parotid gland lesions (tumour, infection, sarcoidosis), trauma
Bilateral lower motor neuron facial weakness 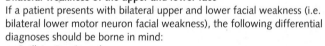	**Bilateral weakness of the upper and lower face** If a patient presents with bilateral upper and lower facial weakness (i.e. bilateral lower motor neuron facial weakness), the following differential diagnoses should be borne in mind: • Guillain–Barré syndrome • Lyme disease • Sarcoidosis • Bilateral Bell's palsy • Myasthenia gravis • Myopathies – dystrophia myotonica, facio-scapulo-humeral dystrophy

Deafness, tinnitus, dizziness and vertigo

Objectives

- Understand the basic anatomy of the auditory and vestibular systems
- Define the Rinne's and Weber's tests and how you may differentiate between conductive and sensorineural hearing loss
- Describe the common causes of deafness and tinnitus
- Understand how you may localize the lesion in a patient with vertigo

DIZZINESS AND TINNITUS

Deafness and tinnitus usually result from diseases of the cochlea and are generally handled at a specialist level by ear, nose, and throat (ENT) surgeons. However, acoustic neuroma is a rare but important 'neurological' cause of deafness, and the eighth (vestibulocochlear) cranial nerve may be involved in other conditions affecting the brainstem or multiple cranial nerves.

The eighth cranial nerve comprises the cochlear nerve, which subserves hearing, and the vestibular nerve, which is concerned with maintenance of balance (Fig. 8.1). Deafness and tinnitus arise from damage to the auditory apparatus and its central connections via the eighth nerve.

THE AUDITORY SYSTEM

Sound waves are channelled through the external auditory meatus to the tympanic membrane and the auditory ossicles to the oval window setting up waves in the perilymph of the cochlea. The waves in the perilymph are transduced into nerve impulses by the end organ of hearing, the spiral organ of Corti (Figs 8.1 and 8.2).

- These nerve impulses travel in the cochlear nerve, which synapses in the cochlear nuclei in the lower pons.
- Fibres from the cochlear nuclei project to and synapse in the inferior colliculus on both sides.
- These fibres project to the medial geniculate nucleus of the thalamus.
- Fibres then pass from the thalamus through the internal capsule to the auditory cortex in the superior temporal gyrus.

- The bilateral nature of the connections ensures that unilateral central lesions do not cause lateralized hearing loss.

DIFFERENTIAL DIAGNOSIS OF DEAFNESS

There are two types of deafness:

1. Conductive: there is failure of transmission of sound from the outer or middle ear to the cochlea.
2. Sensorineural: this is due to disease of the cochlea, cochlear nerve, cochlear nuclei, and their supranuclear connections.

Clinically, conductive and sensorineural deafness can be distinguished by the Rinne and Weber tests.

Rinne's test

The base of a vibrating 128, 256, or 512 Hz tuning fork is held first against the mastoid process, and then, when the tone has disappeared, about 2.5 cm from the external auditory meatus. Normally, the transmission of sound through the outer and middle ear to the cochlea is better than transmission through bone to the cochlea, which bypasses the middle ear apparatus. Thus, in normal ears, air conduction is better than bone conduction.

In conductive deafness, this ability is impaired due to disease of the outer or middle ear and bone conduction is better. In sensorineural deafness, there is impairment of sound perception whether transmitted through air or bone. However, with the latter, the sound may be transmitted through bone to the normal contralateral ear, giving a false positive result.

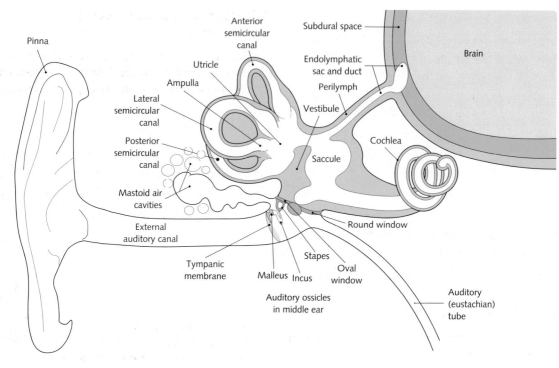

Fig. 8.1 Components of the outer, middle, and inner ear.

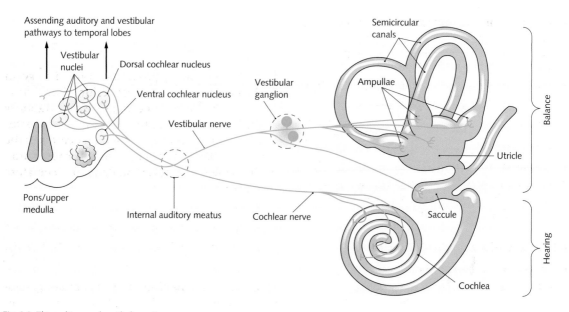

Fig. 8.2 The auditory and vestibular system.

Weber's test

When a vibrating tuning fork is placed in the middle of the forehead, sound is normally heard equally in both ears. In conductive deafness, the sound localizes to the affected ear (due to lack of competitive sounds that would normally be heard on that side). By contrast, in sensorineural deafness, the sound lateralizes to the normal ear.

Conductive deafness

In conductive deafness, there is impaired perception, especially of low-pitched sounds.

Conductive deafness can be caused by:

- Disorders of the outer ear: the build up of wax in the external auditory canal is the commonest cause.
- Disorders of the middle ear: otitis media, cholesteatoma, otosclerosis, rupture of the tympanic membrane.

Sensorineural deafness

In sensorineural deafness, there is often preferential impairment of perception of high-pitched sounds. Sensorineural deafness can be caused by a variety of disorders:

Disorders of the cochlea

- Congenital disorders: from rubella or syphilis in the pregnant mother.
- Infection: purulent meningitis, spread of infection from the middle to the inner ear, mumps, measles.
- Drugs: aminoglycosides, diuretics, salicylates, quinine. (Deafness is transient with the last two but can be permanent with aminoglycosides.)
- Presbycusis: neuronal degeneration in the elderly causing high-frequency hearing loss.
- Noise-induced disorders: high-frequency hearing loss from, e.g. gun blasts, industrial machinery.
- Ménière's disease: vertigo and variable tinnitus and deafness.
- Head injury: fractures through the base of the skull and petrous temporal bone can lead to damage to the cochlea and eighth nerve.

Disorders of the cochlear nerve

- Lesions of the cerebellopontine angle, e.g. acoustic neuroma, other tumours, granulomatous disease, stroke (anterior inferior cerebellar artery).

Disorders of the brainstem

- Multiple sclerosis: plaques of demyelination involving the cochlear nuclei.
- Infarction.
- Neoplastic infiltration.

Disorders of the supranuclear connections

Unilateral lesions of the supranuclear pathways will not cause deafness as the cochlear nuclei on each side have bilateral connections projecting to the temporal cortices.

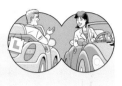

Auditory hallucinations can occur as part of temporal lobe seizures.

Many rare, inherited syndromes are associated with conductive or sensorineural deafness, e.g. mitochondrial disease and Alport's syndrome.

Investigations for deafness

Several audiometric procedures can distinguish deafness caused by cochlear lesions from those caused by lesions of the eighth nerve. Auditory evoked potentials test the integrity of the pathway from the cochlea to the auditory cortex in the temporal lobe; this does not need the cooperation of the patient (i.e. it can be done in a comatose patient).

DIFFERENTIAL DIAGNOSIS OF TINNITUS

Tinnitus is the sensation of ringing, buzzing, hissing, chirping, or whistling in the ear. It is a manifestation of disease of the middle ear, inner ear, or cochlear component of the eighth nerve, and is usually accompanied by some degree of deafness. The causes are summarized in Fig. 8.3. Conductive deafness is associated with low-pitched tinnitus, and sensorineural deafness with high-pitched tinnitus (except Ménière's disease, where the tinnitus is low

Fig. 8.3 Causes of deafness and tinnitus

Site of damage	Cause
Outer ear	Wax, foreign body
Middle ear	Trauma, e.g. fracture of temporal bone Infection, e.g. suppurative otitis media Otosclerosis
Cochlea	Age (presbycusis) Infection, e.g. purulent meningitis Noise induced Drugs, e.g. aminoglycosides Ménière's disease
8th nerve	Lesions of the cerebellopontine angle, e.g. acoustic neuroma Basal meningitis, e.g. TB, sarcoid, malignant infiltration
Brainstem (rare)	Multiple sclerosis Neoplasia Infarction
Cerebral hemisphere (rare)	Bilateral lesions of the temporal lobes, e.g. infarction, neoplasia

pitched). Vibratory mechanical noises in the head can be mistaken for tinnitus. The most common is a bruit from turbulent blood flow in the great vessels of the neck. This may occur as a result of high cardiac output (e.g. febrile or anaemic state) or mechanical obstruction within the lumen of an artery (e.g. arteriovenous malformation or carotid artery stenosis), when the noise heard is in time with the pulse.

THE VESTIBULAR SYSTEM

The sensory feedback from the vestibular, visual, and proprioceptive systems is required to maintain balance. The labyrinth—the vestibular apparatus—lies in each inner ear. It consists of the utricle, saccule, and semicircular canals. There are three semicircular canals (lateral, anterior, and posterior), each positioned perpendicularly with respect to one another (see Fig. 8.2). They respond to rotational acceleration of the head. The utricle and saccule respond to linear acceleration, including gravity.

Afferent information from the labyrinth is relayed by the vestibular component of eighth cranial nerve, the vestibular nerve. The vestibular and cochlear nerves follow the same route from the inner ear through the internal auditory meatus to the cerebellopontine angle before entering the brainstem at the

lower pons. The vestibular fibres synapse in the four vestibular nuclei located at the junction of the pons and medulla. From here there are connections to the:

- Anterior horn cells of the spinal cord, via the vestibulospinal tract.
- Flocculonodular lobe of the cerebellum.
- Third, fourth, and sixth ocular motor nuclei, via the medial longitudinal fasciculus.
- Pontine reticular formation.
- Temporal cortex.

DIZZINESS AND VERTIGO

Dizziness is a very common symptom in GP surgeries and neurology clinics. The term is non-specific and can be used by patients to describe not only vertigo but also feelings of faintness, disorientation, drowsiness, visual disturbance, or even unsteadiness in the legs (imbalance).

It is important to separate all of these from the phenomenon of vertigo, which is best defined as an illusion of movement. This perceived movement may be rotational ('true' vertigo in the pedantic sense) but often it has a swaying, rocking, or heaving quality. All of these feelings of movement are a clear indication of a disorder of the vestibular system, which consists of the:

- Labyrinthine apparatus in the inner ear.
- Vestibular (eighth) nerve from the labyrinth to the brainstem.
- Central connections in the brainstem vestibular nuclei.
- Central projections from the brainstem to the temporal and parietal lobes.

The vestibular apparatus and brainstem nuclei are shown in Figs 8.1 and 8.2.

DIFFERENTIAL DIAGNOSIS OF DIZZINESS AND VERTIGO

Vertigo is the illusion of movement of either the environment or oneself. The movement may be described as to-and-fro, up-and-down, or spinning; it is often associated with nausea and vomiting. The patient might veer to one side when walking and the gait is more unsteady in the dark or with the eyes closed. Nystagmus usually accompanies vertigo. Vertigo may arise from a lesion of the labyrinth, vestibular nerve, cerebellopontine angle, brainstem, cerebellum, or rarely the supranuclear connections (Fig. 8.4).

Clinical features of labyrinthine failure

- Vertigo: occurs in attacks of 1–2 hours duration; there may be accompanying nausea and vomiting.
- Nystagmus: there is horizontal and/or rotary nystagmus with the fast phase opposite to the side of the lesion.
- Gait: the patient may veer towards the side of the lesion when walking.
- Hearing: there may be conductive or sensorineural deafness and tinnitus if the auditory pathway is involved.
- Neurological signs: none apart from nystagmus.

Examples of labyrinthine failure

Ménière's disease

Ménière's disease is characterized by recurrent attacks of vertigo, deafness, tinnitus, and a feeling of pressure or fullness in the ears. It occurs in middle age and the vertigo is usually self-limiting. It is thought to arise from excessive accumulation of endolymphatic fluid and degeneration of the organ of Corti. Permanent deafness may occur after repeated attacks.

Benign paroxysmal positional vertigo (BPPV)

Benign positional vertigo arises from dislocation of particulate material from the otoliths, usually into the posterior semicircular canals. Sudden paroxysms of vertigo occur with movements of the head, particularly lying down, rolling over in bed, bending forward, straightening up, and extending the neck. The vertigo lasts less than a minute and is fatiguable with recurrent movements. The accompanying nystagmus is torsional and similarly fatiguable. Symptoms may be present for several days or months at a time. Some cases follow head trauma or a viral infection of the labyrinth. The Hallpike manoeuvre (see below) can make the diagnosis and a similar manoeuvre can sometimes be therapeutic (Epley's manoeuvre) (Fig. 8.5).

Other causes

Other causes of labyrinthine dysfunction include purulent labyrinthitis following meningitis, motion

Fig. 8.4 Differential diagnosis of vertigo and dizziness

	PERIPHERAL			CENTRAL	
	Labyrinthine failure	Vestibular nerve lesion	Cerebellopontine angle lesion	Brainstem lesions	Cerebellar lesions
Vertigo	Common Short attacks	May be prolonged	Rare	May be prolonged	Brainstem connections involved
Nystagmus	Horizontal and/or rotary	Horizontal and/or rotary	Horizontal	Vertical/horizontal	Horizontal
Fast phase	Opposite to lesion	Opposite to lesion	Towards lesion	Towards lesion	Towards lesion
Gait	Veers towards lesion	Veers towards lesion	Ataxia towards lesion; hemiparetic	Hemiparetic	Ataxia towards lesion
Hearing	Conductive or Sensorineural loss	Sensorineural loss	Sensorineural High-frequency loss early	Unaffected	Unaffected
Other neurological signs	None	± 7th, 5th nerve lesions Ipsilateral cerebellar signs Contralateral 'pyramidal' signs	5th, 7th, 9th, 10th nerve lesions Contralateral 'pyramidal' weakness Ipsilateral ataxia	Ipsilateral cranial nerve palsies	Unilateral cerebellar Signs from an Ipsilateral cerebellar Hemisphere lesion

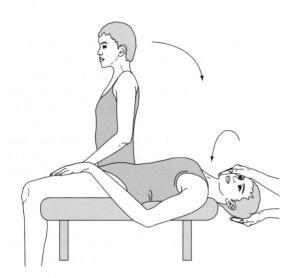

Fig. 8.5 Technique for exhibiting positional nystagmus (Hallpike's manoeuvre).

sickness, and toxic effects from alcohol, quinine, and aminoglycosides.

Vestibular nerve lesions

- Vertigo: this may be severe in vestibular neuronitis (see below).
- Nystagmus: there is horizontal and/or rotary nystagmus with the fast phase opposite to the side of the lesion.
- Gait: the patient may veer towards the side of the lesion.
- Hearing: sensorineural deafness and tinnitus may occur if there is also involvement of the cochlear nerve.
- Neurological signs: depending on the aetiology there may be involvement of adjacent cranial nerves, e.g. fifth and seventh.

The vestibular nerve may be damaged in the petrous temporal bone or the cerebellopontine angle. The latter is dealt with below. Trauma or infection of the petrous temporal bone may involve the seventh and fifth cranial nerves, as may occur with a herpes zoster infection of the nerve or ganglion. Purely vestibular dysfunction occurs in vestibular neuronitis.

Vestibular neuronitis

Vestibular neuronitis manifests as a single severe paroxysm of vertigo without deafness and tinnitus, usually in young or middle-aged adults. Symptoms usually subside within several days but may persist

for weeks. An inflammatory aetiology is presumptive rather than proven but the condition frequently follows an upper respiratory tract infection thus a viral cause has been postulated.

Cerebellopontine angle (CPA) lesions

The CPA is the junction between the pons and cerebellum where the seventh and eighth nerve exits the brainstem. Both brainstem and cranial nerve involvement occurs.

- Vertigo: rarely occurs in the early stages.
- Nystagmus: horizontal, coarse, and towards the side of the lesion.
- Gait: ataxic towards the side of the lesion.
- Hearing: high-frequency deafness is often one of the first symptoms.
- Neurological signs: larger lesions may cause fifth, seventh, ninth, and tenth nerve palsies, ipsilateral cerebellar signs, and contralateral 'pyramidal' weakness.

Causes to consider are acoustic neuroma, other tumours, granulomatous disease, and vascular lesions.

Brainstem lesions

- Vertigo: this may be severe and prolonged.
- Nystagmus: often vertical or multidirectional nystagmus.
- Hearing: usually unaffected since the cochlear and vestibular fibres separate before entering the brainstem.
- Neurological signs: ipsilateral cranial nerve palsies, contralateral 'pyramidal' weakness, and often ipsilateral 'cerebellar' ataxia.

Causes include infarction, demyelination, and neoplastic infiltration.

Episodes of vertigo may arise from transient vertebrobasilar ischaemia but it is rarely the only manifestation of brainstem transient ischaemic attacks. Vertigo prior to a typical headache may be part of migraine with aura.

Cerebellar lesions

- Vertigo: particularly if the lesion is acute and involving brainstem vestibular connections to the flocculonodular lobe.
- Nystagmus: horizontal, coarse, and mainly towards the side of the lesion.

- Gait: ataxia of gait with unsteadiness towards the side of the lesion.
- Hearing: unaffected.
- Neurological signs: unilateral cerebellar signs from an ipsilateral lesion.

Causes of cerebellar dysfunction are considered in Chapter 10.

Vertigo may occur as part of the aura of temporal lobe seizures. Uncommonly, it arises from the neck or from ocular motor disorders (ophthalmoplegia).

Other types of dizziness

Vertigo, as described above, is relatively easily recognized. However, the word 'dizziness' can be used to describe a wide range of other symptoms: light-headedness, a feeling of being on a ship, faintness. Other causes must be considered in the history and examination. The other causes are usually due to pre-syncope, i.e. relative hypoperfusion to the brain and these causes include:

- Anxiety with hyperventilation – 'light-headed'.
- Anaemia – due to hypoxia if chronic and hypovolaemia if acute.
- Postural hypotension: in the elderly, due to drugs, usually antihypertensives, or as part of an autonomic neuropathy.
- Cardiac: low-output cardiac failure, arrhythmias.
- Vasovagal pre-syncope/syncope.
- Iatrogenic: with or without hypotension.

INVESTIGATIONS FOR DIZZINESS AND VERTIGO

Hallpike manoeuvre

The Hallpike manoeuvre is performed with the patient sitting on a bed. The patient's head is positioned 30° to the affected side and taken to 30° below bed level. After a latent period of a few seconds, vertigo is experienced. There is accompanying torsional nystagmus with upper pole beating towards the floor; the direction of vertigo and nystagmus are reversed on sitting up again. With peripheral (labyrinthine) lesions, symptoms and signs last for about 30 seconds and fatigue with repetition such that they cannot then be reproduced (see Fig. 8.5).

Caloric test

The caloric test is a test of vestibular function. With the patient lying supine, the head is raised 30° from horizontal so that the horizontal canals are vertical. Each external meatus is irrigated for 30 seconds with water, first at 30°C, and then, about 5 minutes later, at 44°C. The normal response is summarized by the acronym 'COWS': **C**old water results in nystagmus, with the fast phase **O**pposite to the side irrigated; **W**arm water results in nystagmus, with the fast phase to the **S**ame side irrigated.

Two pieces of information can be obtained from the caloric test:

1. Canal paresis: there is no response to irrigation of the external meatus with either cold or warm water; this occurs in peripheral lesions, i.e. the labyrinth, or vestibular ganglion or nerve.
2. Directional preponderance: cold water in the left ear and warm in the right will both result in nystagmus to the right. If this response is greater than left-sided nystagmus produced by cold water in the right ear and warm in the left, a right directional preponderance exists. This usually implies a lesion of the brainstem vestibular nuclei on the left.

Consider the following when assessing a patient with vertigo:

- Vertigo is either peripheral or central in origin.
- Vertigo from a supranuclear lesion is uncommon, therefore the main differential is between a peripheral (labyrinth, vestibular ganglion/nerve) lesion and a brainstem or cerebellar lesion.
- Vertigo is rarely the sole manifestation of brainstem disease: look for symptoms and signs of additional ipsilateral cranial nerve palsies and contralateral 'pyramidal' limb weakness.
- In vertigo from a cerebellar lesion there might be signs of cerebellar dysfunction; these are absent in vertigo from a lesion of the peripheral vestibular system.
- Vertigo may be the sole symptom of peripheral vestibular dysfunction; this can be confirmed with formal neuro-otological testing.

Dysarthria, dysphonia and dysphagia

Objectives

- Understand the motor pathways responsible for articulation, phonation and swallowing
- Describe the types and common causes of dysarthria, dysphagia and dysphonia

DEFINITIONS

- Dysarthria is a disorder of articulation of speech; there is no difficulty in comprehension or expression of language.
- Dysphonia is a disorder of vocalization, i.e. strength or quality of spoken words.
- Dysphagia is difficulty with swallowing.

Dysarthria, dysphonia, and dysphagia may result from lesions at all levels from the motor cortex down to the numerous muscles involved in articulation, phonation and swallowing. The intervening pathways include the basal ganglia, cerebellum, brainstem, cranial nerves, and the neuromuscular junctions (Fig. 9.1).

Non-neurological local pathology can sometimes account for these symptoms (e.g. dysarthria due to absence of dentures, dysphagia due to oesophageal stricture, dysphonia due to lesions of the vocal cords).

Knowledge of the motor pathways responsible for articulation, phonation, and swallowing enable localization of the site of the lesion.

DYSARTHRIA

Articulation involves the use of the respiratory musculature, larynx, pharynx, palate, tongue, and lips. When a word is heard, signals from the primary auditory cortex are received by Wernicke's area (comprehension of speech), from where the signal is transmitted to Broca's area (expression of speech), and thence to the motor area of the precentral gyrus (primary motor cortex), which controls the speech muscles. The motor pathways for articulation arise from the left (dominant hemisphere in most people)

precentral gyrus and cross to the opposite motor cortex as well, then descend in both corticobulbar tracts to the nuclei of the seventh (motor fibres to the facial muscles, including those of the lips), tenth (nucleus ambiguus: motor fibres to the pharynx, larynx, and soft palate), and twelfth (motor fibres to the tongue) cranial nerves and in the corticospinal tracts to the diaphragm and intercostal muscles. The nuclei of the seventh, tenth, and twelfth cranial nerves receive corticobulbar fibres from both the ipsilateral and contralateral hemispheres. As with all movements, articulation is modulated by the cerebellum and by the basal ganglia (see Fig. 9.1).

Dysarthria can be caused by a lesion at any level in these pathways. Clinical features of lesions at each level are described below.

Upper motor neuron lesions

The muscles of articulation are bilaterally innervated and a unilateral lesion may therefore be asymptomatic. A bilateral lesion is usually required to produce significant dysarthria. This may occur at the same event or at separate times. A lesion may interrupt the corticobulbar tract at the level of the motor cortex, internal capsule, midbrain, or pons before the fibres synapse in the cranial nerve nuclei with the lower motor neurons. An upper motor neuron disorder of articulation is part of a 'pseudobulbar palsy'. This is a disorder of both the right and left corticobulbar fibres supplying the motor nuclei of the brainstem. It results in a spastic dysarthria, slow movements of the face with a staring gaze, and emotional lability due to the loss of the connections from the frontal cortex to the brainstem that suppress emotional output. Facial, palatal and jaw reflexes are brisk, and primitive reflexes are often present. A spastic dysarthria consists of

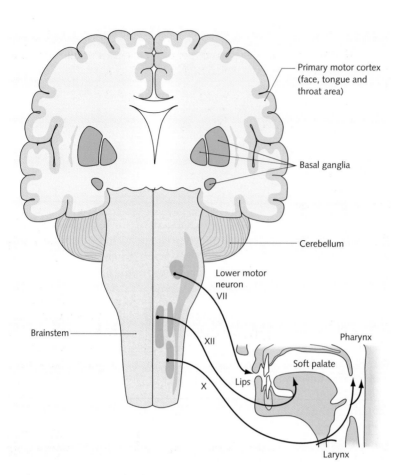

Fig. 9.1 Structures and pathways involved in articulation of speech.

Primary motor cortex (face, tongue and throat area)

Basal ganglia

Cerebellum

Lower motor neuron VII

Brainstem

XII

X

Lips

Soft palate

Pharynx

Larynx

slow, indistinct and strained speech. On examination, the tongue may appear contracted, with limited protrusion. It is often associated with upper motor neuron signs, especially spasticity in the limbs, brisk reflexes, clonus and extensor plantar responses.

Causes of bilateral upper motor neuron lesions include:

- Multiple sclerosis.
- Motor neuron disease.
- Bilateral subcortical ischaemic lesions.
- As part of rare neurodegenerative disorders, e.g. progressive supranuclear palsy.

Lower motor neuron lesions

Lower motor neuron lesions result from damage to the motor nuclei of the seventh, tenth, and twelfth cranial nerves, or their peripheral extensions (the corresponding cranial nerves), and give rise to a 'bulbar palsy'. Speech is slurred and indistinct. Labial and lingual sounds are affected. With bilateral paralysis of the soft palate, the speech gains a nasal quality. The tongue becomes wasted and may fasciculate. The facial muscles may also be weak.

Causes of bilateral lower motor neuron lesions include:

- Guillain–Barré syndrome.
- Motor neuron disease.
- Medullary tumours.
- Syringobulbia.
- Poliomyelitis.

Basal ganglia lesions

Parkinson's disease

The speech in Parkinson's disease is often low volume, monotonous, and without inflection; it often trails off at the end of sentences. There may be alternating acceleration and stuttering pauses in the speech analogous to the 'festinating' gait.

Chorea

The speech in chorea (e.g. Huntington's disease) is hyperkinetic. It is loud and harsh, intonation is variable, and there is poor coordination of the diaphragm and respiratory muscles. This results in short, breathless sentences.

Athetosis

In patients with athetosis, such as in athetoid cerebral palsy, the speech is loud and slow, and consonants are indistinctly pronounced; the speech is sometimes described as 'dystonic'.

With the above syndromes, the diagnosis is often made by the accompanying characteristic movement abnormalities.

Cerebellar lesions

Cerebellar lesions cause ataxic dysarthria. The speech is slow and slurred with abnormally long pauses between syllables. This arises from impaired coordination of articulation, which is evident on attempted rapid side-to-side movements of the tongue. Other cerebellar signs are usually present. If there is also involvement of the corticobulbar tracts, the speech may be 'scanning', with words broken up into syllables, which are spoken with varying force.

Causes of cerebellar lesions include:

- Multiple sclerosis.
- Vascular lesions, e.g. infarcts and haemorrhages.
- Tumours.
- Inherited ataxias, e.g. spinocerebellar dysarthrias.
- Alcoholic cerebellar degeneration.

Myopathies and disorders of the neuromuscular junction

Myopathies and disorders of the neuromuscular junction give rise to a dysarthria similar to that of a bulbar palsy.

In a neuromuscular junction problem there may be evidence of fatiguability, characterized by deterioration of the dysarthria at the end of the day and subsequent improvement the following morning (e.g. myasthenia gravis). If the patient has a myopathic dysarthria there may be a family history of a muscle disorder. There is often prominent wasting and weakness of the facial muscles, involvement of the proximal limbs, and myotonia may be present (e.g. dystrophia myotonica).

Oropharyngeal lesions

Local lesions of the oropharynx can cause difficulty with articulation. Examples include:

- Multiple mouth ulcers, e.g. following chemotherapy.
- Oral candidiasis.
- Quinsy.
- Dental abscess.
- Loose dentures.

Patients who have a cerebellar dysarthria will often suggest that their speech is slurred as if they are drunk without actually being drunk. This can occasionally lead patients into problems with authorities especially if there are other features of cerebellar dysfunction such as imbalance. A written note from a doctor explaining their condition can be a great help for a patient.

DYSPHAGIA

The descending motor pathways for swallowing closely follow those for articulation. Dysarthria is therefore often accompanied by dysphagia. Corticobulbar fibres travel bilaterally to the nuclei of both ninth and tenth cranial nerves. Motor fibres from the tenth nucleus supply the soft palate and pharynx, which are required for swallowing. The adjacent ninth nucleus sends motor fibres to the middle constrictor of the pharynx and stylopharyngeus but the ninth nerve is mostly involved in the sensory component of the swallowing reflex supplies the sensation to the back of the tongue and oropharynx.

Lesions that bilaterally interrupt these pathways will initially cause difficulty with swallowing liquids and subsequently solids. By contrast, lesions causing obstruction of the oesophagus initially tend to cause difficulty with swallowing solids, and then, as the obstruction progresses, difficulty swallowing liquids.

Dysfunction of the swallowing mechanism can be confirmed by videofluoroscopy, when a radio-opaque dye is swallowed and real-time radiographs are taken at each step of swallowing.

Causes of dysphagia overlap with those for dysarthria, and the two symptoms often coexist.

Sites of lesions causing dysphagia

Dysphagia can be caused by lesions of:

- Both cerebral hemispheres (usually vascular or trauma).
- Brainstem (multiple sclerosis, vascular, tumours).
- Cranial nerves (ninth and tenth).
- Neuromuscular junction (myasthenia).
- Muscle (polymyositis).
- Pharynx and oesophagus (local pathology).

DYSPHONIA

Dysphonia is alteration of the volume or quality of vocal sound. Phonation is a function of the larynx and the vocal cords. Sound is produced by air passing over the vocal cords. The pitch is altered by changes in tension of the membranous part of the vocal cords. This is performed by the intrinsic laryngeal muscles, which are supplied by the laryngeal branches of the tenth cranial nerve which arise from the nucleus ambiguus in the medulla. The nucleus ambiguus has bilateral supranuclear innervation from the corticobulbar fibres arising in the primary motor cortex. Lesions in this pathway will cause dysphonia (the voice having a husky quality) or aphonia (the inability to produce any sound). There may be impairment of coughing, which requires normal vocal cord function. Paralysis or a local lesion of the vocal cord can be visualized by indirect laryngoscopy. The paralysed cord fails to abduct and adduct during attempted phonation.

Causes of dysphonia include:

- Medullary lesions involving the nucleus ambiguus: infarction, tumour, demyelination.
- Recurrent laryngeal nerve palsy: following thyroid surgery, bronchial carcinoma, aortic aneurysm.
- Vocal cord lesions: polyps, tumour.
- Functional (psychogenic aphonia).

The proximity of the motor pathways controlling articulation, swallowing, and phonation often leads to impairment of one or more of these functions at the same time (e.g. a patient with a bulbar palsy may present with dysarthria and nasal intonation, drooling due to difficulty swallowing, and a hoarse voice with poor cough).

The causes of dysarthria, dysphagia, or dysphonia are summarized in Fig. 9.2.

It is always wise to inspect the oropharynx first to exclude a local cause for dysarthria/dysphagia.

Fig. 9.2 Causes of dysarthria, dysphagia, and dysphonia

Site	Example
Bilateral upper motor neuron pathways	Primary motor cortex, e.g. motor neuron disease Internal capsule
Basal ganglia Cerebellum (often midline) Brainstem nuclei (VII, X, XII)	Parkinson's disease, Huntington's disease Multiple sclerosis Motor neuron disease
Seventh, tenth, and twelfth cranial nerves Neuromuscular junction Muscle	Bell's palsy Myasthenia gravis Dystrophia myotonica, rare inherited muscle disorders
Oropharynx	Laryngeal tumours

Objectives

- Understand the basic anatomy and function of the cerebellum
- Describe the clinical features associated with cerebellar hemisphere and vermis dysfunction
- Describe the main causes of cerebellar dysfunction

The cerebellum and its connections are responsible for the coordination of skilled voluntary movement, posture, and gait.

The cerebellum can be divided into three functional units (Figs 10.1 and 10.2):

1. The flocculonodular lobe (vestibulocerebellum) and inferior vermis, which are mainly involved in controlling information from the vestibular system.
2. The small anterior lobe and the anterior superior vermis (spinocerebellum), which are mainly involved in receiving proprioceptive information from the limbs.
3. The large posterior lobe and the middle part of the vermis (neocerebellum), which are mainly involved in receiving inputs from the contralateral cerebral cortex via pontine nuclei. It is involved in fine motor control, e.g. finger movements.

Efferent pathways pass from the cerebellum to the deep cerebellar and brainstem nuclei enable coordination of skilled movements.

CLINICAL FEATURES OF CEREBELLAR DYSFUNCTION

Cerebellar dysfunction is characterized by:
- Ataxia of limbs and gait.
- Dysarthria.
- Nystagmus.
- Dysdiadochokinesis (impaired rapid alternating movements).

Incoordination of movement

Cerebellar dysfunction causes impairment of the process of controlling movements once they have been initiated. This gives rise to ataxia (incoordination) as manifested by the following signs:

- Intention tremor: there is no tremor at rest. When the patient moves a limb towards a target a tremor develops, e.g. abnormal finger–nose test.
- Dysdiadochokinesia: the inability to carry out rapid alternating movements with regularity.
- Dysmetria: the inability to control smooth and accurate targeted movements. The movements are jerky, with overshooting of the target as manifested in the finger–nose and heel–shin tests (see p. 244).

Ataxic gait

The patient walks with a staggering gait and may later develop a wide-based gait to improve stability. In mild cases, the unsteadiness may be apparent only when walking heel-to-toe (tandem walking). In a unilateral cerebellar hemisphere lesion, there is unsteadiness towards the side of the lesion. In truncal ataxia, there is difficulty sitting or standing without support.

Ataxic dysarthric speech

Speech can be slow, slurred and scanning in quality. In scanning speech, there is loss of variation of intonation and the words may be broken up into syllables.

Abnormal eye movements

- Jerky pursuits: pursuit movements are slow, with catch-up saccadic movements on attempting

Vermis

Anterior lobe

Dentate and other
intracereberal nuclei

Primary fissure

Fig. 10.1 Posterior aspect of the cerebellum.

Posterior
lobe

Vermis

Tonsil

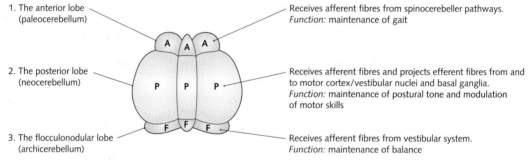

1. The anterior lobe (paleocerebellum) — Receives afferent fibres from spinocerebeller pathways. *Function:* maintenance of gait

2. The posterior lobe (neocerebellum) — Receives afferent fibres and projects efferent fibres from and to motor cortex/vestibular nuclei and basal ganglia. *Function:* maintenance of postural tone and modulation of motor skills

3. The flocculonodular lobe (archicerebellum) — Receives afferent fibres from vestibular system. *Function:* maintenance of balance

Fig. 10.2 The major phylogenetic subdivisions of the cerebellum.

to maintain fixation on the moving target or 'saccadic intrusions'.

- Dysmetria of saccades: when trying to fixate on a target, the eyes overshoot and oscillate several times before fixation is achieved.
- Nystagmus: this is maximal on gaze towards the side of the lesion. Nystagmus results from damage of the vestibular connections of the cerebellum.

Titubation

Nodding tremor of the head may occur. This is mainly in the anterior–posterior plane.

Altered posture

A unilateral cerebellar lesion may cause the head and – when the lesion is recent and severe – the body, to tilt towards the side of the lesion. Head tilt may also be due to a fourth nerve palsy, which can accompany a lesion of the superior medullary vellum (Fig. 10.3).

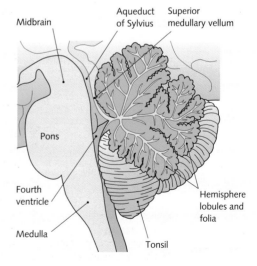

Fig. 10.3 Sagittal section though the cerebellum and brainstem.

62

Hypotonia

Hypotonia is a relatively minor feature of cerebellar disease, resulting from depression of alpha and gamma motor neuron activity. Hypotonia can sometimes be demonstrated clinically by decreased resistance to passive movement (e.g. extension of a limb), by 'pendular' reflexes, or by the rebound phenomenon. This occurs when the patient's outstretched arms are pressed down for a few seconds and then abruptly released by the examiner. The arms rebound upwards much further than would be expected in the presence of cerebellar hypotonia.

The causes of cerebellar dysfunction, and the clinical features resulting from such, are listed in Fig. 10.4.

LOCALIZATION OF A CEREBELLAR LESION

Cerebellar hemisphere

A lesion of the cerebellar hemisphere causes ataxia in the limbs ipsilateral to the lesion. The gait is ataxic,

Fig. 10.4 Causes of cerebellar dysfuntion

Cause	Additional clinical characteristics
Tumours	Type of tumour – metastatic disease, meningioma, acoustic neuroma, medulloblastoma, haemangioblastoma, paraneoplastic syndrome with bronchial and other carcinomas
Multiple sclerosis	Pyramidal, brainstem, and dorsal column signs; optic atrophy
Vascular Haemorrhage	History of hypertension, bleeding disorder, on anticoagulants
Infarction	History of hypertension, ischaemic heart disease, atrial fibrillation, diabetes, hyperlipidaemia
Infections Abscess	Boil or abscess elsewhere, fever, unwell, IV drug abuser
Viral encephalitis	Notably chickenpox within 3 weeks of initial infection
Toxins Anticonvulsants	History of epilepsy; signs of acute toxicity or past history of recurrent toxicity
Alcohol	Acture intoxication; history of chronic abuse, signs of alchoholic liver disease
Metabolic Myxoedema	Myxoedematous facies, dry skin and hair, increased weight, cold intolerance, slow-relaxing reflexes,bradycardia
Trauma	Head injury
Developmental deformities Arnold–Chiari malformation	Pyramidal signs, lower cranial nerve palsies, occipital headache, ± signs associated with a syrinx
Congenital aqueduct stenosis	6th nerve palsies, deafness, papilloedema, intellectual decline
Dandy–Walker syndrome	Large cystic fourth ventricle resulting in hydrocephalus
Inherited cerebellar ataxias Friedreich's ataxias Dominantly inherited ataxias Recessively inherited ataxias	Pes cavus, pyramidal and dorsal column signs, neuropathy, cardiomyopathy, diabetes, optic atrophy

with a tendency to fall towards the affected side. There may be nystagmus maximal towards the side of the lesion and the speech may be slurred.

Cerebellar vermis

Lesions of the midline vermis cause truncal ataxia (imbalance of gait and stance) typically without the classic triad of limb ataxia, dysarthria, and nystagmus.

Lesions of the flocculonodular lobe cause truncal ataxia, vertigo (damage to the vestibular reflex pathways), vomiting (involvement of the floor of the fourth ventricle), and nystagmus.

Space-occupying lesions at midline sites can cause early obstruction of the cerebral aqueduct in the midbrain or the fourth ventricle. This results in hydrocephalus with dilated third and lateral ventricles as well as headache, vomiting, and eventually papilloedema.

Movement disorders

Objectives

- Describe the types of tremor: at rest, with posture and intention
- Define chorea, athetosis, hemiballismus
- Describe the types of generalized and focal dystonia
- Understand the differences between asterixis, myoclonus and tics

The anatomical basis of movement disorders

The basal ganglia are symmetrical groups of grey matter or 'nuclei' deep within the cerebral hemispheres and brainstem. The main components are the caudate nucleus, globus pallidus, putamen, substantia nigra, and subthalamus. These nuclei are mostly concerned with controlling movement, especially the initiation and termination of movement.

- Disease of the basal ganglia often leads to 'extrapyramidal' disorders of movement, including tremor, chorea, athetosis, dystonia, akathisia, and tics.
- Myoclonic jerks (myoclonus) and asterixis are often symptomatic of a range of systemic conditions and specific neurological disorders, although these do not typically affect the basal ganglia they are still considered as movement disorders.

TREMOR

Tremor is a rhythmic oscillatory movement of any part of the body or head. It is described as fast (>6 Hz) or slow (<6 Hz). All tremors disappear during sleep. Tremor may be normal (physiological) or abnormal (pathological). Tremors are 'fine' if they are low amplitude and 'coarse' if they are high amplitude. Tremors can be assessed by observing the patient at rest, during maintenance of a posture (e.g. holding the arms outstretched), and during movements of the limbs or 'intention' (Fig. 11.1).

A physiological tremor affects all muscle groups, although it is most commonly noted in the hands. The tremor is present during waking. It is worse on maintaining a posture, fine in character and fast in rate (8–14 Hz). Patients often do not notice their own tremor.

A pathological tremor often occurs at rest or with movement, is slower (4–7 Hz), coarse in character, proximal as well as distal, and often asymmetrical. This tremor often interferes with everyday activities.

Resting tremor

The most common cause of a pathological resting tremor is Parkinson's disease. The parkinsonian tremor is a coarse 'pill-rolling' tremor and can improve with movement. It is usually observed in the hands and arms on one side more than the other (see Fig. 18.2, p. 114). The tremor may affect other parts of the body, including the jaw and feet. The patient may have other signs of Parkinson's disease (e.g. a shuffling, flexed gait; loss of arm swing; immobile facies as well as rigidity and bradykinesia of the limbs) (see Fig. 18.4, p. 115). There is little correlation between these other features and the degree of tremor. The tremor may respond to anticholinergic drugs but often responds poorly or partially to dopaminergic drugs.

Postural tremor

1. Physiological tremor

Physiological tremor may be exaggerated by:

- Anxiety.
- Metabolic disturbances: hyperthyroidism, phaeochromocytoma.

Fig. 11.1 Summary of movement disorders

Tremor Rhythmic biphasic oscillatory movements of the muscles	Resting	Parkinsonian tremor
	Postural	Physiological, benign essential tremor
	Intention	Cerebellar, red nuclear tremor
Chorea Rapid, irregular, jerky movements		Iatrogenic, e.g. drugs Huntington's chorea Sydenham's chorea
Athetosis Slow, writhing purposeless movements		Wilson's disease Hyperthyroidism Polycythaemia rubra vera
Chorea and athetosis often occur together – choreoathetosis		Systemic lupus erythematosis Senile
Hemiballismus A severe form of chorea Unilateral violent flinging movements of the proximal limb muscles		Infarction of subthalamus Tumour
Dystonia Increased tone producing abnormal posture	Generalized	Dystonia musculorum deformans Iatrogenic Wilson's disease Paroxysmal dystonia
	Focal	Spasmodic torticollis Blepharospasm Oromandibular dystonia Writer's cramp
Tic Repetitive brief contraction of a muscle or group of muscles		simple, e.g. blinking, sniffing complex, e.g. copying someone else's movement or 'echopraxia'
Akathisia Restlessness arising from an irresistible desire to move		Neuroleptic therapy
Myoclonus Brief shock-like muscular contractions that are usually irregular and asymmetrical		Myoclonic epilepsy Essential myoclonus Progressive myoclonus– lipid storage diseases, Creutzfeldt–Jakob disease, hepatic failure Static myoclonus–post-viral, anoxic
Asterixis Arrhythmic flexion movements of the dorsiflexed hands with arms outstretched		Hepatic encephalopathy Uraemic encephalopathy Hypercapnia

- Alcohol withdrawal.
- Drugs: lithium, sodium valproate, sympathomimetics, tea and coffee.

Beta-blockers may diminish a physiological tremor.

2. Essential tremor

Essential tremor may be difficult to distinguish from an exaggerated physiological tremor but it is coarser and slower (8 Hz). It tends to involve the upper limbs and spare the lower limbs. The head and trunk may be involved. It can be inherited in an autosomal dominant manner and presents in childhood or early adulthood; this is called 'familial tremor'. If there is no family history, it is termed 'essential tremor' and often presents insidiously later in middle age. The tremor can progress to be disabling and there is often temporary improvement with alcohol intake. This can be used as a diagnostic manoeuvre.

Essential tremor may partially respond to beta-blockers, anticholinergics (e.g. trihexyphenidyl) and primidone, and sometimes to barbiturates or benzodiazepines.

Intention tremor

1. Cerebellar tremor

Cerebellar dysfunction (see Chapter 10) gives rise to a coarse, often slow (4–6 Hz), action or 'intention' tremor. It is absent at rest and becomes apparent on movement. On performing the finger–nose test, the finger oscillates with increasing amplitude on approaching the target. Rhythmic oscillation of the head and trunk (titubation) may occur and there may be other signs of cerebellar dysfunction.

2. Red nuclear 'rubral' tremor

This is an unusually coarse and often violent ataxic tremor that arises from pathology in the upper brainstem, most often multiple sclerosis. It may also arise from vascular lesions and tumours. Slight movement of the arm may precipitate a wide-amplitude tremor of the limb.

Cerebellar and red nuclear tremors do not respond to anticholinergics or beta-blockers.

Stereotactic surgical lesions of the contralateral ventrolateral thalamus may abolish pathological tremors.

CHOREA AND ATHETOSIS

- Chorea consists of rapid, irregular, jerky movements affecting the face, trunk, and limbs.
- Athetosis refers to slow, writhing movements that can affect any muscle group, particularly those of the face and upper limbs.

These two types of movement disorder often occur together and are then referred to as choreoathetosis. The disorder arises from disease of the basal ganglia.

Causes of choreoathetosis

- Drugs: levodopa, neuroleptics, e.g. phenothiazines, butyrophenones, and oral contraceptives.
- Huntington's chorea.
- Sydenham's chorea.
- Senile chorea.
- Metabolic disorders: Wilson's disease.
- Endocrine disorders: hyperthyroidism.
- Haematological disorders: polycythaemia rubra vera.
- Vascular disorders: systemic lupus erythematosus, small subthalamic infarcts.

Tardive dyskinesia

Long-term treatment with drugs such as phenothiazines and butyrophenones may result in development of choreoathetoid movements of the face, mouth, tongue, and limbs. Withdrawal of the drug is followed by a period of deterioration before improvement is seen. Unfortunately, despite withdrawal, the symptoms frequently persist.

HEMIBALLISMUS

Hemiballismus is similar to severe chorea and is associated with unilateral sudden violent flinging movements of the proximal limb muscles. It results from a lesion of the contralateral subthalamic nucleus (e.g. usually infarction but occasionally tumour).

DYSTONIA

Dystonia is prolonged muscular contraction on attempted voluntary movement, which results in abnormal posturing. Dystonias may be generalized or focal (see Fig. 11.1). The site of the pathology is probably the basal ganglia.

Generalized dystonias

- **Dystonia musculorum deformans:** the disorder is familial (autosomal dominant or recessive). The dystonias may initially be focal and intermittent, but eventually there is constant dystonia of the head, trunk, and limbs.
- **Drugs:** phenothiazines, butyrophenones, levodopa, metoclopramide (focal or generalized).
- **Symptomatic dystonia** (secondary to other diseases): Wilson's disease, cerebral palsy, following hypoxic damage or kernicterus.
- **Paroxysmal dystonia:** familial condition of brief attacks of dystonic posturing provoked by sudden noise, movement, emotional stimuli or exercise.

Focal dystonias

- **Cervical dystonia** ('spasmodic torticollis'): there is involuntary movement of the neck towards one side, in extension (retrocollis) or flexion (anterocollis). The contracting muscles may become painful. The sternomastoid, trapezius and splenius are most affected and may eventually hypertrophy.
- **Blepharospasm:** this comprises a series of involuntary clonic contractions of the eyelid muscles. The eyes may remain closed.
- **Oromandibular dystonia:** involuntary dystonic movements of the mouth, tongue, or jaw can affect women in the sixth decade of life. It may also occur in patients on long-term neuroleptic therapy and the elderly.
- **Writer's cramp:** attempts at writing are prevented by spasm of the muscles of the hand, which may be painful. The symptoms can spread to the forearm and shoulders. On stopping the activity, the spasm resolves. Other focal occupational dystonias occur in musicians and sportsmen.

The most effective treatment for focal dystonias is botulinum toxin injections into the affected muscles at approximately 3 monthly intervals.

Many neurological patients with dystonia, especially generalized dystonia, were given a psychiatric diagnosis in the past. The discovery of mutations in genes associated with some dystonias has revolutionized our understanding of this, often bizarre, disorder. There are still many movement disorders which are considered to be functional and therfore an open-mind and non-judgemental assessment is required for these patients. In another hundred years the molecular basis of these may be uncovered.

Clinically, it can be difficult to differentiate chorea, athetosis, and dystonia because they often occur together.

TIC

A tic is the repetitive brief contraction of a muscle or group of muscles. Multiple tics constitute one of the most notable tic disorders called Gilles de la Tourette syndrome. This is characterized by involuntary snorting, grunting, shouting of verbal obscenities, and aggressive and sexual impulses. It may respond to dopamine-blocking neuroleptic drugs (e.g. sulpiride).

AKATHISIA

Akathisia is characterized by an irresistible desire to move, resulting in continuous restlessness. It is seen in patients on neuroleptic drugs and sometimes in Parkinson's disease. Neurological examination is usually normal when associated with neuroleptic use.

MYOCLONUS

Myoclonic jerks are shock-like asymmetrical muscular contractions that occur irregularly. There is often particular sensitivity to various stimuli, which may precipitate the jerks (e.g. a sudden noise, light, touch, or voluntary movement). The symptoms settle during sleep.

Causes of myoclonus:

- Static myoclonus: postanoxic after cardiorespiratory arrest, postviral.
- Progressive myoclonus (myoclonus with a progressive encephalopathy): lipid-storage diseases (sialidosis, Gaucher's disease), degenerative diseases (Creutzfeldt–Jakob disease, subacute sclerosing panencephalitis), acquired metabolic disorders (hepatic and uraemic encephalopathies).
- Myoclonic epilepsy.
- Essential myoclonus.

Myoclonus may respond to benzodiazepines such as clonazepam. The pathophysiological origin of myoclonus is uncertain but it may arise from pathology at multiple sites in the nervous system, including the cerebral cortex, brainstem and spinal cord.

ASTERIXIS

Asterixis is the sporadic 'flapping tremor' of the hands observed with arms outstretched and hands dorsiflexed. These brief movements occur several times a minute and they are non-rhythmic and not actually a tremor. Asterixis is generally regarded as a form of 'negative' myoclonus, i.e. sudden involuntary relaxation of a muscle group, in this setting the extensor compartment of the forearm. It is seen in metabolic encephalopathies (e.g. hepatic, uraemic, hypoxaemic and hypercapnic) and as a drug induced phenonmenon (e.g. anticonvulsant toxicity).

Limb weakness

Objectives

- Understand the neuroanatomy of the motor system from cerebral cortex to muscle
- Describe the symptoms and signs associated with upper and lower motor neuron syndromes
- Define the lower motor neuron and how lesions along its course are differentiated

Weakness in the limbs can result from:

- Pathology anywhere along the upper motor neuron (UMN) pathway (from motor cortex to the spinal cord).
- A lesion of the lower motor neuron (LMN) pathway (from the anterior horn cell to the peripheral nerve).
- Disorders of the neuromuscular junction.
- Muscular disorders.

The distribution of weakness and other distinctive physical signs usually allow differentiation of the causes of the weakness. Many patients use the word 'weakness' to describe other deficits that are not actually characterized by a lack of power, such as stiffness, slowness, ataxia, fatigue, and clumsiness due to sensory loss.

Neuroanatomy

The upper motor neuron pathway

UMN cell bodies are arranged in a homuncular distribution in the primary motor cortex, at the posterior limit of the frontal lobe (Fig. 12.1).

- The axons of the UMNs descend through the subcortical white matter (corona radiata and then internal capsule).
- The axons descend in the midbrain as the cerebral peduncles and then in the anterior pons and medulla where they cross as the pyramidal decussation.
- During their brainstem course, some of the UMN axons synapse in motor nuclei (cranial nerve nuclei three, four, five, six, seven, ten, eleven, and twelve). These axons are called the corticobulbar

fibres because the motor nuclei in the brainstem are known as the 'bulbar nuclei'.
- The remaining axons form the corticospinal tracts and descend in the lateral white matter of the spinal cord.

The lower motor neuron pathway

- At each spinal level, some of the corticospinal fibres enter the anterior horn of the grey matter and synapse with cell bodies of the LMN, the anterior horn cells or motor neurons.
- When these cell bodies are damaged, the syndrome is referred to as an **anterior horn cell disorder**.
- Each LMN sends out an axon in the ventral (motor) root which joins a dorsal (sensory) root at each spinal level in the intervertebral foramen to form a spinal segmental or mixed nerve. When this nerve is damaged, it is called a **radiculopathy**.
- The spinal nerve in the cervical and lumbosacral regions join other adjacent spinal nerves in a junctional network referred to as a plexus. If these structures are damaged, the clinical syndrome is a **plexopathy**.
- From the plexi emerge peripheral nerves and, when these are damaged, the patient develops a **neuropathy**.
- The axons in the peripheral nerves split into many fibres just before synapsing with muscle fibres.

The neuromuscular junction and muscle pathway

- One axon innervates from 10 to 10 000 muscle fibres, depending on whether fine motor control or a coarser antigravity use of the muscle is required. The group of muscle fibres innervated

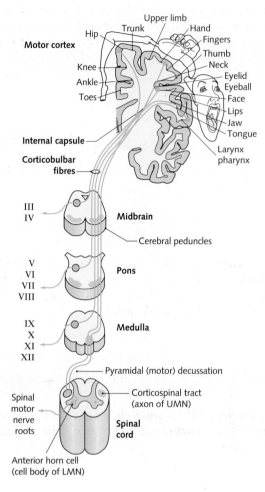

Upper limb
Trunk
Hip   Hand
Fingers
Motor cortex   Thumb
Neck
Knee   Eyelid
Ankle   Eyeball
Toes   Face
Lips
Jaw
Tongue
Internal capsule   Larynx
pharynx
**Corticobulbar
fibres**

III
IV   **Midbrain**

Cerebral peduncles

V
VI   **Pons**
VII
VIII

IX
X   **Medulla**
XI
XII

Pyramidal (motor) decussation

Spinal   Corticospinal tract
motor   (axon of UMN)
nerve
roots   **Spinal
cord**

Anterior horn cell
(cell body of LMN)

Fig. 12.1 Descending motor pathways from the cortex to the brainstem, cranial nerves, and spinal cord.

by one axon is called a motor unit. When the synapses are damaged the condition is called a neuromuscular junction disorder.

• Finally, the muscle itself can be damaged and this is termed a **myopathy** (Fig. 12.2).

Any disorder affecting the UMN, LMN, neuromuscular junction or the muscle can give rise to the symptom of weakness and/or the sign of loss of power.

TERMINOLOGY

Paralysis is the complete loss of voluntary movement. The words 'plegia', 'palsy', and 'paresis' are sometimes used interchangeably to describe weakness, although 'paresis' is the correct term to describe incomplete paralysis. 'Plegia' means complete paralysis and the word 'palsy' is used when the paralysis affects cranial motor nerves (e.g. Bell's palsy, pseudobulbar palsy) or a static weakness (e.g. cerebral palsy). There are several specific terms used to describe the anatomical distribution of weakness.

• **Pyramidal weakness:** loss of power is most marked in the extensor muscles in the arms and the flexors in the legs. This is characteristic of UMN lesions involving the pyramidal tract within the brain or spinal cord (see further details below).
• **Proximal weakness**, affecting the shoulders, hips, trunk, neck and sometimes face. This is characteristic of muscle disease (myopathy) and also a common pattern in myasthenia.

Fig. 12.2 Anatomical sites of weakness

	Site of pathology	Clinical syndrome
UMN pathway	Motor cortex, corona radiata, internal capsule, brainstem Spinal cord (corticospinal tract)	Hemisphere or brainstem (pyramidal weakness) Myelopathy (pyramidal weakness)
LMN pathway	Anterior horn or motor neuron cell body Spinal nerve root Brachial or lumbosacral plexus Peripheral nerve	Motor neuronopathy or 'anterior horn cell disease' Radiculopathy Plexopathy Neuropathy
Neuromuscular junction	Synapse	Neuromuscular junction disorder
Muscle	Muscle	Myopathy

- **Distal weakness**, affecting the hands and feet. This is typical of peripheral motor neuropathy, often affecting the lower limbs first and more severely.
- **Global weakness:** this term is used to describe generalized weakness in a limb (both proximal and distal), which may result from severe pathologies affecting any level within the motor system.

UPPER MOTOR NEURON WEAKNESS

UMN weakness results from damage of the corticospinal tract at any point from the motor cortex to the spinal cord (see Fig. 12.1). If the lesion occurs above the pyramidal decussation at the level of the lower medulla, the weakness is contralateral to the site of the lesion. If it occurs below this level, the signs are ipsilateral to the lesion.

The following clinical features characterize a UMN lesion:

Increased tone (spasticity)

Initially, UMN weakness may be flaccid, with absent or diminished deep tendon reflexes. There is little understanding of the reasons behind this initial flaccidity and it is often referred to as 'shock'. Increased tone of an UMN type is called spasticity. It may develop several hours, days, or even weeks after the initial lesion has occurred. Spasticity is manifested by:

- 'Spastic catch': mild spasticity may be detected as a resistance to passive movement or 'catch' in the pronators on passive supination of the forearm and in the flexors of the hand/forearm on extension of the wrist/elbow.
- The 'clasp-knife' phenomenon: following strong resistance to passive flexion of the knee or extension of the elbow, there is a sudden relaxation of the extensor muscles of the leg and flexor muscles in the arm.
- Clonus: rhythmic involuntary muscular contractions follow an abruptly applied and sustained stretch stimulus, e.g. at the ankle following sudden passive dorsiflexion of the foot.

'Pyramidal-pattern' weakness

The anti-gravity muscles are preferentially spared and stronger (i.e. the flexors of the upper limbs and the extensors of the lower limbs). The patient can develop a characteristic posture of flexed and pronated arms with clenched fingers, and extended and adducted legs with plantar flexion of the feet.

Absence of muscle wasting and fasciculations

Focal muscle wasting and fasciculations are features of a LMN lesion. With chronic disuse, some loss of muscle bulk can occur after an UMN lesion, but this is rarely severe or focal.

Brisk tendon reflexes and extensor plantar responses

The tendon reflexes are brisk. The cremasteric and abdominal or 'cutaneous' reflexes are depressed or absent. The plantar responses are extensor ('upgoing toes' or 'positive Babinski sign').

UPPER MOTOR NEURON SYNDROMES

The common UMN syndromes are hemiparesis and paraparesis. Tetraparesis and monoparesis are less common.

Hemiparesis

Hemiparesis results from unilateral lesions of the contralateral cerebral hemisphere or brainstem (when the face is usually also affected) or from an ipsilateral lesion below the pyramidal decussation in the lower medulla or high cervical cord (when the face is spared) (Fig. 12.3).

The clinical features associated with the hemiparesis usually enable a more accurate localization of the site of the pathology. The most common cause of hemiparesis is a stroke involving the contralateral cerebral cortex or internal capsule (see Fig. 12.3).

Tetraparesis

Pyramidal (UMN) weakness of all four limbs may result from lesions in the brainstem or high cervical cord. When the UMNs are damaged, the condition is called a 'spastic' tetraparesis. Tetraparesis caused by spinal cord pathology is most commonly due to cervical spondylosis, multiple sclerosis, and traumatic cord

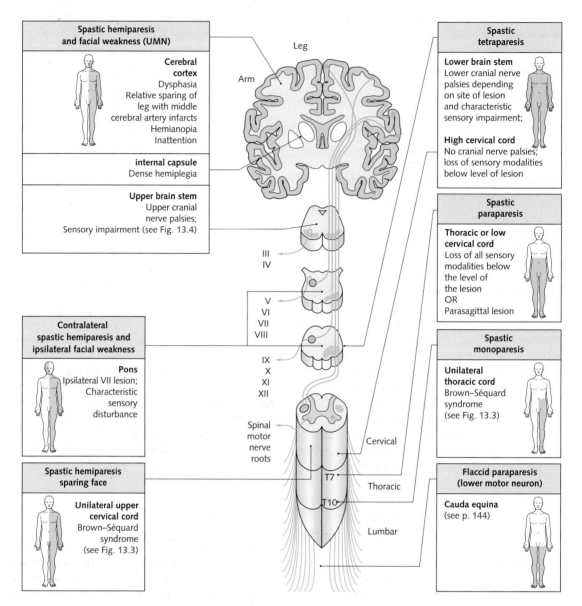

Spastic hemiparesis and facial weakness (UMN)

Cerebral cortex
Dysphasia
Relative sparing of leg with middle cerebral artery infarcts
Hemianopia
Inattention

internal capsule
Dense hemiplegia

Upper brain stem
Upper cranial nerve palsies;
Sensory impairment (see Fig. 13.4)

Contralateral spastic hemiparesis and ipsilateral facial weakness

Pons
Ipsilateral VII lesion;
Characteristic sensory disturbance

Spastic hemiparesis sparing face

Unilateral upper cervical cord
Brown–Séquard syndrome (see Fig. 13.3)

Leg
Arm

III
IV

V
VI
VII
VIII

IX
X
XI
XII

Spinal motor nerve roots

Cervical

T7
T10

Thoracic

Lumbar

Spastic tetraparesis

Lower brain stem
Lower cranial nerve palsies depending on site of lesion and characteristic sensory impairment;

High cervical cord
No cranial nerve palsies; loss of sensory modalities below level of lesion

Spastic paraparesis

Thoracic or low cervical cord
Loss of all sensory modalities below the level of the lesion
OR
Parasagittal lesion

Spastic monoparesis

Unilateral thoracic cord
Brown–Séquard syndrome (see Fig. 13.3)

Flaccid paraparesis (lower motor neuron)

Cauda equina
(see p. 144)

Fig. 12.3 Patterns of motor weakness. Note that these are all upper motor neuron lesions except for pathology in the cauda equina, which damages multiple lumbar and sacral nerve roots.

lesions and less often from neoplasms, arteriovenous malformations (AVMs), or rheumatoid arthritis affecting the atlantoaxial (C1/C2) joint. Cervical spondylotic myelopathy is usually associated with a cervical radiculopathy affecting one or more spinal nerves, usually C6 and/or C7. The patient will therefore have UMN signs in the legs and predominantly LMN signs in the arms, a syndrome referred to as a myeloradiculopathy. Extensive bilateral pathology in the cerebral hemispheres can occasionally cause tetraparesis. Brainstem pathology is usually associ-

ated with additional cranial nerve symptoms such as diplopia, facial numbness, vertigo, dysarthria, dysphagia, and signs such as ocular, facial, or bulbar weakness. The most common brainstem pathologies to cause tetraparesis include stroke, neoplasms, and multiple sclerosis.

Weakness of all four limbs may also result from several LMN disorders, e.g. some types of motor neuron disease and polio, motor neuropathies, disorders of the neuromuscular junction (e.g. myasthenia gravis), and muscle disease (e.g. polymyositis).

Tetraparesis in motor neuron disease is usually due to a combination of UMN (corticospinal pathway) and LMN (anterior horn cell) involvement (see p. 76 for further discussion of LMN lesions; see also Fig. 12.7).

Paraparesis

Paraparesis is usually due to spinal cord disease and is consequently an UMN syndrome, characterized by spasticity, pyramidal weakness, brisk reflexes and extensor plantar responses in the legs. This syndrome is called 'spastic paraparesis'. The most common causes are multiple sclerosis or extrinsic compression in the cervical region between C3 and C6, due to cervical spondylosis, which is a degenerative osteoarthritis associated with osteophytes and other soft tissue changes that compress the cervical cord. Spastic paraparesis is often encountered in clinical exams as well as in the clinic setting, and a systematic approach to the numerous causes is important (Fig. 12.4).

A much rarer cause of bilateral UMN symptoms and signs in the legs, resembling a spinal cord syndrome, is a cerebral lesion involving both cortical leg areas in the parasagittal region of the brain. A parasagittal meningioma classically causes this syndrome but sagittal sinus thrombosis with subsequent venous infarction and the form of cerebral palsy known as 'congenital spastic diplegia' are other causes.

Paraparesis can also be associated with low tone in the legs when it is called 'flaccid paraparesis'. This usually results from lesions in the cauda equina such as central lumbar disc prolapse or infiltrating neoplasms. A cauda equina syndrome is usually associated with severe and early sphincter dysfunction and sensory impairment over sacral and lower lumbar dermatomes or 'saddle anaesthesia' (see Fig. 12.3). The cauda equina is made up of the spinal nerves that exit at the inferior pole of the spinal cord called the conus medullaris. The conus is a highly compacted region of the spinal cord containing many spinal levels. The clinical signs of a conus lesion are therefore often mixed between UMN and LMN such as brisk knee jerks and extensor plantar responses, but with flaccid tone and absent ankle jerks.

Monoparesis

A stroke in one of the distal branches of the middle cerebral artery (MCA) is the most common cause of an isolated upper limb monoparesis. More usually, the MCA is blocked more proximally and there is weakness in the contralateral upper limb with some UMN facial weakness and relative sparing of the leg. This is in contrast to anterior cerebral artery occlusion, which often spares the face and arm and causes contralateral leg weakness.

Other localized cerebral cortical lesions may cause weakness confined to one contralateral limb. This typically affects the leg and foot and occurs with cortical tumours but occasionally with multiple sclerosis, abscesses and granulomas.

A unilateral thoracic cord lesion may also occasionally present with monoparesis of the leg (see Fig. 12.3). There will usually be reflex and sensory findings of a Brown–Séquard syndrome to clarify the diagnosis. This is usually caused by a demyelinating plaque in MS (see Fig. 13.3, p. 84).

Fig. 12.4 Causes of spastic paraparesis

Spinal cord compression	Cervical spondylosis Cervical or thoracic disc herniation Metastatic tumour Primary tumour (meningioma, neurofibroma) Infective (epidural abscess, spinal TB) Epidural haematoma
Inflammatory disorders	Multiple sclerosis Idiopathic transverse myelitis Sarcoidosis Infections (Lyme, zoster, TB, AIDS)
Degenerative disorders	Motor neuron disease Syringomyelia
Vascular	Spinal cord infarction Vasculitis, systemic lupus erythematosus (SLE) Spinal AVM
Trauma	Cord contusion, laceration or transection Displaced vertebral fracture or disc Traumatic epidural haematoma
Metabolic/nutritional	B_{12} deficiency (subacute combined degeneration)
Rare hereditary conditions	Friedreich's ataxia Hereditary spastic paraparesis
Parasagittal brain lesions	Meningioma Cerebral venous sinus thrombosis Congenital spastic diplegia (cerebral palsy).

Upper motor neuron signs are often absent in the earliest stages of a stroke and the patient may have a flaccid hemiparesis. Extensor plantar responses and brisk reflexes often occur within 24–48 hours but spasticity may take weeks to develop. The most important key to the diagnosis is therefore the history of an abrupt onset with possible vascular risk factors.

LOWER MOTOR NEURON WEAKNESS

LMNs extend from the anterior horn cell in the spinal cord to the neuromuscular junction in the muscles. Lesions to the LMNs are characterized by a constellation of typical clinical signs, which vary in their presence and degree by the anatomical site of damage to the LMN in its course from the spinal cord to the muscles. There are typically four different types of LMN lesion (anterior horn cell, spinal nerve, plexus and peripheral nerve – see below). Although the neuromuscular junction and muscle are not strictly a part of the LMN, disorders of these structures are also considered in the differential diagnosis of LMN syndromes because they produce similar signs and symptoms.

LMN syndromes are characterized by the following features:

Decreased tone

Tone is typically reduced, particularly when muscle wasting has occurred.

Focal pattern of weakness and wasting

LMN weakness can occur in individual muscles and in groups of muscles if more than one level of LMN is involved. The denervated muscle becomes atrophied and wasting is evident within days to weeks after the onset. The pattern of weakness and wasting depends on the site of the lesion:

- **Anterior horn cell disease:** eventually causes generalized weakness and wasting; however, it can begin distally in either a hand or foot and

it may mimic a peripheral nerve lesion, e.g. an ulnar neuropathy, common peroneal nerve palsy.
- **Radiculopathies:** result in weakness and wasting in the respective myotomes, i.e. the group of muscles innervated by a single spinal nerve root.
- **Plexopathies:** cause weakness and wasting in the distribution of more than one spinal nerve root, e.g. C8 and T1 in lesions of the lower cord of the brachial plexus.
- **Peripheral neuropathies:**
  - mononeuropathy: a single peripheral nerve is affected, e.g. ulnar mononeuropathy
  - multiple mononeuropathies or 'mononeuritis multiplex': many single nerves are involved, e.g. ulnar, radial and common peroneal nerves
  - polyneuropathy: the longest axons in all the nerves are affected. This typically causes symmetrical distal wasting and weakness affecting the feet, leg, and hands, with loss of all tendon reflexes. If there is also sensory involvement, there will be impairment of sensation in a 'glove and sock' distribution affecting the hands and the legs below the knees.
- **Neuromuscular junction disorders**, such as myasthenia gravis: typically cause weakness in muscles of the head and neck as well as proximal upper limbs. The weakness is characteristically fatigable, i.e. worsens quickly with exercise, and there is little or no muscle wasting (see Chapter 24).
- **Myopathies:** usually cause symmetrical wasting and weakness in the proximal limb girdles (shoulders, hips, and thighs) although distal muscles can be involved, depending on the cause of the myopathy (see Chapter 25).

Fasciculations

Fasciculations are brief, flickering contractions of individual motor units in a denervated muscle. They may be present in weak and wasted muscles but can also occur in muscles that appear unaffected. Fasciculations are particularly prevalent in motor neuron disease and motor neuropathies.

Pain and sensory disturbance

Sensory changes often occur in lesions of the spinal nerve roots, plexii, and peripheral nerves. It should be noted that anterior horn cell disease, diseases of the neuromuscular junction, and myopathies do not have objective sensory signs. Pain accompanies the sensory disturbance when the lesion is caused by infiltrating tumour, vasculitis, or by some toxins, e.g. alcohol. There are no sensory signs in motor neuron disease but patients can experience sensory symptoms such as muscle cramps.

Reduced tendon reflexes and flexor plantar responses

Tendon reflexes are reduced or lost depending on the severity of the LMN lesion. Abdominal and cremasteric reflexes are unaffected. Plantar responses are flexor unless there is severe loss of sensation or power to the big toe when the reflex may be completely absent.

LOWER MOTOR NEURON SYNDROMES

1. **Anterior horn cells**, e.g. polio, motor neuron disease, and syringomyelia.
2. **Spinal nerves** or 'nerve roots', e.g. L5 radiculopathy.
3. **Plexopathy**, e.g. brachial.
4. **Peripheral neuropathy**, e.g. ulnar mononeuropathy or generalized polyneuropathy.

Anterior horn cell disease

There are usually prominent fasciculations, especially in motor neuron disease.
Causes:

- Motor neuron disease, e.g. amyotrophic lateral sclerosis.
- Infective, e.g. poliomyelitis.
- Toxic, e.g. triorthocresyl phosphate.
- Local structural pathology, e.g. syringomyelia or intrinsic cord tumours.

Radiculopathy and plexopathy

A knowledge of the myotomes is necessary to differentiate the site of a radiculopathy or plexopathy. A radiculopathy will cause muscle weakness and wasting in the myotome supplied by the affected single nerve root, with loss of the segmental tendon reflex, if there is one, and sensory loss in the corresponding dermatome (see Fig. 13.2, p. 83).

A plexus lesion will cause weakness and wasting in muscles innervated by several of the spinal nerves that form the plexus, as well as loss of corresponding reflexes. There may be accompanying sensory loss over several dermatomes (see Fig. 12.7). Only part of the plexus is usually involved although characteristic patterns can often be seen.

Brachial plexopathy

The brachial plexus is illustrated in Fig. 12.5 and is discussed in detail in Chapter 22. The following are examples of brachial plexus syndromes:

- Neuralgic amyotrophy.
- Tumour infiltration.
- Radiotherapy-induced plexopathy.
- Pancoast tumour.
- Thoracic outlet syndrome, e.g. cervical rib.
- Erb's palsy (lateral cord: C5, C6).
- Klumpke's palsy (medial cord: C8, T1).

Lumbosacral plexopathy

In general, lesions of the lower plexus cause weakness and wasting of the hamstrings and foot muscles with loss of the ankle jerk and sensory loss on the posterior leg, whereas upper plexus lesions cause failure of hip flexion and adduction with anterior leg sensory loss (Fig. 12.6).
Causes:

- Trauma following abdominal or pelvic surgery, e.g. hysterectomy.
- Infiltration by neoplasia, e.g. cervical, ovarian and colorectal carcinoma, or granulomatous disease.
- Compression from an abdominal aortic aneurysm.

Neuropathy

There are several types of peripheral neuropathy:

- **Mononeuropathy:** disease of a single peripheral nerve, e.g. lesion of the median nerve from compression in the carpal tunnel, lesion of the common peroneal nerve from trauma involving the fibular head.
- **Multiple mononeuropathy** or 'mononeuritis multiplex': this term is used when many single nerves are involved, such as in diabetes, sarcoid, leprosy, and vasculitic disease, especially polyarteritis nodosa, and neoplasia.
- **Polyneuropathy:** this is the more widespread involvement of the peripheral nerves and

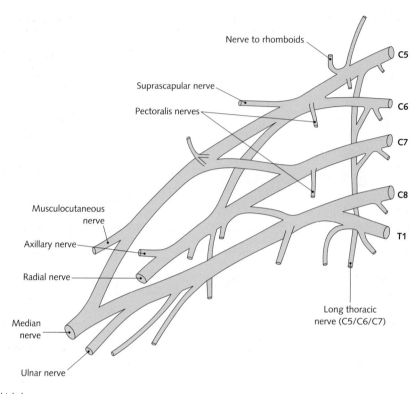

Fig. 12.5 The brachial plexus.

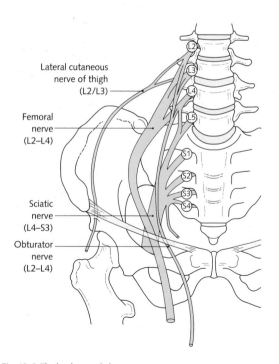

Fig. 12.6 The lumbosacral plexus.

typically occurs in a symmetrical distal distribution in the limbs, e.g. diabetic neuropathy, Guillain–Barré syndrome, vitamin B$_{12}$ deficiency, drugs such as isoniazid. Patterns of weakness caused by these disorders are shown in Fig. 12.7. See also Chapter 23, p. 147.

It can sometimes be difficult to identify the anatomical location of a LMN lesion. The presence or absence of sensory loss can help: if there is lower motor neuron weakness without sensory loss, then anterior horn cell disease, myasthenia or myopathy are probable. Pure motor neuropathies are uncommon, e.g. porphyria, lead poisoning, but Guillain–Barré can mostly affect the motor system and other rare inflammatory neuropathies can be purely motor.

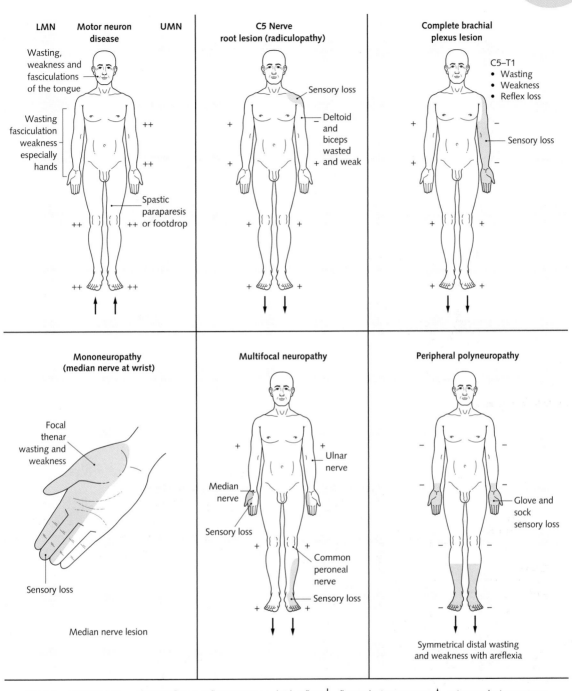

Shading = seonsory loss, −, absent reflex; +, reflex present; ++, brisk reflex; ↓, flexor plantar response; ↑, extensor plantar response

Fig. 12.7 Patterns of weakness and sensory loss due to lower motor neuron lesions. The shaded areas indicate sensory loss.

DISORDERS OF THE NEUROMUSCULAR JUNCTION

These include myasthenia gravis, Eaton–Lambert syndrome, and iatrogenic syndromes.

Myasthenia gravis is the most common disorder of the neuromuscular junction and the extraocular muscles are almost always affected at some point in the disease; they may be the only feature at presentation. There may also be weakness of the bulbar and respiratory muscles as well as proximal muscles especially in the upper limbs.

The characteristic feature is fatigability of muscle strength, which can often be demonstrated clinically. Wasting is uncommon and rarely severe unless the patient has had prolonged immobilization or malnutrition. Reflexes are usually normal and plantar responses are flexor (Fig. 12.8). There is no sensory involvement or fasciculations. See also Chapter 24, p. 157.

MYOPATHY

The limb weakness is usually bilateral and proximal in the shoulder and pelvic girdles and patients complain of an inability to stand from sitting, climb stairs, brush their hair, or reach for objects above their head. Involvement of the face, neck, and trunk occurs in many myopathic disorders. Dysphagia and respiratory muscle weakness might also occur and can be life threatening (e.g. polymyositis). Muscle pain (myalgia) and cramps can occur, especially after exercise. Muscle wasting might be severe and tone is reduced. Reflexes are reduced in advanced myopathy but unaffected in the early stages. Plantar responses are flexor if there is enough power in the big toe to elicit the reflex. There is no sensory disturbance.

Dystrophia myotonica is a genetic disorder involving many organs. It is associated with a myopathy and a distinctive failure of relaxation of muscles following contraction or 'myotonia'. The myopathy is not only proximal but also involves the head and neck as well as forearms and legs. Myopathies are discussed in more detail in Chapter 25, p. 161.

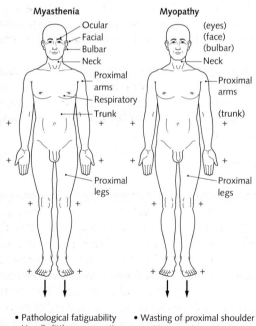

+, reflex present; ↓, flexor plantar response

Fig. 12.8 Pattern of weakness in neuromuscular junction diseases (myasthenia) and in myopathies. In both cases, the tendon reflexes are preserved unless weakness is severe, and sensation is intact.

Limb sensory symptoms

Objectives

- Define the two main neuroanatomical pathways responsible for sensation and the sensory modalities that are transmitted
- Describe how to differentiate between the distribution of sensory symptoms caused by diseases of the peripheral nerves, spinal cord, brainstem and cerebral cortex
- Understand and learn to sketch the clinially important dermatomes (C5, 6, 7, 8, T1 in the arm and L4, 5, S1 in the leg) and the territories of the most commonly affected peripheral nerves (median, ulnar, radial, common peroneal)

Sensory symptoms can arise from lesions at various levels within the central nervous system (cortex, subcortex, thalamus, brainstem, spinal cord) or from lesions of the peripheral sensory pathways (spinal nerve root, plexus, peripheral nerve). The anatomical distribution of sensory disturbance, sometimes its quality and timing, and the finding of other physical signs, usually enable a diagnosis to be made. The knowledge of the anatomy of the main sensory pathways is an essential prerequisite for this diagnostic process.

Nerve endings in skin, joints, ligaments, tendons, and muscle contain different receptors adapted to respond to a variety of sensory stimuli. The sensory information gathered by these receptors is carried back to the spinal cord by sensory nerves. There are two main pathways for the appreciation of different modalities of sensation:

1. Dorsal (posterior) column pathway.
2. Spinothalamic pathway (see Fig. 13.1).

DORSAL (POSTERIOR) COLUMN PATHWAY

The dorsal column pathway carries information concerned with light touch, two-point discrimination, vibration, and proprioception. Fibres carrying this information travel from the cutaneous nerves to the dorsal root ganglia, where their cell bodies lie and relay the information via the dorsal nerve roots to enter the spinal cord. These fibres do not immediately

synapse but ascend the spinal cord ipsilaterally in the dorsal columns and synapse in the gracile and cuneate nuclei of the lower medulla. The fibres decussate in the medulla as the internal arcuate fibres and travel upwards as the medial leminiscus to synapse in the ventral posterolateral thalamus and then the parietal cortex. A somatotopic order is maintained throughout the pathway from the spinal cord to parietal cortex.

When pathology affects the dorsal column pathway, the patient may complain of numbness, 'pins and needles', an illusion of swelling of the limbs, or incoordination of the hands/gait due to loss of proprioceptive information.

Spinothalamic pathway

The spinothalamic pathway carries information about pain and temperature; itch and tickle are also carried by this pathway. The fibres travel within the peripheral nerves to the dorsal root ganglia and dorsal nerve roots (see Fig. 13.1). The fibres ascend or descend in Lissauer's tract for one or two segments before synapsing in the dorsal horn. At this level, they decussate and ascend in the contralateral spinothalamic tract. In the brainstem, the tract becomes the lateral leminiscus and these fibres synapse in the thalamus and ultimately the parietal cortex. A somatotopic order is maintained throughout the central pathway with the sacral fibres being outermost and the cervical fibres innermost.

Clinical manifestations of lesions of this pathway may include parasthaesia, pain, or the acquisition of

81

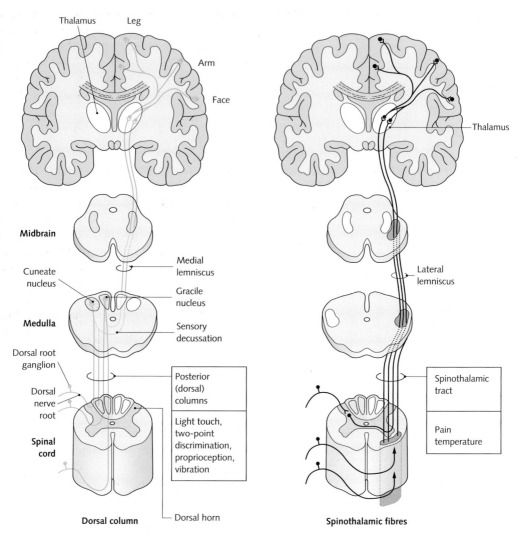

Fig. 13.1 Anatomy of the main sensory pathways in the spinal cord. Note that dorsal column fibres ascend on the ipsilateral side of the spinal cord and decussate in the medulla, whereas spinothalamic fibres cross the central grey matter of the spinal cord (after synapsing in the dorsal horn) and ascend on the opposite side of the cord.

injuries due to impaired pain perception, e.g. burns, excessive wearing of the joints (which may become deformed and then called a 'Charcot joint').

TROPHIC SKIN CHANGES AND ULCERS

When patients lose the sensory supply to limbs, they are less able to prevent trauma and prolonged pressure to their skin. This may result in ulcers especially at pressure points, e.g. heels and sacrum. There is also loss of the autonomic supply to piloerector muscles, sweat

glands, and blood vessels. This can lead to a dry, pale, hairless skin that can become atrophic, swollen and shiny. These associated features are important to recognize in lower motor neuron (LMN) syndromes as they can easily lead to local skin infections that can become systemic and make the patient severely unwell.

SENSORY SYNDROMES

Sensory symptoms may arise from a lesion involving the peripheral nerves, spinal nerves and dorsal roots ganglia, or the central pathways. Lesions of the central pathways can be considered at the level of the spinal cord, brainstem, thalamus, and parietal cortex.

Lesions of peripheral nerves

Mononeuropathy

A lesion affecting sensory fibres in a peripheral nerve is accompanied by sensory impairment of all modalities in the corresponding anatomical distribution (Fig. 13.2). If a mixed motor and sensory nerve is involved, there will also be weakness of the muscles supplied by the nerve (see Chapter 23).

Multiple mononeuropathy

Mononeuritis multiplex involves a number of individual nerves and occurs in diabetes, sarcoidosis, vasculitis, leprosy, amyloidosis, and carcinomatous disease.

Polyneuropathy

A symmetrical impairment of all sensory modalities involving the hands, feet, and legs occurs; this is characteristically termed a 'glove-and-sock' sensory loss. The reflexes are diminished or lost and there may be accompanying muscle weakness. Causes of a polyneuropathy include diabetes, chronic alcohol abuse, vitamin B_{12} deficiency, paraproteinaemia, and drugs (isoniazid, heavy metals, antineoplastic agents), see Chapter 23.

Lesions of the spinal nerve roots, dorsal roots, and ganglia

Each dorsal nerve root carries sensory fibres of all modalities from an area on the skin called a dermatome (Fig. 13.2). The overlap of input from adjacent roots means that lesions of a single nerve root do not result in complete loss of sensation within the defined dermatome. The corresponding tendon reflexes may be diminished or lost. LMN muscle weakness occurs if the anterior roots are also involved and is especially common in plexus lesions.

Reactivation of the herpes zoster virus (shingles) and prolapsed intervertebral discs can cause damage to the spinal nerves and dorsal roots.

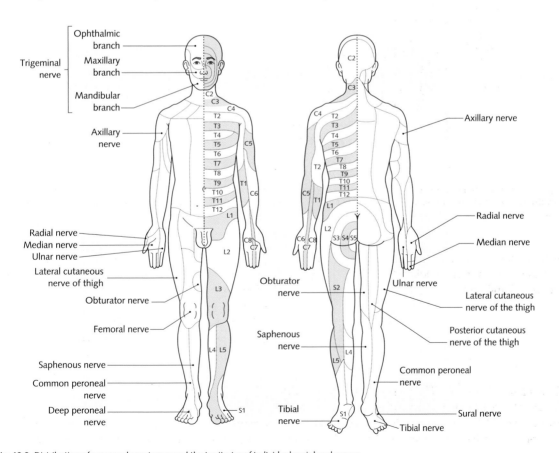

Fig. 13.2 Distribution of sensory dermatomes and the territories of individual peripheral nerves.

Lesions of the spinal cord

Sensory disturbances arising from lesions of the spinal cord are illustrated in Fig. 13.3.

Transection of the cord

Transection of the cord causes bilateral impairment of all sensory modalities below the level of transection (as defined by the dermatomal pattern in Fig. 13.2). There is initially a flaccid, and eventually a spastic paraplegia (thoracic and lumbar cord) or tetraplegia (cervical cord). Traumatic transection following a road traffic accident is the most common cause.

Lesion of the posterior spinal cord

A lesion of the posterior spinal cord affects the dorsal columns, with sparing of the spinothalamic and corticospinal fibres. There is impaired light touch, two-point discrimination, vibration, and proprioception below the level of the lesion. Motor function and perception of pain and temperature are spared unless the lesion progresses to involve the anterior part of the cord. Isolated loss of dorsal column function is rare but can occur in multiple sclerosis, spondylosis or prolapsed intervertebral discs, and vitamin B_{12} deficiency.

Lesion of the anterior cord

A lesion of the anterior cord affects the spinothalamic and corticospinal tracts, with sparing of the dorsal columns. There is bilateral impairment of pain and temperature perception and a spastic paraplegia or tetraplegia below the level of the lesion. Anterior spinal artery occlusion is the commonest cause of this syndrome.

Hemisection of the cord (Brown–Séquard syndrome)

Hemisection of the cord causes impairment of light touch, two-point discrimination, vibration, and proprioception below the level of the lesion on the same

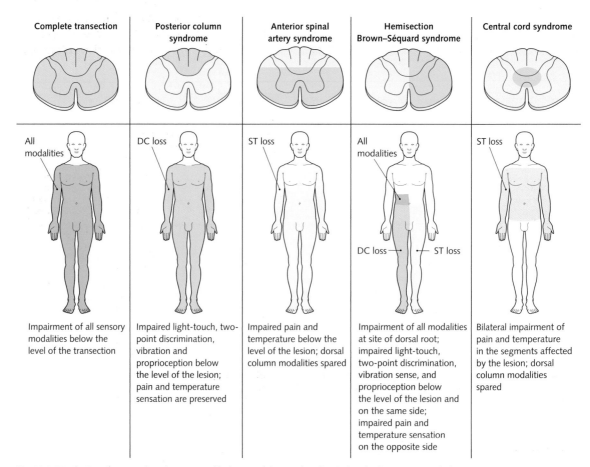

Fig. 13.3 Distribution of sensory disturbance caused by lesions of the spinal cord. DC, dorsal column; ST, spinothalamic.

side; and impaired perception of pain and temperature on the opposite side. Involvement of one or more nerve roots at the site of the lesion will result in impairment of all sensory modalities on that side within the distribution of the dermatomes affected. Upper motor neuron (UMN) weakness is present on the side of the lesion. Tumour deposits and demyelination are the most common causes.

Central cord lesion

A central cord lesion affects the spinothalamic fibres and spares the dorsal columns. There is bilateral loss of pain and temperature perception in the segments affected by the lesion. Only the crossing fibres are involved so that a 'cape-like' distribution of sensory loss occurs, e.g. a syrinx. More commonly, a 'belt' or 'pair of shorts' loss of sensation can occur and is often due to a multiple sclerosis plaque in the thoracolumbar cord. The loss of spinothalamic sensation with preservation of dorsal column function is called a 'dissociated' sensory loss. Wasting and weakness and loss of reflexes may occur from involvement of anterior horn cells and fibres subserving the reflex arc within the cord at the level of the lesion. If the

lesion expands sufficiently it may eventually involve the corticospinal tracts and cause UMN signs below the lesion.

A dissociated pattern of sensory loss between the modalities of pain and temperature and those of light touch, two-point discrimination, vibration, and proprioception occurs in:
- Central cord lesions.
- Hemisection of the cord.
- Lateral medullary lesions.
- B_{12} deficiency.
- Anterior cord syndrome.

Lesions of the brainstem

- Lower medulla: a unilateral lesion of the lower medulla (Fig. 13.4) causes impairment of pain and temperature perception of the face on the side of the lesion, and on the opposite side of the body. Light touch, two-point discrimination,

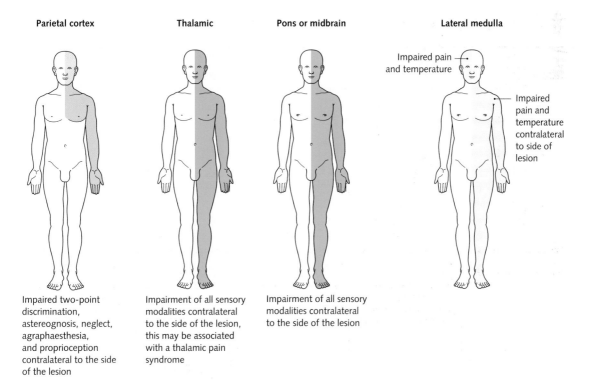

| Parietal cortex | Thalamic | Pons or midbrain | Lateral medulla |

Impaired pain and temperature

Impaired pain and temperature contralateral to side of lesion

Impaired two-point discrimination, astereognosis, neglect, agraphaesthesia, and proprioception contralateral to the side of the lesion

Impairment of all sensory modalities contralateral to the side of the lesion, this may be associated with a thalamic pain syndrome

Impairment of all sensory modalities contralateral to the side of the lesion

Fig. 13.4 Distribution of sensory disturbance caused by cerebral and brainstem lesions.

vibration, and proprioception could be impaired on the side of the lesion but this is usually spared in a lateral medullary infarction. This lesion involves the ipsilateral spinal trigeminal nucleus and tract and the spinothalamic tract subserving contralateral sensation.

- Pons and midbrain: a unilateral lesion of the pons, or midbrain causes impairment of all sensory modalities on the opposite side of the body including the face, because all the sensory tracts have already crossed including the spinal nucleus and tract of the trigeminal nerve.

The brainstem syndromes discussed above can be accompanied by cranial nerve palsies and cerebellar signs ipsilateral to the lesion, and by contralateral hemiparesis. In practice, brainstem lesions are often bilateral and therefore affect sensation in the face and all four limbs.

Lesions of the thalamus

A thalamic lesion (see Fig. 13.4) causes impairment of all sensory modalities on the opposite side of the body, including the face. There may be spontaneous pain and dysaesthesia on the affected side – the 'thalamic pain syndrome'.

Lesions of the parietal lobe

A parietal lobe lesion (see Fig. 13.4) causes:

- Loss of discriminative sensory function of the opposite side of the face and limbs. There is impaired two-point discrimination, lack of

recognition of objects by touch (astereognosis) or figures drawn on the hand (agraphaesthesia), and loss of perception of limb position. However, the primary modalities of pain, temperature, touch, and vibration are relatively preserved.

- Sensory inattention: this is usually caused by lesions of the non-dominant parietal cortex. The patient fails to perceive stimuli on the opposite side of the body when the stimulus is applied bilaterally. However, when applied on the affected side only, the same stimulus is perceived normally. This inattentive defect or 'neglect' may also apply when testing the visual fields, the phenomenon of visual inattention.

When taking the history in a patient with sensory symptoms, asking the patient to precisely locate the anatomical boundaries of their symptoms can be helpful. For instance, the numbness and tingling of carpal tunnel syndrome should not go beyond the wrist but the pain main extend up to the shoulder. The quality of the pain is also important in that complex descriptions, e.g. 'water running down my leg' suggest a central cause, and more simple descriptions, such as 'my feet up to my knees are numb' suggest a peripheral cause.

Objectives

- Define and try to imitate the common abnormalities of gait
- Describe the main causes of gait disorders

The character of a patient's gait will provide clues to the clinical signs and differential diagnosis. When assessing a patient's gait, the following categories should be kept in mind:

- Cerebellar ataxia.
- Spastic paraplegia.
- Hemiparetic.
- Parkinsonian.
- Sensory ataxia.
- Steppage.
- Myopathic.
- Apraxic.
- Antalgic.
- Functional.

The main gait disorders are illustrated in Fig. 14.1.

PRACTICAL APPROACH TO THE ASSESSMENT OF GAIT

Watch the patient walk along a stretch of corridor and observe the characteristics of the gait. Note the following:

- Does the patient walk with an aid? – stick, crutches, rollator.
- Does the patient walk in a straight line? Patients who are ataxic are unsteady and may be unable to tandem walk, i.e. 'heel-to-toe' walking.
- Does the patient have normal arm swing? Arm swing may be reduced in patients who have an extrapyramidal syndrome. This is often more marked on one side than the other, especially in idiopathic Parkinson's disease.

- How well does the patient turn around? Patients who have a extra-pyramidal syndrome or ataxia perform this with difficulty. Patients with idiopathic Parkinson's disease turn in a series of movements or 'en bloc'.
- Ask the patient to walk on the toes (S1) and then heels (L5). Patients with a common peroneal nerve palsy and L5 or S1 radiculopathy will find this difficult, as will patients with a hemiparesis.
- Perform Romberg's test. Ask the patient to stand with feet together and eyes closed. The test is positive if the patient is more unsteady with eyes closed than with eyes open. This occurs in patients with a sensory ataxia who have impaired proprioception. It cannot be tested reliably in patients with a cerebellar disorder or moderate to severe weakness from any cause as the patient will be unsteady irrespective of whether there is a sensory ataxia.

DIFFERENTIAL DIAGNOSIS OF DISORDERS OF GAIT

Gait of cerebellar ataxia

Patients with cerebellar ataxia stand and walk unsteadily, as if they are drunk. They soon begin to compensate for this by adopting a broad base with feet further apart (see Fig. 14.1a). The gait is unsteady, with irregularity of stride. The trunk sways and the patient may veer towards one side. In mild cases, the only manifestation of gait disturbance may be difficulty walking heel-toe in a straight line (i.e. tandem walking).

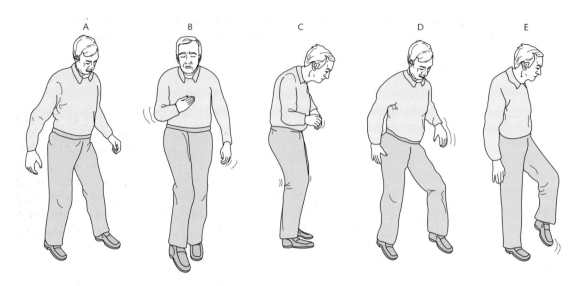

Fig. 14.1 Disorders of gait. (A) Cerebellar ataxia, (B) hemiparetic, (C) parkinsonian, (D) sensory ataxia, and (E) unilateral footdrop.

On neurological examination there may also be nystagmus, dysarthria, and cerebellar signs in the limbs. Ataxia may be absent in the limbs and apparent only in the gait when the lesion is in the midline (cerebellar vermis.), so-called 'truncal ataxia'.

Causes include:

- Multiple sclerosis.
- Vascular disease, e.g. ischaemic, haemorrhagic, AVMs.
- Alcoholic cerebellar degeneration.
- Anticonvulsant therapy, e.g. phenytoin, carbamazepine.
- Posterior fossa tumours.
- Cerebellar paraneoplastic syndrome.
- Hereditary cerebellar ataxias.

Hemiparetic gait

Patients with a hemiparetic gait have a characteristic posture on one side, of flexion and internal rotation of the upper limb and extension of the lower limb (see Fig. 14.1b, and also Fig. 12.3, p. 74). The leg moves stiffly and is swung around in a semi-circle to avoid scraping the foot across the floor. However, such scraping does occur to some extent and the toe and outer sole of the shoe become worn.

Causes include:

- Cortical or internal capsular strokes.
- Cerebral hemispheric tumour.
- Traumatic lesions.

Spastic gait

A spastic gait is seen in patients who have a spastic paraparesis. The legs move slowly and stiffly and the thighs are strongly adducted such that the legs may cross as the patient walks or 'scissor gait'.

Causes include:

- Spinal cord compression.
- Trauma/spinal surgery.
- Birth injuries or congenital deformities: cerebral palsy.
- Multiple sclerosis.
- Motor neuron disease.
- Parasagittal meningioma.
- Subacute combined degeneration of the cord.

Parkinsonian gait

The patient often has a stooped and flexed posture with loss of arm swing, which is almost always more marked on one side in idiopathic Parkinson's disease (see Fig. 14.1c, and also Fig. 18.4, p. 115). The steps are short and the patient shuffles. There may be difficulty starting and stopping. Turning may occur 'en bloc' (i.e. not smoothly but in stiff, stuttering movements). Having started to walk, the patient leans forward and the pace quickens, as though the patient is attempting to catch up on himself (festinant gait).

Gait of sensory ataxia

Sensory ataxia arises from impaired proprioception caused by a lesion of the peripheral nerves, posterior roots, dorsal columns in the spinal cord, or rarely the ascending afferent fibres to the parietal lobes. The gait is unsteady and wide-based, and often 'stamping' (see Fig. 14.1d). Romberg's test is positive and there is impaired perception of joint position on examination of the lower limbs.

Causes include:

- Posterior spinal cord lesions:
  - multiple sclerosis
  - cervical spondylosis
  - tumours
  - vitamin B$_{12}$ deficiency
  - tabes dorsalis (tertiary syphilis).
- Sensory peripheral neuropathies include:
  - hereditary: Charcot–Marie–Tooth disease
  - metabolic: diabetes
  - inflammatory: Guillain–Barré syndrome
  - malignancy: myeloma, paraneoplastic syndrome
  - toxic: alcohol, drugs (e.g. isoniazid).

Steppage gait

Steppage gait arises from weakness of the pretibial and peroneal muscles of lower motor neuron type. The patient has 'footdrop' and is unable to dorsiflex and evert the foot (see Fig. 14.1e). The leg is lifted high on walking so that the toes clear the ground. On striking the floor again, there is a slapping noise. Shoe soles are worn on the anterior and lateral aspects.

Causes include:

- Charcot–Marie–Tooth disease (bilateral footdrop).
- Common peroneal nerve palsy, e.g. from a fibular fracture (unilateral footdrop).

- Anterior horn cell disease, e.g. polio, motor neuron disease (often asymmetrical footdrop).

Myopathic gait

The myopathic gait is often called a 'waddling gait' and is caused by weakness of the proximal muscles of the lower limb girdle. The weight is alternately placed on each leg, with the opposite hip and side of the trunk tilting up towards the weight-bearing side. However, the weak gluteal muscles cannot stabilize the weight-bearing hip, which sways outward, with the opposite pelvis and trunk dropping.

Causes include:

- Muscular dystrophies: Duchenne's, Becker's, limb-girdle, facio-scapulo-humeral.
- Metabolic myopathies: periodic paralysis, hypo- and hyperkalaemia, hypo- and hypercalcaemia.
- Endocrine myopathies: Cushing's disease, Addison's disease, hypo- and hyperthyroidism.
- Inflammatory myopathies: polymyositis and dermatomyositis.

Apraxic gait

Disease of the frontal lobes gives rise to an apraxic gait. The patient walks with feet placed apart and with small, hesitant steps, which may be described as 'walking on ice' or *marche au petit pas*. There is difficulty with initiation of walking and, in advanced cases, it may seem as though the patient's feet are stuck to the floor. There are no abnormalities of power, sensation, or coordination. There may be other signs of frontal cortical dysfunction (e.g. a grasp or rooting reflex); the tendon reflexes may be brisk and the plantar responses extensor.

Causes include:

- Subcortical ischaemic leucoencephalopathy 'small vessel disease'.
- Hydrocephalus including normal pressure hydrocephalus.
- Frontal lobe tumours, e.g. meningioma.
- Frontal subdural haematomas (bilateral).
- Frontal contusions post-head injury.

Antalgic gait

The antalgic gait arises from pain (e.g. a painful hip or knee due to arthritis). The patient tends to bear weight mainly on the unaffected side, only briefly putting weight onto the affected side.

Functional gait

A 'functional', 'hysterical', or 'non-organic' gait arises from psychological or behavioural disturbance. It does not conform to any of the descriptions given above. It can take a number of forms and is variable in character. There are no objective abnormal neurological signs on formal examination. There are often other positive features of an underlying psychiatric disturbance. However, the only manifestation of a midline cerebellar lesion may be severe ataxia of gait, with normal limb signs on formal examination and this can sometimes be mistaken for a non-organic illness.

The character of a patient's gait will provide clues to the clinical signs that might be expected on further neurological examination. The abnormal types of gait are summarized below:

- Ataxic: broad-based and unsteady.
- Hemiplegic: unilateral flexed posture of the upper limb and extended posture of the lower limb.
- Spastic: 'scissoring' posture of the legs.
- Parkinsonian: flexed posture, shuffling small stepped gait with loss of arm swing.
- Sensory ataxia: high stepped 'stamping' gait.
- Steppage: 'footdrop'.
- Myopathic: 'waddling' gait.
- Apraxic: hesitant 'walking on ice' gait.
- Non-organic: bizarre and variable.

DISEASES AND DISORDERS

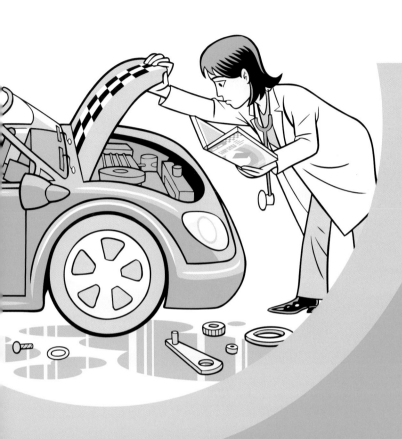

Objectives

- Define the term 'dementia'
- Describe the features in the history and examination that enable the differentiation of dementias
- Understand the investigations required in patients with dementia
- Describe the main primary neurodegeneratives dementias – how would you differentiate these?
- Understand the term 'multi-infarct' dementia

DEFINITION

Dementia is a syndrome and not a single disease entity. Many congenital and acquired diseases cause dementia. Clinically, dementia is associated with a global deterioration of intellect, behaviour, and personality. In the initial stages, there are often focal cortical deficits. Unfortunately, dementia is usually relentlessly progressive and is eventually associated with diffuse involvement of both cerebral hemispheres in the end-stages. The patient is often alert and sometimes even hyperactive in the early and middle stages of the disease. This is in contrast to delirium (acute confusional state), in which alteration of level of consciousness is a defining feature. Impairment of memory is critical to the diagnosis of most dementias.

EPIDEMIOLOGY

The most common causes of dementia are Alzheimer's disease and vascular dementia, and these are predominantly diseases of the elderly.

The prevalence of dementia in persons aged between 50 and 70 years is about 1% and in those approaching 90 years it reaches 50%. The annual incidence rate is 190/100 000 and, with an increasing ageing population, it is expected to rise even further.

GENERAL CLINICAL FEATURES

The earliest feature of dementia, from most causes, is loss of memory for recent events. Subsequent symptoms include abnormal behaviour, loss of intellect, mood changes, and difficulty coping with ordinary routines. Insight may be retained initially but is then usually lost. Ultimately, there is a loss of self-care; disorientation in place, time and person; double incontinence, and behavioural/psychiatric features such as paranoia.

The rate of progression of dementia depends on the underlying cause:

- Alzheimer's disease: slowly progressive over years.
- Vascular dementia: repeated large vessel occlusion causes stepwise deterioration, whereas small vessel disease causes a progresive decline without steps. Both often coexist.
- Prion disease: progressive over months
- Encephalitis: over days to weeks.
- It should be noted that all dementias tend to be accelerated by a change in environment, intercurrent infection, or surgical procedures.

HISTORY AND EXAMINATION

It is essential to obtain a history from a relative or friend, as well as from the patient, to gauge the following:

- Rate of intellectual decline.
- Activities of daily living and social interaction.
- Nutritional status.
- Drug history.

- General health and relevant disorders, e.g. stroke, head injury.
- Family history of dementia.

Neurological examination should specifically look for evidence of:

- Focal signs.
- Involuntary movements.
- Pseudobulbar signs.
- Primitive reflexes, e.g. pout, grasp, and rooting reflexes.
- Gait disorder.

Formal assessment by a clinical psychologist is advisable, but a bedside 'mini-mental' test provides initial information about intellectual function. These tests are designed to test memory, abstract thought, judgement, and specific higher cortical functions, and should include questions similar to those listed in Fig. 34.2 (p. 229).

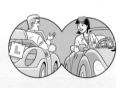

It is vital to take a history from a relative or friend who knows the patient well. Patients with dementia, especially with frontal lobe disease, are often completely unaware of any problem. The relative should ideally be interviewed separately from the patient as personality change, especially when related to disinhibiton, can be difficult for the relative to talk about in front of the patient.

DIFFERENTIAL DIAGNOSES

- Primary neurodegenerative diseases, e.g. Alzheimer's disease, dementia with Lewy bodies, frontotemporal lobar degeneration (including Pick's disease), Huntington's disease.
- Metabolic disorders, e.g. hypothyroidism, vitamin B_{12} and folate deficiency, mitochondrial cytopathies, Wilson's disease and leucodystrophies.
- Infections, e.g. HIV, prion disease and syphilis.
- Vasculitis and inflammatory diseases.
- Normal pressure hydrocephalus.
- Space-occupying lesions, e.g. chronic subdural haematoma.
- Pseudodementia: patients who are depressed may appear demented.

INVESTIGATIONS

It is important to carry out a number of investigations to exclude potentially treatable causes of dementia.

Blood tests

Routine blood tests may be necessary to exclude:

- Hypothyroidism.
- Vitamin B_{12} and folate deficiency.
- Syphilis.

Specific blood tests should be performed to screen for rarer causes of dementia:

- Metabolic disorders, e.g. Wilson's disease, leucodystrophies.
- HIV: 'AIDS dementia'.
- Vasculitis and inflammatory diseases.

Cranial imaging

Cranial imaging can be performed using computed tomography (CT) or magnetic resonance imaging (MRI). Variable degrees of cerebral atrophy with enlarged ventricles are seen with most forms of dementia (Fig. 15.1).

It is important to exclude:

- Space-occupying lesions: especially chronic subdural haematoma in the elderly following a fall.
- Normal-pressure hydrocephalus: enlarged ventricles without cortical atrophy. This presents with dementia, urinary incontinence, and gait apraxia. It is diagnosed by therapeutic lumbar puncture and removal of up to 50 mL of CSF, which should cause improvement in the clinical state. If this procedure is successful then it can be treated more permanently by ventriculoperitoneal shunting.

MRI can now be used to calculate the volume of brain tissue in various parts of the CNS. This can demonstrate bilateral hippocampal and temporal lobe atrophy in Alzheimer's disease and asymmetrical anterior hippocampal, amygdala, and temporal lobe atrophy in frontotemporal lobar degeneration (FTLD).

Neuropsychometry

Neuropsychologists have been trained to test the domains of cognitive function in a lot more detail

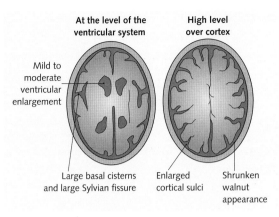

At the level of the ventricular system

High level over cortex

Mild to moderate ventricular enlargement

Large basal cisterns and large Sylvian fissure

Enlarged cortical sulci

Shrunken walnut appearance

Fig. 15.1 CT scan appearances of atrophy of the brain with enlarged ventricles. This is a non-specific finding in many causes of dementia.

than most doctors are able to perform. Formal neuropsychometry is especially useful when performed at intervals. This enables comparison of intellectual function within a patient over time. It can be a reliable indicator of either progression in disease (suggesting an organic dementia) compared to improvement or plateau in decline of intellectual function which can be seen in patients with treated depression or functional memory loss.

Electroencephalography (EEG)

EEG traces rarely demonstrate specific changes in dementia. The most common finding is wide-spread delta waves. These changes can be seen earlier in Alzheimer's disease than in FTLD. There is often a loss of the responsive alpha rhythm in Alzheimer's disease which is often preserved in FTLD.

Periodic complexes on the EEG tracing may indicate prion disease such as Creutzfeldt–Jakob disease. This group of disorders is associated with a rapidly progressive course, which is usually an important diagnostic feature.

Muscle biopsy

Muscle biopsy should be undertaken to look for the presence of ragged, red fibres and other features typical of mitochondrial cytopathies if the clinical history and examination is suggestive of mitochondrial disease.

Genetic testing

The following genetic diseases can be associated with dementia.

- Huntington mutation: Huntington's chorea.
- Amyloid precursor protein (APP), presenilin 1 and 2, and apoliprotein E4 mutations: Alzheimer's disease.
- Prion protein gene mutation: familial Creutzfeldt–Jakob disease.
- Tau and progranulin mutations: FTLD.

Brain biopsy

Brain biopsy is rarely performed but is indicated when a treatable cause of dementia is suspected but other investigations fail to reach a diagnosis (e.g. cerebral vasculitis).

MANAGEMENT

Amenable causes of dementia should be treated. Some of these are potentially reversible or their clinical course can be stabilized (e.g. vasculitis, hydrocephalus, and depressive pseudodementia).

In non-treatable cases (e.g. Alzheimer's disease), depression and any underlying systemic disorders should be treated to maximize cognitive function. The use of centrally acting cholinergic drugs for primary neurodegenerative dementias is discussed below.

Neuroleptic medication may be required for behavioural disturbance but can exacerbate extrapyramidal features, such as slowing of movements.

Management of most cases of dementia requires careful advice and counselling of the patient and family, and shared care involving the family, carers, hospital specialists, GP, and community psychiatric services. Long-term residential care is often required.

PRIMARY NEURODEGENERATIVE DEMENTIAS

Alzheimer's disease

Alzheimer's disease (AD) is the most common cause of dementia in the developed world. There are approximately 500 000 cases in the UK at any one time. It is rarely seen in persons under the age of 45 years, except in familial cases, and the incidence increases dramatically with age, especially in patients over 70 years.

Familial Alzheimer's disease is uncommon. Mutations in the the amyloid precursor protein (APP) gene on chromosome 21 is associated with young-onset AD. There is also an association of late-onset disease with the apolipoprotein E4 genotype. Recently, mutations in the genes presenilin 1 and 2 have been described.

Individuals with Down syndrome develop the full neuropathological and clinical changes of Alzheimer's disease by their fourth to fifth decade of life, probably as a consequence of the excessive APP produced by a 50% increase in gene dosage due to the extra chromosome 21.

Pathology

Alzheimer's disease is identified by the presence of senile plaques and neurofibrillary tangles in the brain. Senile plaques consist of dystrophic neurites clustered round a core of β-amyloid protein, which is derived from the larger precursor protein, APP.

Neurofibrillary tangles are derived from the microtubule-associated protein tau, which is in an abnormally hyperphosphorylated state. The majority of the pathology affects the hippocampus, temporal and parietal lobes.

Clinical features

Alzheimer's disease presents with features of progressive episodic (knowledge of events) memory loss and evolves over many years. Dysphasia, apraxia and topographical disorientation are common early features reflecting involvement of the parietal lobes. Seizures and myoclonus are relatively common in late disease. Pyramidal and extrapyramidal features rarely occur.

Diagnosis

A definite diagnosis of Alzheimer' disease can be made only from pathological findings. In practice, a typical history with progressive episodic memory loss and negative routine tests will allow a diagnosis of probable Alzheimer's disease.

CT scans show non-specific generalized cerebral atrophy with enlarged ventricles due to loss of brain tissue rather than hydrocephalus. The temporal lobes may be more severely atrophic (see Fig. 15.1). Serial volumetric analysis of the temporal lobes and hippocampi using MRI may enable a more specific diagnosis.

Drug treatment

The acetylcholinesterase inhibitor tacrine is licensed in the USA and France, and donepezil, galantamine and rivastigmine have been licensed in the UK. In general, these arrest symptoms by approximately 6 months but do not alter the course of the neuro-degenerative process. They can be used in patients with mild to moderate disease and need to be monitored carefully for cholinergic side-effects (e.g. bowel disturbance).

Memantine has also been demonstrated to improve symptoms in advanced disease and may have an additional benefit in combination with anti-cholinesterase inhibitors.

Current pharmaceutical research is directed towards inhibition of the hyperphosphorylation of the protein tau, which underlies the neurofibrillary tangles, removal of β-amyloid and neuroprotective agents.

Prognosis

In spite of recent advances in our understanding and treatment, the prognosis of Alzheimer's disease is very poor, with relentless progression to death, which is often due to bronchopneumonia. The mean survival is 8 years from the onset of the disease.

Dementia with Lewy bodies (DLB)

DLB has only been recognized as a separate clinical entity within the past 15 years. It is associated with prominent early visual hallucinations, memory disturbance and fluctuations in the clinical course even from day to day. The extrapyramidal features in DLB are similar to those in idiopathic Parkinson's disease, except the characteristic resting tremor is absent, there is a poor response to L-dopa therapy and the clinical signs are often symmetrical. In contrast to dementia seen in the later stages of idiopathic Parkinson's disease, the dementia occurs early in DLB. The neuropathology is a mixture of that seen in Parkinson's disease with Lewy bodies in the substantia nigra but also in the cerebral cortex, as well as amyloid plaques and neurofibrillary tangles. The patients often develop prominent psychiatric side-effects with dopamine agonists, such as confusion and hallucinations. Clinical trials have shown that acetylcholinesterase inhibitors can produce significant improvement in the symptoms of DLB.

Frontotemporal lobar dementia (FTLD)

FTLD is a relatively rare cause of dementia. It is accompanied by marked cerebral atrophy in the frontal and anterior temporal lobes with relatively sparing of the parietal lobes in contrast to Alzheimer's disease. The neuropathology of FTLD is heterogeneous. Some cases demonstrate argyrophilic inclusions (i.e. pieces of protein that stain with silver) which are called Pick bodies. They are found within the neuronal cytoplasm and contain the protein, tau. Some cases have inclusions which contain tau but are not Pick bodies and other cases contain inclusions which are ubiquitin positive and tau negative.

The disease is more common in women, at least 50% are genetic (associated with numerous mutations in tau and a protein called progranulin). It tends to occur between the ages of 40 and 60 years, which is younger than sporadic Alzheimer's disease.

FTLD is often associated with prominent frontal features which leads to behavioural and psychiatric features at presentation and misdiagnosis. The EEG is usually normal in the early stages of the disease, and CT scans show prominent frontotemporal atrophy.

No specific treatment has been found, and the disease progresses to death over 2–5 years.

FTLD is one a several neurodegenerative disease associated with accumulation of tau. Other examples include corticobasal degeneration and progressive supranuclear palsy. These diseases are collectively known as the 'tauopathies'.

VASCULAR DEMENTIA

Large-vessel disease

Strategically localized single brain lesions may profoundly affect specific cognitive functions (e.g. language or memory) without causing global dementia. When the cognitive changes are accompanied by other classical symptoms and signs of stroke such as acute onset hemiparesis, diagnostic problems do not usually arise. 'Silent' strokes, especially in the frontal lobes, may lead to cognitive changes without the other typical features of common stroke syndromes.

Multi-infarct dementia

Multi-infarct dementia is the second most common cause of dementia, and often coexists with Alzheimer's disease. It is caused by the accumulation of bilateral multifocal ischaemic events. It occurs mainly after the age of 50 years and with a history of atherosclerotic (larve vessel) and arteriosclerotic (small vessel) risk factors, especially hypertension. Dementia may occur in a stepwise fashion, with each successive stroke, or may relentlessly progress after many 'silent infarcts'. The pathology usually involves both cortical (large vessel) and subcortical (small penetrating vessel) infarcts. There is also often evidence of other vascular disease (e.g. ischaemic heart disease, peripheral vascular disease). Sometimes there is little radiological evidence of large vessel stroke but prominent subcortical, basal ganglia and pontine small vessel disease leading to a frontal apraxia, pseudobulbar palsy, and parkinsonism. This is called 'subcortical ischaemic leucoencepahlopathy'.

Diagnosis

The diagnosis of multi-infarct dementia is made based on the history and the presence of multiple areas of large vessel infarction and/or prominent small vessel disease on CT or MRI.

Treatment

Primary prevention for patients at risk, to prevent the onset of multiple strokes (see Chapter 26).

Secondary prevention of atherosclerosis in established cases with good control of hypertension, hyperlipidaemia and antiplatelet agents such as aspirin, and dipyridamole or clopidogrel in patients with a history of dyspepsia.

Vasculitis

Vasculitis is an uncommon cause of dementia, but should be recognized, as most cases are amenable to treatment. They include:

- Polyarteritis nodosa.
- Primary granulomatous angiitis: isolated vasculitis of the central nervous system.
- Systemic lupus erythematosus.
- Giant-cell arteritis.
- Thrombotic microangiopathies.

DEMENTIA AS A PART OF OTHER DEGENERATIVE DISEASES

In the following conditions, dementia may be a prominent finding with other neurological features:

- Parkinson's disease (frontotemporal).
- Huntington's disease (frontal/subcortical).
- Progressive supranuclear palsy (frontal).
- Motor neuron disease (frontotemporal).

PSEUDODEMENTIA

Depression in the elderly can mimic the initial phases of dementia and is termed 'pseudodementia'. Pseudodementia is amenable to antidepressant medications.

It is vital to take a good social and psychiatric history in patients with dementia. The social circumstances surrounding a patient with dementia are critical for optimal management, e.g. familiar environments and routine. Remember that the carers also need social support. Even when depression is not the main cause of memory difficulties, its treatment can still lead to significant stabilization in the patient's symptoms.

Epilepsy

Objectives

- Describe the main types of seizure
- Describe the aetiological factors associated with epilepsy
- Understand which drugs are used in the common epilepsy syndromes and their side-effects
- How would you manage status epilepticus?
- Understand the social implications of being diagnosed with epilepsy

DEFINITIONS

Seizures result from abnormal, paroxysmal, synchronous and rapid electrical discharges arising from cerebral neurons. These discharges are usually self-terminating but have a tendency to recur.

- **Epileptic seizure:** can be defined clinically as an intermittent, stereotyped disturbance of consciousness, behaviour, emotion, motor function, or sensation, arising from abnormal neuronal discharges.
- **Epilepsy:** the condition in which seizures recur, usually spontaneously.
- **Status epilepticus:** a state of continued or recurrent seizures, with failure to regain consciousness between seizures over 30 minutes. This is a medical emergency and has a mortality rate of 10–15%.
- **Prodrome:** premonitory changes in mood or behaviour; these may precede the attack by some hours.
- **Aura:** the subjective sensation or phenomenon that may precede and mark the onset of the epileptic seizure. It may localize the seizure origin within the brain.
- **Ictus:** the attack or seizure itself.
- **Postictal period:** the time after the ictus during which the patient may be drowsy, confused, and disorientated. The patient may also have residual focal neurological signs, e.g. Todd's paralysis.

CLASSIFICATION

The International Classification of Epileptic Seizures (ICES) was proposed in 1981 to replace older classifications (Fig. 16.1).

EPIDEMIOLOGY

Between 3 and 5% of the population suffer one or two seizures during their lives. Recurrent seizures occur in 0.5% of the population and 90% of these cases are well controlled with drugs and have prolonged remissions.

Epilepsy more commonly presents during childhood or adolescence, but can occur at any age. Incidence rates vary with age, being between 20 and 70 cases per 100 000 persons a year; the prevalence rate ranges between 4 and 10 per 1000. There are two peaks in the incidence of grand mal seizures. The first occurs in children and adolescents, in whom no cause can be found. The second occurs in patients in their fifties and sixties, in whom the disease is probably caused by subcortical ischaemic changes secondary to hypertension.

AETIOLOGY

Epilepsy is a symptom of numerous disorders but in over 50% of patients with epilepsy, no apparent cause is found, in spite of full investigation.

Fig. 16.1 International classification of epileptic seizures

Partial seizures (seizures beginning focally)

— **Simple** (consciousness not impaired)
  With motor symptoms
  With somatosensory or special sensory symptoms
  e.g. taste/smell.
  With autonomic symptoms
  With psychological, e.g. 'jamais vu' or
  'deja vu' symptoms

— **Complex** (with impairment of consciousness)
  Beginning as a simple partial seizure and progressing
  to a complex partial seizure
  Impairment of consciousness at onset

— **Partial seizure becoming secondarily generalized**

Generalized seizures

— **Absence** seizure
  Typical (petit mal)
  Atypical

— **Others**
  Myoclonic seizure
  Clonic seizure
  Tonic seizure
  Tonic-clonic seizure (grand mal)
  Atonic seizure

Of the symptomatic causes in adults, vascular disease (especially stroke), alcohol abuse, cerebral tumours, and head injury are the most common.

Factors that may predispose to seizures are described below.

Family history

There is an increased liability to seizures in relatives of patients with epilepsy. This is especially true in the case of absence seizures, where up to 40% of cases have a family history. No single genetic trait can account for the vast heterogeneity of all epileptic syndromes. The mechanism probably involves factors that alter membrane structure or function, which may lead to a lowered seizure threshold.

Prenatal and perinatal factors

Intrauterine infections such as rubella and toxoplasmosis, as well as maternal drug abuse and irradiation in early gestation, can produce brain damage and neonatal seizures. Perinatal trauma and anoxia, when sufficiently severe to cause brain injury, may also result in epilepsy.

Trauma and surgery

Severe closed or open head trauma is often followed by seizures. These can be within the first week ('early'), or may be delayed up to several months or years ('late'), when the likelihood of chronic epilepsy is greater. Surgery to the cerebral hemispheres is followed by seizures in about 10% of patients.

Metabolic causes

Many electrolyte disturbances can cause neuronal irritability and seizures such as hyponatraemia and hypernatraemia, hypocalcaemia, hypomagnesaemia, and hypoglycaemia. Other metabolic causes include uraemia, hepatic failure, acute hypoxia, and porphyria. Chronic metabolic encephalopathies can produce permanent grey-matter injury.

Toxic causes

Drugs such as phenothiazines, monoamine oxidase inhibitors, tricyclic antidepressants, amphetamines, lidocaine, and nalidixic acid may provoke fits, either in overdose or at therapeutic levels in patients with a lowered seizure threshold.

Withdrawal of antiepileptic medication and benzodiazepines may also cause seizures especially when it is done rapidly.

Chronic alcohol abuse is a very common cause of seizures. These may occur while drinking, during a withdrawal phase, secondary to hypoglycaemia or trauma.

Other toxic agents capable of causing seizures include carbon monoxide, lead, and mercury.

Infectious and inflammatory causes

Seizures may be the presenting feature or part of the course of encephalitis, meningitis, cerebral abscess, or neurosyphilis, and usually indicate a poorer prognosis in these conditions. High fevers secondary to non-cerebral infections in children over 6 months and under 6 years of age are a common cause of generalized seizures ('febrile convulsion'). These are usually self-limiting, and seizures do not tend to recur in adult life.

Vascular causes

Up to 15% of patients with cerebrovascular disease experience seizures, especially with large areas of infarction or haemorrhage. Less common vascular causes of seizures include cortical venous thrombosis and arteritis (e.g. polyarteritis nodosa) as well as vascular malformations.

Intracranial tumours

Sudden onset of seizures in adult life, especially if partial, should always raise the possibility of an intracranial tumour.

Hypoxia

Seizures can develop during or following respiratory or cardiac arrest secondary to anoxic encephalopathy.

Degenerative diseases

All patients with degenerative corticoneuronal diseases of the brain have an increased risk of seizures (e.g. Alzheimer's disease).

Photosensitivity

Some seizure types are precipitated by flashing lights, or flickering television or computer screens.

Sleep deprivation

Sleep deprivation often precipitates seizures in susceptible patients.

Failure to comply with medication is a very common cause of seizures, including status epilepticus. Usually, the patient fails to comply because of side-effects of the anti-convulsants or difficulty coming to terms with their condition psychologically. It is therefore important to ask about troublesome side-effects and discuss alternatives with the patient and the GP.

PATHOPHYSIOLOGY

Electrical discharges between neurons are usually restricted, and produce the normal rhythms recorded on the electroencephalogram (EEG).

When a seizure occurs, large groups of neurons are activated repetitively and 'hypersynchronously', with dysfunction of the inhibitory synaptic contact between neurons. This produces the high-voltage spike-and-wave activity on the EEG typical of a seizure.

The onset of the epileptic discharge may include the whole cortex ('primary generalized'), may be confined to one area of the cortex ('partial'), or may start focally and then spread to involve the whole cortex ('secondary generalization of a partial seizure').

CLINICAL FEATURES

The diagnosis of epilepsy is primarily a clinical one. A detailed history is therefore essential and usually requires eyewitness reports, particularly when consciousness is lost during the event.

If an aura preceded the attack, the patient may be able to describe this, which may help localize the focus. The aura may not be rememebered by the patient especially if there is secondary generalization.

Simple partial seizures

Simple partial seizures involve focal symptoms. Motor and sensory seizures, arise in the frontal motor or parietal sensory cortex and affect the contralateral face, trunk, or limbs. Simple partial seizures can occur in any region of the cerebral cortex, e.g. bad tastes or smells, *jamais vu/deja vu* with temporal lobes seizures or abnormal behaviour in frontal seizures. There is no loss of consciousness unless there is a subsequent spread of activity ('secondary generalization'). A structural brain lesion must be excluded (e.g. stroke, tumour, or abscess).

Complex partial seizures

Complex partial seizures usually originate in the temporal or frontal lobe and cause a disturbance of consciousness usually without loss of postural control, i.e. the patient remains standing. The actual attack varies between and within individuals. In temporal lobe complex partial seizures the patient may experience *déjà vu*, depersonalization, epigastric fullness, strange tastes or smells, fidgeting with fingers and lip smacking (limb and oral automatisms), and altered emotion. Typically, witnesses suggest that the patient either wanders in a confused state and is only partly responsive or stops what they were doing and stares meaninglessly with repetitive oral and hand movements. Complex partial seizures typically last up to 10 minutes but can continue for several hours as a part of 'non-convulsive status epilepticus'.

Absence seizures (petit mal)

Absence seizures have an onset between 4 and 12 years of age. The attacks may occur several times a day, with a duration of 5–15 seconds. The patient suddenly stares vacantly. There may be eye blinking and myoclonic jerks. They are often diagnosed following complaints about an inattentive child with a deteriorating performance at school.

Tonic-clonic seizures (grand mal)

Tonic-clonic seizures start with a sudden loss of consciousness and fall to the ground. This is followed by the 'tonic' phase, which lasts for about 10 seconds, when the body is stiff, the elbows are flexed, and the legs extended. Breathing stops and the patient may turn cyanotic.

The tonic phase is followed by the 'clonic phase', which usually lasts for 1–2 minutes, and during which there is violent generalized rhythmical shaking. The eyes roll back, the tongue may be bitten, and there is a tachycardia. Bladder and bowel control may be lost. Breathing recommences at the end of this phase. Following a tonic-clonic seizure, the patient often cannot be roused for several minutes and awakes with confusion, headache, myalgia, and some retrograde amnesia.

HISTORY AND INVESTIGATIONS TO AID DIAGNOSIS

The diagnosis of a seizure is based on the clinical history; additional information can be provided by brain imaging, the EEG, or blood tests. The use of neuroimaging is more important in cases with a late onset (over the age of 25 years), that are partial, refractory to treatment, are associated with persisting abnormal clinical signs, or when the presentation is with status epilecticus.

Clinical features during an attack that support the diagnosis of a seizure include pupil dilatation, raised blood pressure and heart rate, extensor plantar responses, and central and peripheral cyanosis.

In generalized seizures, the pO_2 and pH are lowered, the creatine phosphokinase (CPK), or creatine kinase (CK) is elevated, and there is a marked elevation of serum prolactin.

The EEG is extremely useful if recorded during an attack and may show spike and wave activity. Interictal EEGs are often normal but may show focal spikes or slow waves suggesting subclinical seizure activity. In some cases, abnormal activity can be provoked by hyperventilation or photic stimulation (flashing light). This is especially true for absence seizures, in which there is the characteristic three-per-second spike-and-wave pattern in all leads.

Computed tomography (CT) or magnetic resonance imaging (MRI) may reveal structural lesions that have caused the seizures, especially if there is a partial onset. In complex partial seizures of temporal lobe origin, the MRI may demonstrate hippocampal sclerosis.

It is important to distinguish epilepsy from other causes of transient focal dysfunction or loss of consciousness, as there are social and economic implications when a diagnosis of epilepsy is made, e.g. the patient is unable to drive or operate certain machinery.

The most common differentials of a convulsive seizure include:

- Syncope (vasovagal attacks, arrhythmias, carotid sinus hypersensitivity, postural hypotension): there is usually prodromal pallor, nausea, and sweating. Palpitations may be experienced with arrhythmias.
- Non-epileptic seizures or 'pseudoseizures': psychologically determined, feigned seizures are surprisingly common, especially in patients with known epilepsy. The following features help to differentiate a pseudoseizure from an epileptic seizure: pupils, blood pressure, heart rate, pO_2, and pH remain unchanged; plantar responses are flexor; serum prolactin levels are normal; the EEG shows no seizure activity during the episode and no postictal slowing.
- Transient ischaemic attacks (TIAs): these can include transient loss of consciousness – among other brainstem symptoms – when the posterior circulation is involved but this is very uncommon and often overdiagnosed.
- Hypoglycaemia: this can cause behavioural disturbance and seizures.

DRUG TREATMENT

Antiepileptic treatment should be considered when two or more unprovoked seizures have occurred within a short period. Whenever possible, treatment should involve only one drug, to avoid interaction between the anticonvulsants and additive side-effects. Treatment is aimed at making the patient seizure free, but this is not always possible.

The most common anticonvulsants in current clinical use are carbamazepine, sodium valproate, lamotrigine, and phenytoin. Second-line drugs include gabapentin, topiramate, levetiracetam, and phenobarbitone. In general, the first-line drugs for primary generalized epilepsy in adults are sodium valproate or lamotrigine, for absence epilepsy in children is ethosuximide or sodium valproate, and for partial seizures is carbamazepine or lamotrigine. Many patients still take phenobarbitone and phenytoin for generalized seizures but these are less commonly prescribed because of their side-effect profile. Some patients may still be taking vigabatrin but this is used rarely now because it can cause progressive and irreversible visual field defects.

Whichever drug is used, the dose should be built up slowly. Measurement of blood drug concentrations is important for phenytoin, as it displays zero-order kinetics and small increases in dose can cause it to reach toxic levels. For other drugs, therapeutic drug monitoring, if available, can be used to check compliance or to confirm clinically diagnosed toxicity. If the patient is seizure and side-effect-free and has a slightly high serum anticonvulsant level then it is usually more appropriate not to change the drug dosage. Phenobarbitone is still used in refractory epilepsy and status epilepticus and levels should be monitored.

Pharmacokinetics of antiepileptic drugs

Phenytoin, phenobarbitone, topiramate and carbamazepine are well known to induce enzymes within the liver that metabolize other drugs. This effect is most important when using several antiepileptic drugs together and when the patient is on the combined oral contraceptive pill. Many of the antiepileptic drugs also block pathways within the liver for metabolism of drugs, e.g. sodium valproate prolongs the half-life of lamotrigine. Care must be taken when prescribing these drugs, especially in combination, to avoid toxic levels and other adverse reactions.

Adverse effects of antiepileptic drugs

All antiepileptic drugs can produce acute, dose-related, idiosyncratic or chronic toxicity, and variable degrees of teratogenicity (damage to the developing fetus).

Acute toxicity

All anticonvulsants can cause drowsiness and slowed cognition especially at higher doses. Some antiepileptic drugs cause a non-specific encephalopathy when blood levels are high. This is associated with sedation, nystagmus, ataxia, dysarthria, and confusion. If any of these features is present, blood levels must be measured.

Idiosyncratic toxicity

Allergic skin reactions occur in up to 10% of patients on phenytoin and in up to 15% on carbamazepine. Lamotrigine can be associated with a particularly severe skin rash. These can be reduced by introducing these drugs slowly, at low doses, and building up to therapeutic levels. Bone marrow aplasia is a rare idiosyncratic complication of carbamazepine.

Chronic toxicity

Chronic toxicity is especially associated with phenytoin and includes the development of coarsened facies, acne, hirsuitism, gum hypertrophy, and possibly peripheral neuropathy. All anticonvulsants appear to have some effect on cognitive function and can cause drowsiness. This is especially a problem with phenytoin. Carbamazepine and phenytoin can cause a sometimes-irreversible cerebellar ataxia in a dose-related manner. Generally, carbamazepine and sodium valproate have fewer chronic effects than phenytoin. Lamotrigine is being increasingly used for many types of epilepsy because of its low side-effect profile, to date, including low levels of teratogenicity. Levetiracetam is also being used more frequently because of a relatively lower incidence of side-effects and absence of effect on hepatic metabolism.

Teratogenicity

Phenytoin increases the risk of major fetal malformation including hair lip, cleft palate, and cardiovascular anomalies by a factor of two to three times. The use of sodium valproate and carbamazepine in pregnancy is associated with neural tube defects. Folate supplements and early screening using ultrasound and amniocentesis (to test for alpha-fetoprotein) are indicated in such cases.

Patients with epilepsy and on treatment who wish to become pregnant should seek specialist advice before conception and require regular follow-up by a neurologist during the pregnancy.

Withdrawal of antiepileptic drugs

In view of the many adverse reactions associated with anticonvulsants, a patient who has achieved remission for over 2 years should be considered for drug withdrawal. However, there is the risk of recurrence of seizures, especially in some forms of epilepsy, and this has important consequences for driving, employment, and self-esteem. Thus, the final decision to attempt withdrawal must be made by the patient and, if undertaken, must be carried out very slowly, with gradually decreasing doses.

STATUS EPILEPTICUS

'Serial epilepsy' is defined as a succession of tonic-clonic seizures without regaining of consciousness between attacks. The patient has 'status epilepticus' when the seziures continue for greater than 30 minutes without stopping. If left untreated, this can lead to irreversible brain damage as the patient becomes hypoxic and eventually death ensues.

Patients with status epilepticus require immediate resuscitation. This involves establishing an airway and administering oxygen. The circulation should be assessed and an infusion set up with normal saline.

Blood tests comprise blood gases, glucose, electrolytes, renal and liver function, and anticonvulsant levels.

If hypoglycaemia is suspected in a patient with a possible history of alcohol abuse or malnutrition then thiamine must be given with intravenous glucose, as glucose alone can precipitate Wernicke's encephalopathy.

Drug treatment

It is helpful to plan therapy in a series of progressive phases:

- Premonitory stage (0–10 minutes): rapid treatment may prevent the evolution to status. Lorazepam, diazepam, midazolam, or paraldehyde can be used at this stage.
- Early status (10–30 minutes): a dose of fast-acting intravenous benzodiazepines such as lorazepam. This can be repeated once if seizures are not terminated. Repeated doses of benzodiazepines may lead to an accumulation and an increased risk of respiratory depression especially with diazepam.
- Established status (30–60 minutes): phenobarbitone or phenytoin is usually given at this stage with intravenous loading doses.
- Refractory status (after 60 minutes): by this stage, anaesthesia is required, with ventilation and intensive care treatment. The most common agents used are intravenous thiopentone or propofol. EEG monitoring is very helpful to confirm when status has been aborted. In all cases, neuromuscular blockade should be avoided if possible, because if the seizures return, the patient's muscles will be paralysed and therefore the return of seizure activity may go unnoticed.

Despite the best medical management, there is still 5–10% mortality with status epilepticus, especially when the cause is due to a catastrophic intracerebral event.

NEUROSURGICAL TREATMENT OF EPILEPSY

The indication for surgical treatment requires the accurate identification of a localized site of onset of seizures or the ability to disconnect epileptogenic zones and prevent spread as a palliative procedure.

The majority of the procedures undertaken in centres worldwide involve some form of temporal lobe surgery. Less commonly, extratemporal cortical excisions, hemispherectomies, and corpus callosotomies are carried out.

For temporal lobe surgery, the two conditions with the best surgical outcome are mesial temporal sclerosis (Ammon's horn sclerosis) or an indolent glioma of the medial temporal region. Development anomalies such as dysembryoplastic neuroepithelial tumours (DNET) are increasingly being diagnosed as the cause of partial epilepsy and some are amenable to surgical removal.

THE SOCIAL CONSEQUENCES OF EPILEPSY

Considerable social stigma is often attached to a diagnosis of epilepsy. There are implications for employment, not only in the ability to carry out certain jobs (e.g. driving or using machinery) but also because many employers are unwilling to take on people with epilepsy.

The aim is to allow patients to lead as unrestricted a life as possible but bearing in mind some precautions, such as to avoid swimming alone or engaging in dangerous sports such as rock climbing. They should also be advised about simple domestic precautions such as not locking the bathroom door.

DRIVING AND EPILEPSY

The DVLA can revoke a British driving licence in any individual felt to be unsafe to himself/herself and/or the public. Patients who have had one or more seizures need to contact the DVLA regarding the length of period they are not allowed to drive. As a guide, the following conditions need to apply before the patient can return to driving with or without treatment:

- Patients cannot drive for 1 year after a single seizure.
- Patients who have only nocturnal seizures may drive if they are seizure free during the daytime for 3 years.
- For single seizures with a specific provocative cause that is unlikely to recur, e.g. encephalitis or acute drug toxicity, the ban on driving may be for only 3–6 months.
- Patients who are driving and taking antiepileptic drugs but who wish to stop epileptic medication are recommended to stop driving during cessation and for 6 months following the last dose of their drug.

Headache and craniofacial pain

Objectives

- Understand the main headache syndromes and their management
- Describe the features that would enable differentiation of a primary and secondary headache
- Understand the types of brain shift that occur in raised intracranial pressure

Headache is one of the most common symptoms in medicine and may account for up to 40% of neurological consultations. The most important role of the general physician is in determining whether the patient has a primary or secondary headache.

TENSION-TYPE HEADACHE

Tension-type headache is possibly the most common form of headache and is experienced by most people at some point in their lives. It is increasingly recognized that in many patients the development of persistent daily headache arises from a transformation of increasingly frequent migraine, rather than a primary tension headache syndrome, often in the context of overuse of analgesics. These patients have 'chronic migraine' and may respond to antimigrainous treatments.

The patient often complains of a diffuse, 'band-like', dull headache, which may be accompanied by scalp tenderness and be aggravated by noise and light. The headache may last hours to days and occur infrequently or everyday. There are no abnormal physical signs.

Treatment is with reassurance, short term analgesia (anti-inflammatories and paracetamol), physical treatments (massage, relaxation therapy), and, in selected cases, tricyclic agents. Chronic opiate use should be avoided (see below). In most patients, the headache will be self-limiting and reassurance that a more sinister cause is unlikely may be satisfactory for the patient. In patients who have refractory daily headache, a small dose of amitriptyline, lower than the doses used for depression, or sometimes a selective serotonin reuptake inhibitor (SSRI) can be tried, although there is less convincing evidence for the SSRIs.

Paradoxically, these headaches can be exacerbated by analgesic overuse. These 'analgesic' headaches are especially caused by chronic use of codeine-containing drugs. In patients who probably have a mixture of analgesic and tension-type headache, the first aim should be to wean the patient off their opiate-based analgesia and concurrently commence a small dose of amitriptyline and occasional paracetamol or anti-inflammatories (e.g. Aspirin, ibuprofen) for acute exacerbations of the headache.

MIGRAINE

Migraine is a common, often familial, condition characterized by an episodic unilateral throbbing headache lasting up to 24 hours. The patient often complains of photophobia, phonophobia, and occasionally osmophobia, as well as nausea and sometimes vomiting. Patients with migraine often cannot bear to do anything apart from lying quietly in a dark room until their headache subsides. Exacerbation of pain by movement is a prominent feature of migraine. It is more common in young women and the headache is often preceded by a visual aura with fortification spectra or flashing lights or a sensory aura with numbness and tingling in the fingers and/or face.

The headache is thought to have a vascular component and to be related to the release of vasoactive substances. The level of serum 5-hydroxytryptamine (5-HT) rises with the prodromal symptoms and falls during the headache. The headache may follow abnormal electrical activity within the cortex or 'spreading depression' and subsequent brainstem activation leads to alterations in cranial vascular tone.

There are various subdivisions of migraine, although migraine with aura (classical) and without aura (common) are the most frequently encountered forms.

Migraine with aura or 'classical migraine'

Patients with a classical migraine complain of an aura, which usually consists of moving white lights or spectra in the shape of fortifications ('fortification spectra'). Some patients experience a sensory aura which involves paraesthesias or numbness that spreads up a limb or part of the face. These precede the migrainous headache by up to 40 minutes and usually last about 20 minutes, rarely more than 60 minutes. The gradually spreading nature of the visual or sensory symptoms is important for making the diagnosis. The aura may extend into the headache phase.

Common migraine

There is no aura in common migraine but the headache is similar to classical migraine.

Basilar migraine

In basilar migraine, the aura symptoms result from dysfunction in the territory of the posterior cerebral circulation, which supplies the brainstem, cerebellum, and most of the occipital cortices. The aura can consist of bilateral visual symptoms, ataxia, dysarthria, vertigo, limb paraesthesia, and weakness. There may be loss of consciousness before, during or after the onset of headache, which often causes diagnostic confusion.

Hemiplegic migraine

Hemiplegic migraine is rare and involves hemiplegia that can persist for days after the headache has settled. In some cases, there is an autosomal dominant transmission and in 50% of these, it is associated with defects in a gene that codes for a calcium channel.

Cerebral autosomal dominant arteriopathy with subcortical infarcts and leucoencephalopathy

CADASIL (cerebral autosomal dominant arteriopathy with subcortical infarcts and leucoencephalopathy) is characterized by a history of migrainous headaches in middle-aged patients (30–60 years), associated with cerebrovascular disease progressing to dementia, and diffuse white matter deficits on MRI. The pathological hallmark of CADASIL is electron-dense granules in the media of arterioles that can often be identified by electron microscopic evaluation of skin biopsies. More than 90% of cases have mutations in the NOTCH 3 gene.

Differential diagnosis

The diagnosis is made from the history, as there are usually no clinical findings in the more common forms of migraine.

The headache needs to be differentiated from meningitis and subarachnoid haemorrhage (SAH), as both these require prompt treatment. The onset of migraine is usually subacute over a few hours and not associated with a pyrexia and disturbance of consciousness. Meningitis is also usually of subacute onset over hours but is usually associated with a swinging pyrexia, uncontrollable vomiting that is persistent with the headache, and ultimately a clouding of consciousness. SAH is associated with a hyperacute onset of the worst headache the patient has ever had followed by neurological deficit and clouding of consciousness. In practice, it can still be difficult to differentiate these types of headaches during the first attack. A previous history of recurrent similar attacks is suggestive of migraine.

Hemiplegic migraine must be differentiated from stroke or transient ischaemic attacks (TIAs). In a patient who presents for the first time with hemiplegia and headache it must be initially assumed that the patient has had a stroke or TIA unless there is a family history of hemiplegic migraine.

Management

The patient needs to be reassured that there is no evidence of an underlying neoplasm. The avoidance of any precipitating dietary factors (e.g. chocolate, cheese) may be helpful. For patients taking oral contraceptives/HRT, changing the brand or stopping the drug may be required. Patients who develop aura should stop hormonal therapy as there is growing evidence that there is an increased incidence of stroke in these patients. The risk is especially high in smokers with aura.

During an attack

Antiemetics are often required to allow ingestion of other drugs such as simple analgesics (e.g. paracetamol) or stronger analgesics (e.g. NSAIDs). Rectal preparations of antiemetics, e.g. domperidone, are often helpful.

Attacks may be terminated by the use of 5-HT agonists (sumatriptan, naratriptan, zolmitriptan, rizatriptan, eletriptan). There are now preparations that can be given subcutaneously or nasally which bypass the need for gastric absorption. Ergotamine is still used for acute attacks, but relatively infrequently because of liability to side-effects.

NSAIDs are often as effective as triptans and high-dose aspirin can be taken regularly throughout the attack. Gastrointestinal side-effects such as dyspepsia may be limiting. Patients should avoid regular codeine because of the risk of induction of a chronic 'analgesic' headache.

Prophylaxis

For frequent and severe attacks that occur more than twice per month, regular daily treatment may be required to prevent headaches. Drugs include:

- Propranolol (beta-adrenergic receptor blocker).
- Tricyclic agents, e.g. amitriptyline, dothiepin.
- Pizotifen (5-HT antagonist).
- Sodium valproate or topiramate (anticonvulsants).
- Verapamil (calcium antagonist).
- Methysergide (5-HT antagonist): rarely used now because it can cause retroperitoneal fibrosis.

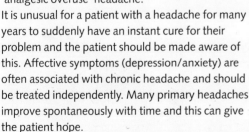

Patients with chronic headache often have chronic migraine or 'analgesic overuse' headache.

It is unusual for a patient with a headache for many years to suddenly have an instant cure for their problem and the patient should be made aware of this. Affective symptoms (depression/anxiety) are often associated with chronic headache and should be treated independently. Many primary headaches improve spontaneously with time and this can give the patient hope.

CLUSTER HEADACHE

Cluster headache occurs more commonly in men, with an onset in early middle life. Features of cluster headache comprise severe unilateral pain localized around the eye with unilateral conjunctival injection, lacrimation, rhinorrhoea, and sometimes a transient Horner's syndrome.

The headache and associated features last between 10 minutes and 2 hours, typically occurring one to three times daily in clusters lasting weeks or a few months at a time. Intervals between clusters may extend to several years. Onset of an attack is often in the early hours of the morning, waking the patient from sleep. There may be migrainous features, but movement sensitivity is not typical and in fact patients with cluster headache often want to pace around rather than stay still.

Treatment

Treatments used in migraine, particularly sumatriptan and ergotamine, are usually effective for acute symptomatic relief of cluster headache, and oxygen inhalation can also be a helpful measure.

Specific preventive treatments include a course of corticosteroids (e.g. 60 mg of prednisolone tapering over 10–20 days) and verapamil, often in high doses. Methysergide can be used for resistent cases but this should be under hospital supervision because it can cause retroperitoneal fibrosis. Lithium can be used during an acute cluster but is particularly useful if the symptoms are more chronic. Lithium therapy requires careful monitoring of plasma levels.

GIANT-CELL ARTERITIS (TEMPORAL ARTERITIS)

Giant-cell arteritis is a granulomatous arteritis that usually affects the branches of the external carotid artery, including the palpable superficial temporal artery, in those over 60 years of age.

The majority of patients experience pain over thickened, tender, often non-pulsatile, temporal arteries.

The headache is accompanied by:

- A raised erythrocyte sedimentation rate (ESR): often highly elevated (60–100).
- Visual loss (25% of untreated cases): amaurosis fugax (a TIA involving the retinal vessels) or permanent visual loss due to inflammation or occlusion of the posterior ciliary vessels.
- Jaw claudication and scalp tenderness.

- Systemic features include proximal muscle pain in the form of polymyalgia rheumatica in up to 50% of cases, weight loss, lassitude.
- Rarer complications: brainstem ischaemia, cortical blindness, cranial nerve lesions, aortitis, involvement of coronary and mesenteric arteries.

Diagnosis

The diagnosis is made from the history and a raised ESR, although in rare cases the ESR is normal. The diagnosis is confirmed by a biopsy of the temporal artery. At least 1 cm of the artery needs to be excised as the disease process may be patchy.

Treatment

Treatment is with high-dose corticosteroids (e.g. prednisolone 60 mg per day). There is a risk of blindness if treatment is delayed, and therefore the steroids should be started immediately and not be delayed until after the biopsy.

The dose of steroids is gradually reduced as the ESR falls. It is usually possible to withdraw steroids slowly after several months to years.

Patients with temporal arteritis may have a normal temporal artery biopsy. If the ESR is very high and the clinical story is compatible, then even with a negative biopsy a trial of steroids should be given. If there is a dramatic response to treatment then the diagnosis can be made. If there is no response to steroids then other causes of a raised ESR should be sought.

HEADACHE OF RAISED INTRACRANIAL PRESSURE

The headache of raised intracranial pressure, caused by an intracranial tumour, abscess or other space-occupying lesion, has certain characteristic features:

- There is a generalized ache.
- It is aggravated by bending, coughing, or straining which all raise intracranial pressure.
- It is worse in the morning or after prolonged recumbency.
- It may awaken the patient from sleep.
- The severity gradually progresses.

It is often accompanied by:

- Vomiting.
- Visual obscurations (transient loss of vision with sudden changes in intracranial pressure).
- Progressive focal neurological signs.
- Risk of herniation: there is a risk that tonsillar herniation will occur in rapidly expanding or chronic untreated space-occupying lesions. When this happens, the cerebellar tonsils herniate through the foramen magnum and can result in brainstem compression and death or otherwise known as 'coning'. This usually occurs with lesions in the posterior fossa (cerebellum and brainstem) or following untreated supratentorial herniation (Fig. 17.1). Supratentorial lesions usually cause lateral and central tentorial herniation initially. This is associated with reduced level of consciousness, third nerve palsy, especially loss of pupillary reflexes and pupillary dilatation, and ipsilateral hemiparesis due to pressure on the contralateral cerebral peduncle. If left untreated, transtentorial herniation will progress to tonsillar herniation.

Imaging of the brain with computed tomography or magnetic resonance imaging is essential. Contrast may be required to visualize the lesion. See Chapter 27 for further management of intracranial masses.

Worsening or change in patients with a chronic primary headache disorder must be independently assessed as these patients can develop a new pathology causing secondary headache in addition to their original condition.

OTHER NEUROLOGICAL CAUSES OF HEADACHE AND CRANIOFACIAL PAIN

These include:

- Stroke, especially intracranial haemorrhage: see Chapter 26.
- Meningitis: see Chapter 28.
- Trigeminal and postherpetic neuralgia: see Chapter 19.

Brain shift — types

Tentorial herniation (lateral): a unilateral expanding mass causes tentorial (uncal) herniation as the medial edge of the temporal lobe herniates through the tentorial hiatus. As the intracranial pressure continues to rise, 'central' herniation follows

Subfalcine 'midline' shift: occurs early with unilateral space-occupying lesions. Seldom produces any clinical effect, although ipsilateral anterior cerebral artery occlusion has been recorded

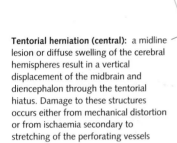

Tentorial herniation (central): a midline lesion or diffuse swelling of the cerebral hemispheres result in a vertical displacement of the midbrain and diencephalon through the tentorial hiatus. Damage to these structures occurs either from mechanical distortion or from ischaemia secondary to stretching of the perforating vessels

Tonsillar herniation: a subtentorial expanding mass causes herniation of the cerebellar tonsils through the foramen magnum. A degree of *upward* herniation though the tentorial hiatus may also occur. Clinical effects are difficult to distinguish from effects of direct brainstem/midbrain compression

Fig. 17.1 Types of brain shift in a coronal section.

NON-NEUROLOGICAL CAUSES OF HEADACHE AND CRANIOFACIAL PAIN

Local causes

- Sinus disease.
- Ocular-glaucoma, refraction errors.
- Temporomandibular joint dysfunction.
- Dental disease.

Systemic causes

Headache can accompany any febrile illness or may be a presenting feature of metabolic disease, e.g. hypoglycaemia or malignant hypertension. Certain drugs may also cause headache (e.g. nitrates, nifedipine, carbamazepine, lansoprazole, caffeine).

Parkinson's disease, other extrapyramidal disorders, and myoclonus

Objectives

- Define akinetic-rigid syndrome and dyskinesias
- Describe the main clinical features of the akinetic-rigid syndromes
- Understand the differentiation of idiopathic Parkinson's disease from other parkinsonian syndromes
- Define chorea, tremor, dystonia, athetosis, ballism, tic and myoclonus

Extrapyramidal conditions cause disorders of movement that can be broadly divided into two categories:

1. Those where there is diminished movement with an increase in tone: akinetic-rigid syndromes.
2. Those in which there are added movements outside voluntary control: dyskinesias.

These two categories can exist within the same disease (e.g. Parkinson's disease patients treated with long-term L-dopa).

AKINETIC-RIGID SYNDROMES

These conditions are caused by lesions of the basal ganglia and their connections. The basal ganglia consist of the caudate nucleus, globus pallidus, putamen, substantia nigra, and subthalamic nucleus. The caudate and putamen are collectively known as the 'corpus striatum'.

Parkinson's disease

Parkinson's disease was first described by James Parkinson in 1817, who named it the 'shaking palsy'. It is the most common of all the akinetic-rigid syndromes. The disease is equally common throughout the world, with increasing incidence with age. The prevalence is 1 in 200 in those over 70 years. It is more common in men than in women.

Pathology

There is progressive degeneration of cells within the pars compacta of the substantia nigra in the midbrain (Fig. 18.1). These neurons are dopaminergic. Eosinophilic inclusions called Lewy bodies can be found in the surviving neurons of the substantia nigra. The nigral cells projecting to the striatum are mostly affected – the 'nigrostriatal' pathway. This causes a loss of dopamine in the striatum. Pathological changes may also be seen in other non-dopaminergic brainstem nuclei such as locus ceruleus. The involvement of the non-dopaminergic system may account for the lack of response of some features of Parkinson's disease to dopamine replacement therapy.

Aetiology

The cause of Parkinson's disease is unknown. Twin studies have provided conflicting information about the possible genetic component of Parkinson's disease. Recently, several family pedigrees have been described with familial Parkinson's disease. These include mutations in alpha-synuclein and Parkin genes.

A consistent environmental factor has not been elucidated. Increased interest in exogenous toxins as a cause arose with the finding that drug addicts taking heroin contaminated with 1-methyl-4-phenyl-1,2,3,6-tetrahydropyridine (MPTP) developed a similar condition, with selective destruction of the nigral cells and their striatal connections. There is also some evidence that pesticides and herbicides may increase the risk of developing Parkinson's disease.

Clinical features

Clinical features of Parkinson's disease comprise the classical triad of tremor, rigidity, and bradykinesia, in association with changes in posture and gait.

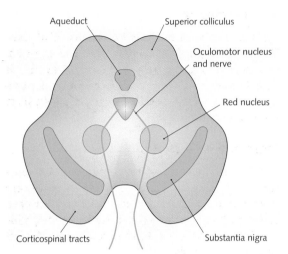

Fig. 18.1 Cross-section of the midbrain.

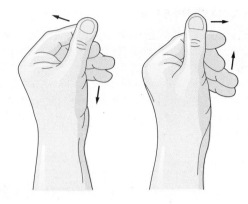

Fig. 18.2 Pill-rolling tremor.

An important and characteristic feature of Parkinson's disease is the striking asymmetry of the clinical signs. Tremor, rigidity, and bradykinesia can occur in other disorders of the basal ganglia and lead to a parkinsonian syndrome. If a patient presents with symmetrical parkinsonian clinical signs then they are unlikely to have idiopathic Parkinson's disease.

Tremor

This is a characteristic coarse resting tremor (4–7 Hz), which is usually decreased by use of the tremulous limb and increased with emotion and distraction, e.g. walking or using the contralateral limbs. The tremor disappears during sleep. It is often 'pill-rolling' in nature. The thumb moves rhythmically backwards and forwards on the palmar surface of the fingers (Fig. 18.2). The resting tremor can affect any part of the body including the chin, tongue, and feet.

Rigidity

There is stiffness of the limbs, which can be felt throughout the range of movement and equally in the flexors and extensors. This is termed 'lead-pipe' rigidity. When combined with the tremor, which can be subclinical, there is a jerky element ('cog-wheel' rigidity). The increase in tone can be felt most easily when the wrist is rotated in both directions and can be made more apparent when the patient is asked to voluntarily move the opposite limb (synkinesis). The rigidity is usually asymmetrical in the limbs.

Both rigidity and spasticity produce an increase in tone, but there are important differences (Fig. 18.3).

Bradykinesia, hypokinesia, and akinesia

Slowing and poverty of movement is the most disabling feature of Parkinson's disease. Bradykinesia and hypokinesia affect not only the limbs but also the muscles of facial expression to give mask-like facies known as hypomimia. The muscles of mastication, speech, and voluntary swallowing, and some of the axial muscles can also be involved. There is particular difficulty in initiating and terminating movements.

Fig. 18.3 The differences between spasticity and rigidity

Spasticity	Rigidity
Lesion in upper motor neuron	Lesion in basal ganglia and connections
Increased tone more marked in flexors in arms and extensors in legs	Increased tone equal in flexors and extensors
Increased tone most apparent early during movement ('clasp-knife effect')	Increased tone apparent throughout range of movement (lead pipe rigidity)
Reflexes brisk with extensor plantars	Normal reflexes with flexor plantars

Postural changes

The posture is characteristically stooped (Fig. 18.4), with a shuffling, flexed, festinant gait with poor asymmetrical arm swing. Falls are common later in the disease process, as the normal righting reflexes are affected. When the patient tries to turn either when walking or lying (e.g. in bed), there are great difficulties and the patient is said to move 'en bloc'.

Other features

Speech is altered, producing a monotonous, hypophonic dysarthria, due to a combination of bradykinesia, rigidity, and tremor. Power is usually preserved, although in advanced disease the slowness (bradykinesia) and rigidity make testing power difficult. Sensory examination is also normal, although patients can often describe discomfort and sensory abnormalities in the legs. Handwriting reduces in size and becomes spidery (micrographia). Constipation is usual and urinary difficulties are common, especially in men. Depression is common.

Cognitive function is preserved in the early stages but dementia is a common complication later in the disease probably due to Lewy body disease in cortical neurons.

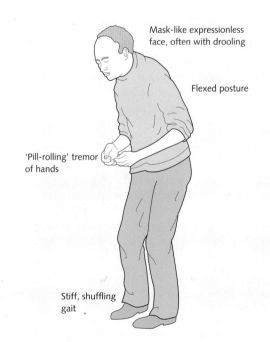

Mask-like expressionless face, often with drooling

Flexed posture

'Pill-rolling' tremor of hands

Stiff, shuffling gait

Fig. 18.4 Parkinsonian posture.

Natural history

Parkinson's disease progresses over a period of years. The rate of progression is very variable, with the mildest forms running over several decades. The course is usually over 10–15 years with progressive immbolity, falls and cognitive decline. Death is usually from bronchopneumonia.

Differential diagnosis

Parkinson's disease is a clinical diagnosis. A distinction must be made between 'idiopathic Parkinson's disease' and 'parkinsonism'. Parkinsonism denotes a syndrome that appears clinically similar to idiopathic Parkinson's disease but has a different pathological or aetiological basis.

Causes of parkinsonism include:

- Drugs: especially dopamine antagonists, e.g. phenothiazines, reserpine, haloperidol.
- Trauma: especially repetitive head injury, e.g. boxing.
- Cerebrovascular disease: especially lacunar infarcts of the basal ganglia and small vessel disease of the cerebral white matter.
- Toxins such as MPTP.
- Other akinetic-rigid syndromes, e.g. multisystem atrophy and progressive supranuclear palsy (see below).

Hypothyroidism and retarded depression may superficially mimic Parkinson's disease but will have no physical signs of parkinsonism.

Treatment

The main aim of drug treatment is to restore the dopamine levels within the striatum. Downstream effects of reduced striatal dopamine results in excessive acetylcholine, and anticholinergics have a small role in the treatment of Parkinson's disease, especially in the management of tremor.

Levodopa (L-dopa)

L-dopa forms the mainstay for the symptomatic treatment of most patients with Parkinson's disease. It is given in a combined form with a peripheral decarboxylase inhibitor (benserazide – as Madopar™; carbidopa – as Sinemet™) to prevent peripheral conversion of the inactive L-dopa to the active form, dopamine. This reduces the peripheral side-effects of nausea, vomiting, and hypotension. The conversion to dopamine still occurs within the CNS because benserazide and carbidopa can not cross the blood–brain barrier, but L-dopa can easily cross into the brain.

Treatment is commenced gradually and increased slowly until either a good clinical effect is achieved or side-effects limit further increases. L-dopa improves bradykinesia and rigidity, but has a lesser effect on tremor.

Initially, the majority of patients with Parkinson's disease, but not other parkinsonian syndromes, have a dramatic improvement with L-dopa and can lead to an almost normal life for several years. However, with time, the duration of action of the drug reduces and marked fluctuations in symptoms occur. Patients often experience swings in mobility from overactivity to underactivity called the 'on–off syndrome'. These swings occur due to L-dopa-induced improved mobility, the 'on period', followed by a period of immobility, called the 'off period'. As the disease progresses, these swings become more severe and unpredictable. The 'on periods' can become associated with dyskinesias, which can be troubling, and the 'off periods' can become associated with sudden and unpredictable periods of immobility called 'freezing'. Some of these freezing and dyskinetic periods can have no relationship to the timing of the L-dopa dose, which makes it even harder for patients to plan their life. Consequently, L-dopa therapy should not be started until necessary and many patients now commence therapy with a dopamine agonist. These are less likely to be associated with the severe motor fluctuations that occur with L-dopa.

Dopamine agonists

Dopamine agonists are analogues of dopamine and directly stimulate the dopamine receptors. The most effective anti-parkinsonian dopamine agonists stimulate D2 receptors predominantly, but other types of dopamine receptor stimulation are probably important.

Dopamine agonists have varying selectivity and include pergolide, ropinirole, carbergoline, pramipexole, and apomorphine. Apomorphine is administered as individual subcutaneous injections or as a subcutaneous infusion and is usually reserved for patients at the end-stages of the disease. The dopamine agonists are usually prescribed alone as the first-line treatment of Parkinson's disease, especially in younger patients, to delay L-dopa usage. They rarely produce the same dramatic motor response as L-dopa and most patients require this to be added to their regime sooner or later. In the elderly, dopamine

agonists can have particularly severe psychiatric side-effects and they are often avoided. There are growing concerns that the older agonists (pergolide, cabergoline) are associated with a long-term risk of pleuropulmonary fibrosis.

Anticholinergic drugs

Anticholinergic drugs include benzhexol (trihexyphenidyl) and bentropine, which are antimuscarinic agents that penetrate the central nervous system. They are most effective in reducing tremor, although not so effective for rigidity and bradykinesia. Side-effects such as dry mouth, constipation, urinary retention, visual blurring, hallucinations, and confusion often prevent their use, especially in the elderly. They are often reserved for younger patients who have only a troublesome tremor.

Selegiline

Selegiline is an inhibitor of monoamine oxidase B (MAO-B), which acts to block the degradation of dopamine in the CNS. Early use can delay the need for L-dopa, but there may be an increased risk of cardiovascular morbidity in advanced cases. Rasagiline is a newer MAO-B inhibitor which may have fewer side-effects.

COMT (catechol-O-methyltransferase) antagonists

COMT antagonists are a new group of drugs. Dopamine is broken down peripherally by both dopa decarboxylase and by COMT. The rationale of these drugs is therefore to prevent the additional COMT-mediated breakdown and increase dopamine availability centrally. They are used in conjunction with L-dopa to reduce the L-dopa dose. Entacapone is the most widely used drug in this group. Tolcapone is being cautiously reintroduced into clinical use after previous incidence of a few cases of hepatic failure.

Surgery

Surgery is not extensively carried out but this does have a place in severe cases and younger patients. The techniques used in the past have included stereotactic thalamotomy for severe tremor, pallidotomy and transplantation of fetal substantia nigra into the patient's striatum. The surgical ablation procedures have now been largely supplanted by the technique of deep brain stimulation, usually with implanted wires in the subthalamic region.

'Parkinson's plus' syndromes

'Parkinson's plus' syndromes represent other much less common neurodegenerative disorders that are also associated with some or all of the extrapyramidal features of idiopathic Parkinson's disease. In general, they tend to have more symmetrical parkinsonian signs and less resting tremor. They usually respond poorly and inconsistently to L-dopa therapy and each has its own specific neurological features in systems other than the extrapyramidal system.

Progressive supranuclear palsy ('PSP' or Steele–Richardson–Olszewski syndrome)

Progressive supranuclear palsy may mimic Parkinson's disease in its early stages. However, there is marked axial rigidity and a striking supranuclear gaze palsy that initially affects vertical gaze but subsequently may affect all eye movements. There is usually a history of falls early in the disease and PSP should be strongly considered in any patient with parkinsonian signs who suffers frequent falls within the first few years of onset. A pseudobulbar palsy develops insidiously with dysarthria, dysphagia, and emotional lability, and the patient often has a staring, immobile face. There is usually little response to L-dopa but some of the stiffness and bradykinesia may show a partial response. There is relentless progression towards complete immobility and the median survival is less than 6 years from diagnosis.

Multisystem atrophy (MSA)

There are three main variants of multisystem atrophy:

- Striatonigral degeneration: this produces a picture similar to Parkinson's disease but is usually more symmetrical and without the tremor. There is usually no response to medication and the patient may have 'pyramidal', i.e. upper motor neuron, signs within the limbs, although at onset may only be extrapyramidal features.
- Shy–Drager syndrome: this comprises parkinsonism combined with severe autonomic failure. The parkinsonian features may respond well to L-dopa, but the resulting postural hypotension often forces withdrawal of the drug.
- Olivopontocerebellar atrophy (OPCA): this term is applied to patients who present with a predominantly cerebellar motor syndrome, often followed later by parkinsonian features.

It has recently been recognized that these three clinical syndromes are very similar pathologically and hence they are all now a part of the diagnosis of 'multisystem atrophy', in which parkinsonian features may occur with varying degrees of autonomic failure, pyramidal signs, and cerebellar features.

Corticobasal degeneration

This rare degenerative disorder is characterized by strikingly asymmetrical involvement of the limbs especially the arm. Patients may experience the 'alien limb' phenomenom where their arm performs actions that the patient is unaware of. The arm may eventually become functionally useless. Initial symptoms typically begin at the age of 60 years. Eventually, both sides are affected as the disease progresses. Parkinsonian symptoms and signs are often prominent initially but other symptoms such as cognitive and visuospatial impairments, apraxia, myoclonus, and dysphagia may also occur. Patients usually become bed bound through immobility and die within 6–8 years. Treatment is mainly supportive and L-dopa has little clinical response. Post-mortem examination of the brain demonstrates tau inclusions.

Other parkinsonian syndromes

Drug-induced parkinsonism

All drugs that have dopamine antagonist effects can cause a parkinsonian syndrome, usually with bradykinesia and rigidity but little tremor. The neuroleptics (e.g. phenothiazines), are a common cause. Other drugs include reserpine, butyrophenones, metoclopramide, and prochlorperazine. Some of the effects may be irreversible even on stopping the offending drug.

Cerebrovascular disease

The pathological basis of cerebrovascular disease causing parkinsonism is usually multifocal small-vessel disease, particularly subcortical ischaemia and lacunar infarcts. Patients often have a degree of cognitive impairment and pyramidal signs in the limbs with symmetrical bradykinesia and rigidity but without resting tremor. It typically affects the lower limbs and gait and is sometimes called 'lower limb parkinsonism'. Treatment is aimed at secondary prevention by treating cardiovascular risk factors especially hypertension.

Wilson's disease

Wilson's disease is an inherited autosomal recessive disorder of copper metabolism resulting in low levels of the copper binding protein, caeruloplasmin. This causes elevated levels of free copper in the blood, which results in copper deposition in the brain, particularly in the basal ganglia, in the Descemet's membrane in the cornea (Kayser–Fleischer rings) and in the liver, which causes cirrhosis. Patients typically present in their teens or early adult life with atypical parkinsonism, tremor, dystonia, and marked dysarthria. The diagnosis is made by measuring low levels of caeruloplasmin and total copper in the serum, with high free copper in the urine and serum. The disease is treatable with copper-binding agents such as penicillamine and trientine, and the neurological damage is partly reversible on successful treatment.

Idiopathic Parkinson's disease can be differentiated from other parkinsonian syndromes by:

- An excellent response to L-dopa.
- Asymmetrical onset of the bradykinesia, rigidity and usually tremor.
- Absence of other neurological system involvement, e.g. pyramidal system.

The diagnosis of an akinetic-rigid syndrome can still be unclear and a 'DAT' scan, which is a measure of the number of dopaminergic terminals in the putamen, can be helpful. The passage of time and progression of the disease often makes the diagnosis more clear.

DYSKINETIC SYNDROMES

Dyskinesias means 'abnormal movements' and can be further subdivided into:

- **Tremor:** rhythmic oscillation of a body part, produced by either alternating or synchronous contractions of reciprocally innervated antagonistic muscles.
- **Dystonia:** a disorder dominated by sustained muscle contractions, which frequently cause twisting and repetitive movements or abnormal postures. Dystonic movements may be slow and writhing. When they are distal, they are termed athetosis.
- **Chorea:** from the Greek word for 'a dance', this consists of irregular, unpredictable, brief, jerky movements that flit from one part of the body to another in a random sequence. Patients may turn the movement into a purpose, such as brushing their hand through their hair. When the movements are slower and more flowing, the term choreoathetosis is applied.
- **Ballism:** the least common of the dyskinesias, and derived from the Greek word 'to throw', this involves wide-amplitude, violent, flailing movements. There is prominent involvement of proximal muscles and the movements can be regarded as a severe form of chorea.
- **Tics:** abrupt, transient, stereotypical, coordinated movements or vocalizations, which vary in intensity and are repeated at irregular intervals.

Many conditions incorporate one or more of the above dyskinesias. Only the most common or important of these will be discussed below.

Tremor

Benign essential tremor

Benign essential tremor is a common condition, often inherited as an autosomal dominant trait. It causes tremor at 5–8 Hz, which is usually worse in the upper limbs. The head and trunk may also be tremulous. It is most apparent on posture (e.g. holding a glass), or with intense emotions and can interfere with activities. It is not usually present at rest. Treatment is not always necessary, but the tremor may respond to a beta-blocker. Other less effective agents include primidone, clonazepam, and gabapentin.

Dystonia

Dystonia can be classified as:

- Generalized: affecting multiple parts of the body.
- Focal: affecting a single part of the body, e.g. writer's cramp, spasmodic torticollis.
- Segmental: involving several contiguous parts of the body.

This classification system is often not that helpful clinically.

In practice, generalized dystonia tends to have a genetic basis whereas focal dystonia tends to be idiopathic or secondary to lesions often within the basal ganglia.

Early-onset generalized dystonia

Historically, this is also known as idiopathic torsion dystonia and dystonia musculorum deformans. It is the most common hereditary form of dystonia and is caused by mutations in the gene DYT1 with autosomal dominant inheritance and incomplete penetrance as only 40% of patients with a mutation develop the disease.

It is characterized clinically by the twisting and jerking of the limbs, trunk and neck caused by spasms or contractions of the muscles.

Treatment consists of the anticholinergics and sometimes patients are given a trial of L-dopa. Surgery is often confined to patients who are severely affected and consists of lesions to the thalamus and globus pallidus as well as deep brain stimulators to the subthalamic nuclei, which have been used with great effect recently in some cases.

Dopa-responsive dystonia

Dopa-responsive dystonia is a progressive dystonia that initially affects the lower limbs usually in early childhood. The most commonly identified forms of dopa-responsive dystonia are dominantly inherited conditions caused by mutations in genes involved in the production of endogenous dopamine.

There is marked diurnal variation, with symptoms worsening as the day progresses and amelioration occurs with sleep. There is a striking response to small doses of L-dopa, which treats many of the symptoms of the disease.

Cervical dystonia ('spasmodic torticollis')

In cervical dystonia, dystonic spasms gradually develop around the neck, usually in the third to fifth decades of life, causing the head to turn laterally (torticollis), although the head can be drawn backwards (retrocollis) or forwards (anterocollis). The sternocleidomastoid, upper trapezius, and scalenii muscles are often involved. The patient's intermittent jerking movements of the neck can appear to be like a tremor and is sometimes called a 'dystonic tremor'. Patients often demonstrate a 'geste antagonist', which is a manoeuvre that stops the involuntary movement (e.g. gentle pressure with the hand on the side of the jaw). Response to anticholinergics is often poor. Locally injected botulinum toxin can provide good relief.

Writer's cramp

Writer's cramp is the most common form of occupational focal dystonia. There is a specific inability to perform a previously highly developed skilled movement, in this case writing, due to dystonic posturing of the affected limb. It occurs particularly in those who spend many hours writing. Other skilled functions of the hands are usually normal. Some patients respond to anticholinergics or to selective botulinum injections to affected muscles.

Blepharospasm and oromandibular dystonia

Blepharospasm and oromandibular dystonia (Meige's syndrome) are related conditions and consist of spasms of forced blinking and involuntary movement of the mouth and tongue (e.g. lip smacking and protrusion of the tongue). Speech and swallowing may also be affected. Blepharospasm may be reduced with regular injections of botulinum toxin into the orbicularis oculi muscles.

Chorea

Causes of chorea

- Drug-induced, e.g. chronic levodopa use, tricyclic antidepressants, oral contraceptive pill.
- Stroke, vasculopathy, and blood dyscrasias, e.g. lacunar infarction of the basal ganglia, systemic lupus erythematosus, polycythaemia.
- Postinfective, e.g. Sydenham's chorea (poststreptococcal infection).
- Hereditary, e.g. Huntington's disease.
- Hyperthyroidism.
- Senile chorea: idiopathic chorea in the elderly.
- Wilson's disease.

Huntington's disease (Huntington's chorea)

Huntington's disease is a hereditary condition caused by an expanded trinucleotide repeat (CAG) on chromosome 4. It is clinically characterized by progressive personality changes, movement disorders including chorea, and eventually dementia. These symptoms develop in middle age, and progress to death within 12–15 years. There is neuronal loss initially in the caudate nucleus as well as other areas such as the cerebral cortex. A reduction in inhibitory neurotransmitter, GABA (gamma-aminobutyric acid), and acetylcholine levels have been found. There is no effective treatment, although phenothiazines may reduce the chorea by causing parkinsonism. Patients often have an affective disorder that may also require treatment. A genetic test is available for prenatal diagnosis. The use of the test in relatives of sufferers requires careful counselling.

It is now considered essential to counsel patients prior to performing genetic tests. The patients should understand what the implications of a positive and negative test has on them and their families. Many patient's relatives decide not to undergo presymptomatic testing.

Tics

Simple tics (e.g. twitching of the eyelids) are very common and usually benign.

Gilles de la Tourette syndrome

Gilles de la Tourette syndrome is a rare syndrome in which there is the occurrence of multiple motor tics accompanied by sudden explosive grunting and involuntary utterance of sexually related obscenities called vocal tics. It develops in childhood or adolescence and usually affects patients for life. The caudate nuclei have been implicated in the pathology. Treatment with haloperidol and other neuroleptics is sometimes helpful.

Hemiballism

Hemiballism comprises violent flailing movements of one side of the body, caused by infarction or haemorrhage in the contralateral subthalamic nucleus.

DRUG-INDUCED MOVEMENT DISORDERS

Acute dystonic reactions

Dystonia develops in 2–5% of patients on neuroleptics or antiemetics (metoclopramide and prochlorperazine). This reaction is unpredictable and can occur even after single doses of the drugs. The range of dystonias includes torticollis, oculogyric crisis, and trismus. They respond rapidly to intravenous injection of an anticholinergic drug (e.g. procyclidine or benztropine). Some patients on neuroleptics who develop these reactions are also treated or cotreated with an oral anticholinergic.

Drug-induced parkinsonism

See p. 117.

Akathisia

Akathisia is a restless, repetitive, and irresistible need to move, usually caused by neuroleptics. It ceases with drug withdrawal.

Tardive dyskinesia

Tardive dyskinesia is a movement disorder involving the face, mouth and tongue causing lip smacking, grimacing, and facial contortions. Choreoathetoid limb movements can also occur. It develops after chronic exposure to neuroleptics, can be irreversible and may be temporarily worsened when the offending drug is stopped. It can be avoided by 'drug holidays' where the offending drug is stopped for a period of time before being recommenced at a lower dose or by changing the neuroleptic. It is thought to be due to drug-induced supersensitivity of the dopamine receptors.

MYOCLONUS

Myoclonus comprises sudden, brief, shock-like involuntary movements of single muscles or groups of muscles. These movements can arise from dysfunction of the brain or spinal cord. They do not tend to originate in the extrapyramidal system and are therefore considered separately from other movement disorders.

Myoclonus occurs as part of the normal sleep startle or hypnogogic myoclonic jerk, but also occurs as part of a wide range of disorders. Myoclonus can be symptomatically treated with benzodiazepines such as clonazepam, but an underlying cause should always be sort. Myoclonus can become worse with auditory, tactile or visual stimuli.

Myoclonic epilepsy

Myoclonus may be a feature of many different forms of epilepsy (e.g. juvenile myoclonic epilepsy, Lennox Gastaut syndrome).

Progressive myoclonic epilepsy

Myoclonus may be combined with epilepsy and progressive dementia in several rare inherited metabolic diseases, e.g. Lafora body disease, lipid-storage diseases (Gaucher's disease).

Postanoxic action myoclonus or 'Lance Adams' syndrome

Postanoxic action myoclonus occurs following severe cerebral anoxia (e.g. after cardiorespiratory arrest), and is sensitive to drugs that increase 5-HT levels. These usually have severe side-effects and anticonvulsants such as clonazepam, piracetam, or levetiracetam are now used.

Subacute sclerosing panencephalitis

Subacute sclerosing panenecephalitis (SSPE) occurs many years after contracting measles and represents an abnormal immunological response to the measles virus. There is progressive dementia, myoclonic jerking, spasticity, and rigidity. It usually leads to death within 1–2 years.

Creutzfeldt–Jakob disease

Sporadic Creutzfeldt–Jakob disease (CJD) is caused by a prion (an infective protein), leading to a spongiform encephalopathy with progressive dementia, myoclonus, ataxia, and death within 2 years (see Chapter 28).

Cranial nerve lesions

Objectives

- Define the twelve cranial nerves and their functions
- Describe the common pathologies affecting the cranial nerves
- Understand how the differnet pathologies affecting each nerve can be differentiated by associated clinical symptoms and signs

The most common cranial nerve lesions and the symptoms and signs associated with them are summarized in Fig. 19.1.

OLFACTORY NERVE (FIRST, I)

The most common causes of either hyposmia or anosmia are nasal and sinus disease, often in association with smoking. Head injury can also cause anosmia secondary to trauma to the cribriform plate and the delicate olfactory sensory axons that pass through it. A tumour or other space-occupying lesion of the frontal lobe may occasionally cause anosmia by compression of the olfactory bulb and tract (e.g. meningioma of the olfactory groove).

OPTIC NERVE (SECOND, II)

Visual field defects

Lesions at various points in the visual pathway cause characteristic patterns of visual field loss (see Fig. 5.2, p. 28).

Papilloedema

Papilloedema is swelling of the optic disc. Initially, there is redness of the disc, with blurring of the margins and loss of retinal venous pulsation. Then there is loss of the physiological cup and the disc becomes engorged. In severe papilloedema, there may be retinal haemorrhages around the disc.

Raised intracranial pressure, caused by space-occupying lesions such as tumours, abscesses, tuberculomas and benign intracranial hypertension,

is a common cause of papilloedema. Strictly speaking, optic neuritis causes a papillitis (i.e. swelling of the optic nerve head due to inflammation), rather than papilloedema, which is caused by swelling due to raised pressure around the optic nerve.

On clinical examination of papilloedema there is an enlarged blind spot, but usually no visual disturbance unless the disc swelling is caused by local inflammation (i.e. 'papillitis'), infiltration of the optic nerve head, or acute ischaemia of the optic nerve. If papilloedema is severe, prolonged and untreated then there is often constriction of the visual fields and blindness due to infarction secondary to pressure on the blood vessels that supply the optic nerve.

Optic neuritis

Optic neuritis is an inflammatory optic neuropathy that is most often due to multiple sclerosis but which can have many other causes (Fig. 19.2).

In contrast to papilloedema, there is early severe visual loss, especially to colour, and there is often a central scotoma (visual field defect) in optic neuritis. There is also often pain in or behind the eyes, but not in papilloedema. Anterior optic neuritis may cause swelling of the optic disc, but often the inflammatory process is in the posterior part of the nerve and is named 'retrobulbar neuritis'. The optic disc will be normal on ophthalmoscopy in retrobulbar neuritis. When optic neuritis is caused by multiple sclerosis, the prognosis for recovery of vision is very good. There is usually gradual improvement in vision over a few days, weeks, or months, and patients often return to near normal visual acuity. However, there is often a relative loss of colour

Fig. 19.1 Summary of the cranial nerves and the clinical features resulting from lesions of individual nerves

Cranial nerve number	Cranial nerve name	Symptoms and signs caused by lesions
1	Olfactory nerve	• Loss of smell/taste
2	Optic nerve	• Papilloedema/papillitis • Visual field defect
3	Oculomotor nerve	• Ophthalmoplegia with diplopia • Pupillary dysfunction • Ptosis • Divergent strabismus
4	Trochlear nerve	• Diplopia (superior oblique palsy)
5	Trigeminal nerve	• Loss of sensation to the face • Weakness of muscles of mastication • Loss of corneal reflex
6	Abducens nerve	• Diplopia (lateral rectus palsy) • Convergent strabismus
7	Facial nerve	• Weakness of muscles of facial expression • Loss of taste (anterior two-thirds of the tongue) • Hyperacusis • Loss of tears
8	Vestibulocochlear nerve	• Loss of hearing and imbalance
9	Glossopharyngeal nerve	• Loss of taste (posterior one-third of the tongue) • Difficulties swallowing (motor and sensory loss) • Carotid sinus dysfunction
10	Vagus nerve	• Weakness of palate, vocal cords with swallowing difficulties
11	Accessory nerve	• Weakness of shrugging shoulders and head turning
12	Hypoglossal nerve	• Weakness of tongue movement

Fig. 19.2 Causes of optic nerve lesions

• Optic nerve compression, e.g. local fracture or cerebral tumour, aneurysm
• Papilloedema: chronic and untreated
• Infiltration, e.g. glioma, lymphoma
• Inflammation (optic neuritis), e.g. multiple sclerosis, sarcoidosis, Behçet's
• Ischaemic, e.g. anterior ischaemic optic neuropathy (AION), especially temporal arteritis
• Metabolic, e.g. vitamin B_{12} deficiency
• Toxins and drugs, e.g. tobacco–alcohol amblyopia, methanol, ethambutol
• Hereditary, e.g. Leber's optic neuropathy (mitochondrial cytopathy) Friedreich's ataxia
• Infective, e.g. direct spread from paranasal sinuses or orbital cellulitis, syphilis
• Trauma

Optic atrophy

Optic atrophy is usually seen on ophthalmoscopy as a pale featureless disc and it may follow many different pathological processes including any of the causes of optic neuropathy in Fig. 19.2. It represents the end stage of damage to the optic nerve and patient's vision can be very poor (e.g. Leber optic neuropathy) or near normal (e.g. multiple sclerosis).

OCULOMOTOR (THIRD, III), TROCHLEAR (FOURTH, IV), AND ABDUCENS NERVES (SIXTH, VI)

The oculomotor, trochlear, and abducens nerves are considered together because they innervate the muscles responsible for movement of the eye. Lesions of these nerves cause the clinical sign of ophthalmoplegia, which is weakness or paralysis of these muscles and the symptom of double vision or 'diplopia'.

The individual supply of these nerves is as follows:

• **Trochlear nerve** (fourth, IV): superior oblique muscle.
• **Abducens nerve** (sixth, VI): lateral rectus.
• **Oculomotor nerve** (third, III): supplies all the other muscles (medial, superior and inferior recti, inferior oblique).

Conjugate gaze

Conjugate horizontal gaze (i.e. movement of the eyes so that the visual axes are aligned) requires

vision and the visual evoked potentials show delay in conduction of signals from the eye to the occipital cortex. The other causes of optic neuritis may result in permanent visual loss.

the coordinated contraction of both third and sixth nerves. For example, looking to the left requires the functioning of the left lateral rectus (sixth nerve) and the right medial rectus (third nerve). The medial longitudinal fasciculus (MLF) is a white matter tract that connects the sixth nerve nucleus in the lower pons on one side to the third nerve nucleus in the midbrain on the other side (Fig. 19.3).

Internuclear ophthalmoplegia

Internuclear ophthalmoplegia results from a lesion in the medial longitudinal fasciculus of the brainstem. When bilateral, it is almost pathognomonic of demyelinating disease such as multiple sclerosis. Unilateral lesions are often also caused by multiple sclerosis but may also be caused by small brainstem infarcts or other focal pathology of the pons.

A horizontal conjugate eye movement is initiated in the cortex and the signal stimulates the appropriate sixth nerve nucleus to abduct one eye. If there is a lesion of the MLF then the signal cannot travel from the sixth nerve nucleus to the contralateral third nerve nucleus and therefore abduction of the ipsilateral eye occurs without adduction of the contralateral eye. For example, a lesion of the right medial longitudinal fasciculus causes a right internuclear ophthalmoplegia and results in failure of adduction of the right eye on attempted left lateral gaze. There may also be coarse jerky horizontal nystagmus of the abducting eye that is trying to compensate for the misalignment of the visual axes (Fig. 19.4).

Isolated oculomotor (third) nerve lesions

The principal causes of a third nerve palsy are listed in Fig. 19.5.

Signs of a complete oculomotor nerve palsy are:

- Unilateral complete ptosis.
- Ophthalmoplegia causing a divergent strabismus with the affected eye deviated in a 'down and out' position.
- Affected pupil fixed and dilated.

There is often only partial involvement, and therefore the clinical signs may not include all of the features indicated above (e.g. partial ptosis, pupil-sparing).

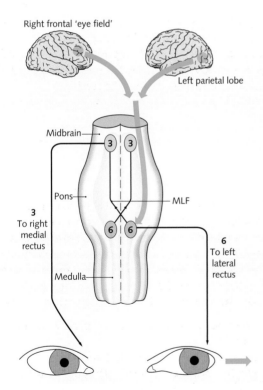

Fig. 19.3 The pathway for lateral conjugate gaze. To look left, impulses from the right frontal cortex pass to the left pontine centre for lateral gaze which also receives input from the vestibular nuclei and occipital cortex. Impulses generated here pass to both the ipsilateral (left) sixth nerve nucleus (lateral rectus, abduction), which in turn coordinates activation of the contralateral (right) third nerve nucleus (medial rectus, adduction) via the medial longitudinal fasciculus. 3, third nerve nucleus; 6, sixth nerve nucleus; MLF, medial longitudinal fasciculus.

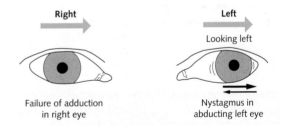

Fig. 19.4 Right internuclear ophthalmoplegia. On attempted left lateral gaze, there is failure of adduction of the right eye and coarse nystagmus of the left eye in abduction. The lesion is in the right medial longitudinal fasciculus.

Fig 19.5 Common causes of an oculomotor nerve lesion

- Aneurysm of the posterior communicating artery (or internal carotid artery) – usually painful
- Mononeuritis multiplex – any of the possible causes, especially diabetes (often pupil-sparing)
- Midbrain infarction, tumour or part of Weber's syndrome
- Herniation of the uncus of the temporal lobe

'Pupil-sparing' (i.e. the pupil is a normal size and reacts normally but there is ptosis and ophthalmoplegia), occurs because the parasympathetic fibres are on the outer surface of the nerve and are not involved in some pathologies. This is a common finding with infarction of the nerve in diabetes mellitus, but is much less likely with extrinsic compressive lesions, which often cause early pupillary abnormalities with initial sparing of eye movements.

In a patient with a third nerve palsy, visible intorsion of the eye on attempted downwards and inwards gaze indicates that the fourth nerve is spared. If the fourth nerve is involved as well as the third nerve, then the paretic eye deviates in an 'out' position only, secondary to unopposed abducens action, and not in the 'down and out' position.

Isolated trochlear (fourth) nerve palsy

An isolated fourth nerve palsy causes a superior oblique palsy and is very rare in isolation. The normal function of the superior oblique is to depress and intort the eye when it is adducted, such as when going downstairs or reading a book. When it occurs in isolation, it results in defective depression and intorsion of the adducting eye. The head is held tilted away from the side of the affected eye in an attempt to correct the diplopia. Trochlear palsies usually occur in conjunction with third or sixth nerve palsies.

Isolated abducens (sixth) nerve palsy

A sixth nerve palsy results in failure of abduction of the affected eye due to weakness of the lateral rectus muscle. Diplopia is maximal on attempting to look laterally away from the side of the lesion. A convergent strabismus may be evident in the primary position, but becomes more apparent on abduction of the affected eye.

The abducens nerve has an extremely long intracranial route from the nucleus to the lateral rectus muscle and is often damaged by compression against the tip of the petrous bone when there is raised intracranial pressure. This is called a false localizing sign because it does not mean the main pathology is affecting the sixth nerve or the pons but has caused the sixth nerve lesion usually through mass effect from anywhere in the skull.

The principal causes of a sixth nerve palsy are listed in Fig. 19.6.

Combined ocular palsies

Many conditions can cause combinations of third, fourth, and sixth nerve palsies, with variably affected pupils and ptosis. Some of the more common causes are listed in Fig. 19.7, including conditions that are not neuropathies but which produce similar clinical pictures.

TRIGEMINAL NERVE (FIFTH, V)

The sensory fibres of the trigeminal (fifth) nerve supply sensation to the face including the cornea. The motor fibres supply the muscles of mastication. The sensory fibres are divided into three branches:

- Ophthalmic (V_1): which also supplies the cornea and is the afferent part of the corneal reflex.
- Maxillary (V_2).
- Mandibular (V_3).

Fig. 19.6 Common causes of an abducens nerve palsy

- Mononeuritis multiplex – any of the possible causes, especially diabetes
- Multiple sclerosis (brainstem)
- Raised intracranial pressure (false localizing sign)
- Neoplasia – brainstem or local infiltration from a nasopharyngeal carcinoma
- Brainstem infarction (pontine)

Fig. 19.7 Conditions causing combined ocular palsies

Brainstem lesions	Multiple sclerosis Encephalitis Tumour, especially glioma
Multiple cranial neuropathies	Basal meningitis (TB, sarcoid, neoplastic, syphilis) Tumours (meningioma, lymphoma, chordoma) Cavernous sinus thrombosis
Neuromuscular disorders	Myasthenia gravis Botulinum toxin injection
Ocular muscle disorders	Thyroid eye disease Orbital myositis Infiltration, e.g. lymphoma Rare ocular myopathies Local trauma

A lesion of the trigeminal nerve involving all segments will cause unilateral touch, pain, and temperature sensory loss to the face, tongue, and buccal mucosa, with reduction in the corneal reflex on the affected side. There will also be deviation of the jaw towards the side of the lesion when the mouth is opened if the motor component is involved.

The causes of a trigeminal nerve palsy are listed according to anatomical site in Fig. 19.8.

Trigeminal neuralgia ('tic douloureux')

Trigeminal neuralgia occurs mostly in the elderly and consists of severe paroxysms of electric-shock-like pain, usually in the V_2 and V_3 divisions of the trigeminal nerve. The paroxysms of pain are usually stereotyped and can be triggered by certain stimuli (e.g. washing the face, shaving, cold wind or eating), or by touching a particular position on the face. Physical examination is normal. The pain can be described as 'lancinating' and causes the patient severe distress to the point of precipitating a reactive depressive illness.

The mechanism in most cases is believed to be local irritation of the nerve by an adjacent ectatic arterial vessel.

Spontaneous remissions for months or years can occur. Medical treatment usually consists of carbamazepine, gabapentin, or phenytoin, which act as membrane stabilizers and therefore reduce the frequency of spontaneous nerve impulses within the nerve. These do not always work and surgical intervention may be required. Many surgical techniques can be used, including obliteration of the trigeminal ganglion and root with a sclerosant – phenol may be used but glycerol tends to give fewer side effects. Radiofrequency thermocoagulation involves finding the source of overactivity within the ganglion and then making a lesion at the point. More novel techniques include microvascular decompression of the vessels at the cerebellopontine angle, which might be irritating the fifth nerve.

Postherpetic neuralgia

Herpes zoster (shingles) may involve the trigeminal nerve, especially the ophthalmic division (V_1). The resolution of the vesicular erruptions may subsequently be followed by pain within the distribution of the affected divisions.

FACIAL NERVE (SEVENTH, VII)

The muscles of the upper part of the face are supplied bilaterally from the motor cortex. An upper motor neuron lesion (i.e. above the level of the facial nucleus in the pons), such as a stroke or tumour, will cause contralateral weakness of the lower half of the face and spare eye closure and forehead movement. Weakness unilaterally of all the facial muscles (upper and lower face) is caused by a lower motor neuron lesion i.e. facial nucleus or facial nerve (see Fig. 34.8, p. 239).

The facial nerve carries mainly motor fibres supplying the muscles of facial expression. It also has a sensory component, subserving taste from the anterior two-thirds of the tongue, and a parasympathetic component to the lacrimal, submaxillary, and submandibular glands (lacrimation and some of salivation). The most common cause of facial weakness is a supranuclear lesion (e.g. in the cerebral hemisphere) such as stroke or tumour, causing an upper motor neuron type of weakness.

The causes of lower motor neuron-type facial weakness are listed anatomically in Fig. 19.9.

Bell's palsy

Bell's palsy consists of an acute lower motor neuron facial palsy, which is usually unilateral. The exact cause and site of the pathology is uncertain but it may be related to inflammation of the facial nerve within

Fig. 19.8 Causes of trigeminal nerve palsy according to site

Brainstem (nuclei and connections)	Multiple sclerosis Infarction Brainstem gliomas Syringobulbia
Cerebellopontine angle	Acoustic neuroma Meningioma
Cavernous sinus	Internal carotid aneurysm Meningioma Cavernous sinus thrombosis Carotico-cavernous fistula Extension of pituitary tumour
Gasserian (trigeminal) ganglion	Herpes zoster (shingles) Neoplastic infiltration Idiopathic trigeminal neuropathy Sjörgen's

Fig. 19.9 Causes of facial weakness (lower motor neuron) according to site

Pons (there may be associated sixth nerve palsy [lateral rectus palsy], 'centre of lateral gaze' [failure of conjugate gaze towards the lesion], and corticospinal tracts [contralateral hemiparesis])	• Demyelination – multiple sclerosis • Vascular lesions • Pontine tumours, e.g. glioma • Motor neuron disease
Cerebellopontine angle	• Acoustic neuroma • Meningioma • Basal meningitis (TB, sarcoid, syphilis, Lyme disease, neoplastic)
Within the petrous temporal bone	• Bell's palsy • Middle ear infection • Trauma • Herpes zoster (Ramsay–Hunt syndrome) • Tumours, e.g. glomus tumour
Within the face (the branches emerge from the stylomastoid foramen and pierce the parotid gland to supply the muscles of facial expression)	• Parotid gland tumours • Mumps • Sarcoidosis • Guillain–Barré syndrome • Mononeuritis multiplex
Other causes of facial weakness (often bilateral)	**Neuromuscular junction** • Myasthenia gravis **Myopathies** • Myotonic dystrophy • Facio-scapulo-humeral muscular dystrophy

the petrous temporal bone. Herpes viruses have been implicated in some studies. Bell's palsy may be preceded by a history of aching around the ear in the 24 hours before onset. The palsy is usually complete within a few hours. There should be no sensory loss in the face.

In most cases, the cause is not found. In the minority, the causes include mononeuritis multiplex, sarcoidosis, and Lyme disease.

The prognosis is usually extremely good, with 80% of patients making a full recovery within 2–8 weeks. If recovery is delayed, the ultimate degree of recovery is often incomplete and may be accompanied by synkinesis or 'crocodile tears' due to aberrant reinnervation.

The use of a short course of high-dose steroids within the first week is controversial but the current trials suggest that this may speed the recovery. Treatment with acyclovir has been proposed but conclusive evidence is lacking. Surgery may be required to treat corneal exposure and synkinesis.

Acoustic neuromas often spare the motor fibres of the seventh nerve. Unfortunately surgical removal of the tumour often involves sacrificing the seventh nerve and patients are then left with severe facial weakness post-operatively.

VESTIBULOCOCHLEAR NERVE (EIGHTH, VIII)

The vestibulocochlear (eighth) nerve is responsible for hearing and balance. Lesions cause deafness, tinnitus, loss of balance, vertigo with or without vomiting, and the clinical sign of horizontal gaze-evoked jerky or rotary nystagmus.

Causes of deafness and vertigo are listed in Fig. 19.10.

Cerebellopontine angle lesions

The most common lesions in the cerebellopontine angle are an acoustic neuroma (a benign schwannoma of the vestibular part of the eighth cranial nerve), and a meningioma. Other causes include metastases and other primary tumours. Bilateral acoustic neuromas may be found in association with neurofibromatosis type 2.

Fig. 19.10 Neurological causes of deafness and vertigo

Brainstem	Demyelination (multiple sclerosis) Infarction
Eighth nerve	Acoustic neuroma Basal meningitis Trauma
End organ disease	Degenerative syndromes Vascular including vasculitis Ménière's syndrome Infection (herpes zoster, mumps, etc.) Benign positional vertigo

There is often involvement of the fifth and seventh cranial nerves, cerebellar connections, and sometimes the sixth nerve in addition to the eighth nerve because of their closely related anatomy as they leave the pons (see Fig. 27.2, p. 184). This results in the clinical picture of unilateral progressive sensorineural deafness, occasional tinnitus, vertigo with or without nystagmus, loss of facial sensation including the corneal reflex, weakness of muscles of facial expression (which suggests a malignant cause as benign lesions usually spare the seventh nerve in the early stages), cerebellar ataxia, and sometimes diplopia due to damage to the sixth nerve.

To make the diagnosis requires imaging focused on the internal auditory meatus and brainstem, preferably using magnetic resonance imaging because this provides far more detail than computed tomography in this region. The treatment is surgical for large tumours and radiotherapy for smaller tumours.

Ménière's disease

Ménière's disease comprises paroxysmal attacks of disabling vertigo, transient impairment of hearing, tinnitus and a feeling of pressure in the ears. Ultimately, the vertigo diminishes but deafness often becomes permanent. In some cases the condition may remit at an earlier stage. Treatment is with episodic use of vestibular sedatives (e.g. cinnarizine, cyclizine, or prochlorperazine). Thiazide diuretics and a low-salt diet may also reduce the excess of endolymphatic fluid that contributes to the symptoms.

Benign paroxysmal positional vertigo

Benign paroxysmal positional vertigo comprises transient vertigo precipitated by head movements, usually due to particulate material in the posterior semicircular canal. The syndrome may follow viral infection, trauma, or age-related degenerative change in the labyrinth. Symptoms can be reproduced using Hallpike's manoeuvre, which involves tilting the patient backwards from a sitting position and turning the patient's head suddenly to one side when they are horizontal (see Fig. 8.5, p. 54). Treatment is usually with specific repositioning manoeuvres, e.g. Epley's, or a programme of vestibular exercises.

LOWER CRANIAL NERVES (GLOSSOPHARYNGEAL, VAGUS, ACCESSORY, AND HYPOGLOSSAL)

Isolated palsies of the lower cranial nerves are rare. Combined palsies, especially involving the ninth, tenth, and twelfth nerves, produce 'bulbar palsies' and are found with:

- Motor neuron disease.
- Tumours: brainstem, nasopharyngeal carcinoma, glomus tumour.
- Polyneuropathy, e.g. Guillain–Barré syndrome.
- Trauma, especially to the base of skull.

Diseases affecting the spinal cord (myelopathy)

- Understand the anatomy of the spinal cord and be able to sketch a cross-section of the cord showing the central grey matter and major surrounding tracts
- Describe the syndrome of motor, sensory and sphincter dysfunction that arises from a spinal cord lesion
- Understand the clinical features arising from spinal cord compression, transverse myelitis, metabolic cord disease, intrinsic cord lesions or complete transection of the spinal cord
- Understand the causes of mixed upper and lower motor neuron signs in the limbs

The spinal cord extends from the top of the C1 vertebra to the bottom of the body of the L1 vertebra in adults. There is an expansion in the diameter of the cord in the cervical and lumbar regions due to increased numbers of anterior horn motor cells to the arms and legs. The lower end of the spinal cord is known as the conus medullaris (Fig. 20.1). The spinal cord is continuous with the medulla oblongata superiorly and the filum terminale, which is a fibrous band containing little neural tissue, inferiorly.

The spinal cord, cauda equina, and filum terminale, down to the S2 level, is surrounded by a thick covering of dura mater, which is separated from the fine arachnoid mater by the potential subdural space. The arachnoid mater is separated from the pia mater, which invests the spinal cord and nerve roots, by the subarachnoid space.

A representative part of the spinal cord in cross-section is shown in Fig. 20.2. It contains the central grey matter, consisting of neuronal cell bodies, and the peripheral white matter, which contains the ascending and descending axonal pathways. The ascending pathways relay sensory information from the periphery to the brain, brainstem, and cerebellum and the descending pathways relay motor instructions from the brain. There are three main white matter tracts. The two main ascending tracts are the spinothalamic tract and dorsal columns and the main descending pathway is the lateral corticospinal tract (see Fig. 20.2 and Fig. 13.1, p. 82).

Most of the main sensory and motor pathways cross to the contralateral side during their course in the CNS. It is important to know these sites of decussation because clinically different syndromes result from interruption of the pathways at various levels.

MAJOR PATHWAYS WITHIN THE SPINAL CORD

Pain and temperature

The dorsal nerve roots subserving pain and temperature enter the spinal cord and the fibres synapse within the dorsal horn. The second-order neurons immediately cross over to the opposite side of the cord and join the spinothalamic tract, which ascends to the thalamus. This pathway runs anterolaterally in the spinal cord (see Fig. 20.2).

A lesion of the spinothalamic tract on one side will result in loss of pain and temperature below the level of the lesion on the contralateral side.

Proprioception (joint-position sense) and vibration

Fibres carrying information regarding proprioception and vibration enter the spinal cord in the dorsal root and do not synapse but join the ipsilateral dorsal (posterior) columns. The posterior columns lie posteromedially in the spinal cord and ascend to synapse in nuclei at the lower end of the medulla (see Fig. 20.2 and Fig. 13.1, p. 82). The second-order neurons

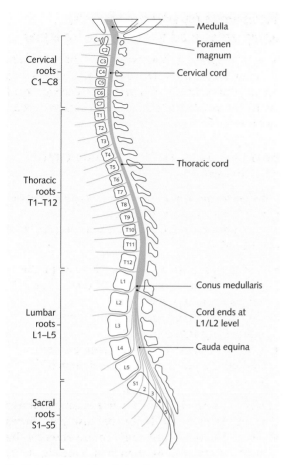

Fig. 20.1 Anatomy of the spinal cord.

cross over in the medulla to form the medial leminiscus, which ascends to the thalamus.

A lesion of the dorsal columns on one side will result in loss of proprioception and vibration below the level of the lesion on the ipsilateral side.

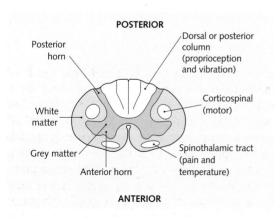

Fig. 20.2 A cross-section of the spinal cord, showing the positions of the major pathways.

Motor pathways

The corticospinal tracts begin in the motor area of the cerebral cortex as upper motor neurons and their axons descend ipsilaterally through the corona radiata and the internal capsule. The axons then cross in the medulla as the 'pyramidal decussation' and descend laterally in the spinal cord (see Fig. 20.2). The axons in the tracts enter the anterior horn of the spinal cord (see Fig. 12.1, p. 72) and synapse on the lower motor neuron cell body or 'anterior horn cell'. Weakness can therefore be caused by lesions of either the upper motor neuron (UMN) or the lower motor neuron (LMN) (see Fig. 12.1, p. 72). These two types of weakness have distinct clinical signs and symptoms that usually allow them to be differentiated and therefore enable gross anatomical localization of the lesion.

A lesion of the corticospinal tract on one side of the spinal cord will cause an ipsilateral upper motor neuron defect (spastic hemi- or monoparesis, clonus, brisk reflexes, and an extensor plantar response).

The clinical syndromes of spinal cord disease

There are three main motor syndromes associated with spinal cord disease

- Paraparesis (UMN involvement of legs only).
- Tetraparesis (UMN involvement of all four limbs).
- Brown–Séquard syndrome (unilateral lesion causing UMN involvement of one side).

These three patterns of weakness are often associated with sensory signs. They may develop rapidly or slowly, and over days to months to years, depending on the cause. Any lesion involving the spinal cord results in a syndrome called a 'myelopathy'. If the lesion damages the anterior horn cells as well as the white matter tracts then the patient will have UMN signs below the level of the lesion and LMN signs at and about the level of the lesion. If a myelopathy occurs together with a radiculopathy (i.e. root involvement), then the condition is called a 'myeloradiculopathy'. For example, the most common cause of compression of the cervical spinal cord is due to 'wear and tear' osteoarthritis and degenerative changes within the cervical vertebrae or 'cervical spondylosis'. This leads to damage to the white matter tracts in the cervical cord, resulting in UMN signs in the legs (paraparesis) and sensory loss below the level of the lesion (sensory level) (i.e. 'myelopathy'), as well as LMN signs in the arms due to damage of spinal roots at the level of the spondylotic lesion, i.e. 'radiculopathy'.

Paraparesis (spastic paraparesis or paraplegia)

Paraparesis indicates bilateral upper motor neuron damage involving the axons that innervate the legs from both corticospinal tracts. The clinical signs include increased tone with spasticity, pyramidal distribution of weakness, increased reflexes with clonus, and extensor plantar responses. The abdominal and cremasteric reflexes or 'cutaneous reflexes' may be absent (Fig. 20.3). There is often also involvement of the two sensory pathways from the level below the lesion. This is called a 'sensory level'. Sphincter dysfunction is also typical of spinal cord disease and occurs early with intrinsic spinal cord lesions and later in the course of extrinsic spinal cord lesions.

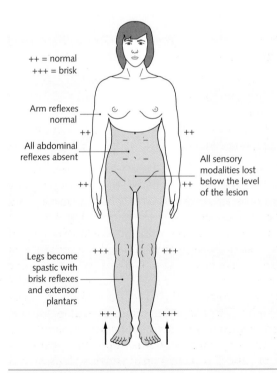

++ = normal
+++ = brisk

Arm reflexes normal

All abdominal reflexes absent

All sensory modalities lost below the level of the lesion

Legs become spastic with brisk reflexes and extensor plantars

−, Absent reflex; +, Reduced reflex; ++, Normal
+++, Pathologically brisk reflex; ↑, Extensor plantar

Fig. 20.3 Clinical signs of cord compression caused by a lesion of the thoracic cord at the T7 level.

Tetraparesis (spastic tetraparesis, tetraplegia, quadriparesis, quadriplegia)

Spastic tetraparesis produces the same clinical picture as paraparesis but involves both arms and legs; it is usually caused by a lesion in the high cervical cord but is occasionally due to brainstem or bilateral cortical damage.

Brown–Séquard syndrome (unilateral cord lesion)

Brown–Séquard syndrome is rare in its pure form but partial forms are more common.

The pure Brown–Séquard clinical picture (Fig. 20.4) consists of:

- Ipsilateral spastic leg and sometimes arm if the lesion is above C5, with brisk reflexes and an extensor plantar response.
- Ipsilateral loss of joint-position sense and vibration (dorsal columns).
- Contralateral loss of pain and temperature (spinothalamic tracts cross at their level of entry).

The sensory level is often a few segments lower than the level of the lesion because pain fibres ascend a few spinal segments before entering the dorsal horn to synapse then cross (see Fig. 13.1, p. 82).

There are other less common clinical syndromes affecting the spinal cord which will be discussed below.

CAUSES OF SPINAL CORD DISEASE

Transection of the cord

Spinal cord transection is usually the result of trauma following anterior dislocation of one vertebra on another. The forces required to do this often result in associated fractures. It causes loss of all motor, sensory, and autonomic function, including the sphincters, below the level of the lesion either immediately, if the transection is complete, or within hours if the damage is partial but later results in secondary oedema causing involvement of the whole spinal cord at the level of the partial lesion.

Fig. 20.4 Clinical signs of a Brown–Séquard lesion at level C7 on the left.

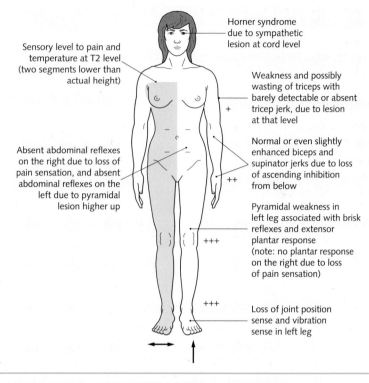

Sensory level to pain and temperature at T2 level (two segments lower than actual height)

Horner syndrome due to sympathetic lesion at cord level

Weakness and possibly wasting of triceps with barely detectable or absent tricep jerk, due to lesion at that level

Normal or even slightly enhanced biceps and supinator jerks due to loss of ascending inhibition from below

Absent abdominal reflexes on the right due to loss of pain sensation, and absent abdominal reflexes on the left due to pyramidal lesion higher up

Pyramidal weakness in left leg associated with brisk reflexes and extensor plantar response (note: no plantar response on the right due to loss of pain sensation)

Loss of joint position sense and vibration sense in left leg

−, Absent reflex; +, Reduced reflex; ++, Normal
+++, Pathologically brisk reflex; ↑, Extensor plantar

With any severe, acute spinal cord lesion there are usually two clinical stages:

- **Spinal shock:** initially, there is loss of all reflex activity below the level of the lesion, with flaccid limbs, atonic bladder with overflow incontinence, atonic bowel, gastric dilatation, and loss of genital reflexes and vasomotor control.
- **Heightened reflex activity:** this occurs after about 1–2 weeks and is associated with spasticity of the limbs, brisk reflexes and extensor plantar responses. Patients develop a spastic bladder (small capacity with urgency, frequency, and automatic emptying) and hyperactive autonomic function (sweating and vasomotor changes).

Bilateral upper motor neuron signs in the legs (with or without arm involvement) with no cranial nerve signs usually indicates spinal cord pathology. The lesion must be above the body of L1, because the spinal cord ends at this level and lesions below this level involve the cauda equina and so cause lower motor neuron signs.

Differential diagnosis

In the absence of trauma, similar symptoms and signs of a very severe cord lesion should make one consider the following:

- Ischaemic infarction of the cord: occlusion of a major segmental artery, dissecting aortic aneurysm, vasculitis, anterior spinal artery thrombosis.
- Haemorrhage into the spinal cord from an arteriovenous malformation, epidural or subdural haemorrhage.

The supply to the diaphragm is via the phrenic nerve (C3, C4, and C5) and therefore any cord lesion above C3 may cause neuromuscular respiratory failure.

- Acute or subacute necrotizing or demyelinating myelopathy.
- Epidural abscess.
- Acute vertebral collapse-usually associated with neoplastic disease of the vertebrae

Treatment

Complete transection of the spinal cord has a very poor neurological outcome. It is more usual for incomplete cord transection to occur. In this scenario, it is vital to treat any spinal fracture and instability with orthopaedic or neurosurgical input as this may prevent secondary damage to the intact cord from the spinal injury. The reduction of spinal cord oedema with immediate administration of high-dose corticosteroids may help.

Spinal cord compression

The clinical picture is determined by the site of compression. Lesions affecting the cord below T1 will not involve the arms, whereas lesions between C5 and T1 cause LMN and sometimes UMN signs in the arms, and UMN signs in the legs. Lesions above C5 cause UMN signs in the arms and legs. Compressive lesions may spare sphincter function until the patient has severe disease. Therefore, any patient with sphincter involvement needs urgent investigation.

Causes

- Trauma (see above).
- Spondylotic/disc disease.
- Tumours: metastatic or myeloma.
- Inflammatory lesions: epidural abscess, tuberculoma, granuloma.
- Epidural haemorrhage.

Disc protrusion

The most common cause of disc disease is spondylosis. These are the degenerative changes within vertebrae and intervertebral discs that occur during ageing or secondary to trauma or rheumatological disease. Damaged discs usually protrude laterally and cause compression of the nerve roots, resulting in a lower motor neuron lesion. The most common pathologies involve the C5/C6 and C6/C7 discs, causing C6 and C7 radiculopathies (damage to the spinal segmental nerves) in the upper limbs, and L4/L5 and L5/S1 discs, involving the L5 and S1 spinal nerves in the lower limbs (see Fig. 22.2). However, discs can protrude centrally and posteriorly. This results in cord

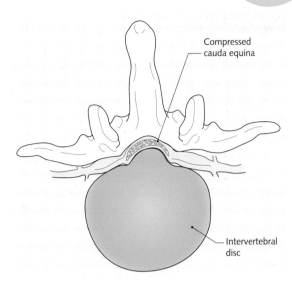

Fig. 20.5 Central disc protrusion compressing cauda equina below L1.

compression when it occurs above the level L1 and causes a spastic paraparesis (usually a low cervical or thoracic disc) or tetraparesis (high cervical disc), with variable sensory loss and sphincter dysfunction.

If central disc protrusion occurs below the L1 vertebral level then the cauda equina will be affected and the patient will have a lower motor neuron syndrome affecting the legs and bladder (see Fig. 20.5).

Spinal cord tumours

Spinal cord tumours can be:

- **Intramedullary** (within the spinal cord): these are usually malignant, e.g. glioma, ependymoma causing an intrinsic cord lesion (see p. 137).
- **Intradural** but extramedullary, i.e. on the surface of the cord arising from the meninges (meningioma) or spinal root (neurofibroma) but within the dural sac. These are usually benign and present with spinal cord compression.
- **Extradural** (in the epidural space): these are usually manifestations of multifocal systemic neoplasia, e.g. metastatic carcinoma, lymphoma, myeloma, or can be other mass lesions, e.g. abscess, lipoma. These also present with spinal cord compression.

Inflammatory lesions

- Epidural abscess.
- Tuberculoma.

Epidural abscesses are most often caused by *Staphylococcus aureus*. The organism usually reaches the cord via the bloodstream but may spread directly (e.g. from osteomyelitis in a vertebra). There is fever, severe back pain with paraparesis (or tetraparesis), with or without spinal nerve lesions. Diagnosis is made with magnetic resonance imaging (MRI) and lumbar puncture. Treatment is with appropriate antibiotics and surgical drainage. The treatment of the underlying source of infection is also important.

Tuberculoma is a frequent cause of cord compression in areas where tuberculosis (TB) is common, (e.g. India, Pakistan, Africa, and in areas with high immigrant populations from these places). It often occurs in the absence of pulmonary disease. There may be destruction of vertebral bodies and spread of infection along the extradural space. This results in cord compression and paraparesis or 'Pott's paraplegia'. The clinical signs of TB meningitis may coexist. Diagnosis requires a high index of suspicion. The tuberculoma can be picked up on MRI, and *Mycobacterium tuberculosis* may be seen or grown from samples of cerebrospinal fluid. Treatment is with antituberculous therapy, as guided by the local microbiology sensitivities, but triple and often quadruple therapy is often needed. This is continued for at least 9 months and may be used in conjunction with the judicious use of corticosteroids for coexisting oedema.

Epidural haemorrhage and haematoma

Epidural haemorrhage and haematoma are rare sequelae of anticoagulant therapy, bleeding diatheses, and trauma, including lumbar puncture. They often result in a rapidly progressive cord or cauda equina lesion.

Patients frequently do not clinically improve after decompression for cervical spondylosis although myelopathic pain usually decreases with time. The main aim of decompression is to prevent progression of disease. This needs to be highlighted when discussing possible cervical decompressive surgery with patients.

Vascular cord lesions

Anterior spinal artery occlusion

This is described in Chapter 26 (p. 169).

Transverse myelitis

Transverse myelitis is a broad term used to describe inflammation of the cord with resultant paraparesis (or tetraparesis), arising from a wide range of diseases:

- Multiple sclerosis (MS) and rarely Devic's disease.
- Postviral demyelination, e.g. Epstein–Barr virus, varicella zoster.
- Sarcoidosis.
- Viral infection.
- Connective tissue diseases, e.g. systemic lupus erythematosus, Sjorgen's.
- Syphilis.

Metabolic and toxic cord disease

Subacute combined degeneration of the cord

Subacute combined degeneration of the cord (SCDC) is the most important example of metabolic disease affecting the spinal cord and is caused by deficiency of vitamin B_{12}. The deficiency may result from nutritional deficiency (especially in vegans), pernicious anaemia, gastrectomy, or disease of the terminal ileum (e.g. Crohn's disease, 'blind-loop' syndrome). Up to 25% of patients with neurological damage caused by vitamin B_{12} deficiency do not have haematological abnormalities (i.e. macrocytic megaloblastic anaemia).

Treatment is with vitamin B_{12}, but this may not significantly improve the spinal cord damage. The condition can be made dramatically worse by giving folic acid without vitamin B_{12}.

Vitamin B_{12} deficiency can also cause damage to the peripheral nerves. The resulting syndrome is of a peripheral neuropathy, with a sensory ataxia due to loss of joint-position sense, and a spastic paraparesis. The full clinical picture of an upper motor neuron lesion in the legs is modified by the peripheral neuropathy (i.e. there is usually loss of ankle jerks but the plantar responses are usually extensor). Patients can also develop optic atrophy and a mild dementia.

There are only a few common causes of absent ankle jerks (i.e. lower motor neuron) and extensor plantar responses (i.e. upper motor neuron). These include:
- Combined pathology, e.g. cervical spondylosis and peripheral neuropathy.
- Motor neuron disease.
- Conus medullaris lesions.
- Subacute combined degeneration of the cord (B_{12} myelopathy).
- Friedreich's ataxia.
- Tabes dorsalis (tertiary neurosyphilis).

Intrinsic cord lesions

The signs of an intrinsic cord lesion are usually caused by MS. Much rarer causes include an intrinsic tumour or a syrinx (syringomyelia).

Syringomyelia and syringobulbia

Syringomyelia (relatively common) and syringobulbia (very rare) are caused by a fluid-filled cavity (syrinx) within the spinal cord and brainstem, respectively.

The cavitation of the cervical cord is associated, in the majority of cases, with a congenital abnormality of the foramen magnum, which is usually an Arnold–Chiari malformation. This causes the cerebellar tonsils to lie in the posterior foramen magnum and potentially they can compress the brainstem. A syrinx can also arise due to an intrinsic tumour or following trauma.

Clinically, there is an evolving picture as the expanding cavity damages the various neurons and pathways (Fig. 20.6):

- Pain in the upper limbs is often an early feature, which may be exacerbated by coughing or straining if associated with an Arnold–Chiari malformation.
- Dissociated spinothalamic sensory loss (i.e. loss of pain and temperature but preservation of vibration and joint position sense) in a 'cape-like' or 'suspended' distribution (i.e. the dermatomes above and below the level of the syrinx are spared).
- There is unilateral or bilateral Horner's syndrome (meiosis, ptosis, and anhydrosis) due to damage to sympathetic fibres within the spinal cord down to T1.
- There is wasting and weakness of the small muscles of the hand due to damage of the anterior

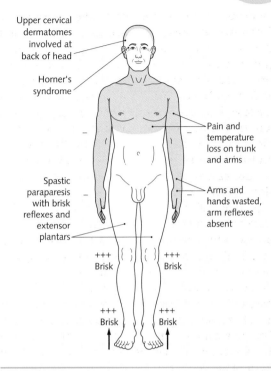

Upper cervical dermatomes involved at back of head

Horner's syndrome

Pain and temperature loss on trunk and arms

Spastic paraparesis with brisk reflexes and extensor plantars

Arms and hands wasted, arm reflexes absent

+++ Brisk   +++ Brisk

+++ Brisk   +++ Brisk

−, Absent reflex; ++, Normal; +++ Brisk ; ↑, Extensor plantar

Fig. 20.6 The evolving pattern of an intrinsic cord lesion at T1. This pattern may be seen with syringomyelia and intrinsic cord tumours, e.g. glioma, ependymoma, and astrocytoma.

horn cells at the level of T1 (a common site for a syrinx).
- Spastic paraparesis develops only after the cavity is markedly distended and compresses on the corticospinal tracts.
- Ultimately, the posterior columns may also become affected.

With syringobulbia, there is also:

- Bilateral wasting and weakness of the tongue.
- Hearing loss.
- Vestibular involvement with nystagmus.
- Facial sensory loss.

Intrinsic cord lesions usually cause sacral sparing, i.e. preservation of pain and temperature sensation in the sacral deramatomes, because the ascending spinothalamic fibres from the sacrum lie peripherally and tend to be the last that are affected by the expanding lesion.

Motor neuron disease

21

Objectives

- Define: 'upper motor neuron', 'lower motor neuron' and 'motor unit'
- Describe the types of MND
- Understand how the diagnosis of MND is made
- Understand the mangement of MND

The motor neuron cell bodies within the primary motor cortex and their axons, which descend down to synapse with the motor nuclei of the cranial nerves and the anterior horn cells, are called the upper motor neurons (UMNs); the cell body of the anterior horn cell and its axon that projects to muscle is the alpha lower motor neuron (LMN) (see Figs 12.1, p. 72 and 12.3, p. 74). Features of upper and lower motor neuron defects are listed in Fig. 21.1. Each alpha motor neuron extends peripherally to innervate a variable number of skeletal muscle fibres (from 20 to over 1000). The alpha motor neuron, and the muscle fibres it supplies, is known as a 'motor unit'.

In addition to the alpha motor neurons, smaller cell bodies innervate the intrafusal muscle fibres of muscle spindles. These are called gamma motor neurons and they are involved in the control of muscle contraction.

TYPES OF MOTOR NEURON DISEASE

Motor neuron disease (MND) is a disease in which there is progressive degeneration of motor neurons in the motor cortex and in the anterior horns of the spinal cord. There is also degeneration of the cells within the somatic motor nuclei of the cranial nerves within the brainstem. There is usually relentless progression of the disease to death within 1–5 years.

MND is subdivided into three main clinical groups and a possible, more controversial, fourth. These categories do not represent distinct aetiological or pathological mechanisms, and often with disease progression the clinical features of all the groups merge.

Amyotrophic lateral sclerosis

Amyotrophic lateral sclerosis (ALS) is often used synonymously with MND in the USA and in Europe. In the UK, it is used to represent a particular form of MND with a mixture of UMN and LMN signs in the limbs, head, and neck, e.g. spastic tetraparesis with brisk reflexes (UMN), in association with marked wasting and fasciculations of the tongue and intrinsic hand muscles (LMN) (Fig. 21.2).

Progressive muscular atrophy

Progressive muscular atrophy (PMA) is associated with LMN signs (wasting, weakness, and fasciculations, although tendon reflexes are usually preserved), which often begin asymmetrically in the small muscles of the hands or feet and spread. This form often progresses to include UMN signs with time.

Progressive bulbar and pseudobulbar palsy

'Bulbar' refers to the brainstem motor nuclei. 'Bulbar' palsy refers to involvement of the LMN. 'Pseudobulbar' palsy involves the UMN bilaterally as a unilateral UMN lesion has little effect in the head and neck muscles apart from the face where the lower half only receives unilateral UMN innervation.

The lower cranial nerve nuclei and their supranuclear connections are involved in these variants of the disease. Patients present with dysarthria, dysphagia, nasal regurgitation, choking, and dysphonia ('Donald Duck' voice). They may have wasting and fasciculation of the tongue.

Fig. 21.1 Features of upper and lower motor neuron lesions

Upper motor neuron	Lower motor neuron
Spastic paralysis	Flaccid paralysis
No wasting	Muscle wasting
No fasciculations	Fasciculations present
Brisk reflexes	Reduced or absent reflexes
Clonus	No clonus
Extensor plantar response (Babinski)	Plantar response flexor or absent

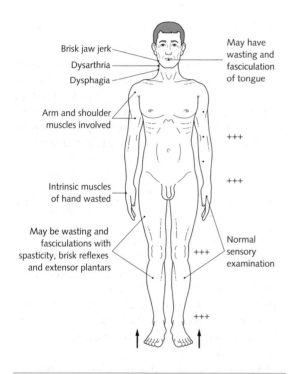

++, Normal; +++, Pathologically brisk reflex; ↑, Extensor plantar

Fig. 21.2 Clinical findings in a patient with classic amyotrophic lateral sclerosis with a mixture of upper and lower motor neuron signs. There is often a mixed bulbar and pseudobulbar picture, e.g. wasted, fasciculating tongue with a spastic palate, which may remain isolated or be the presenting feature of amyotrophic lateral sclerosis.

Primary lateral sclerosis

Primary lateral sclerosis is somewhat more controversial as a subgroup of MND. This is a purely UMN disease and the diagnosis can only be made once other conditions are excluded. Patients often progress to a more classic ALS-type picture with time.

Eye movements and sphincter involvement are never affected in MND and their abnormality virtually excludes the diagnosis. Respiratory muscles may be involved and occasionally patients present with type 2 respiratory failure from the onset. Patients may complain of sensory symptoms, including pain in the limbs, but have no sensory signs. They may also experience troublesome cramps, especially at night.

EPIDEMIOLOGY

The majority of cases of MND are sporadic with no family history. Familial cases account for between 5 and 10% of patients. The most common familial form is due to abnormal expression of the superoxide dismutase-1 gene (SOD-1) found on chromosome 21. In the remaining familial cases, the mutation is unknown.

Sporadic MND has an incidence of about 1 in 100 000. The incidence increases with age, with a peak between 60 and 70 years of age. There are endemic areas where the incidence is much higher (e.g. Guam), but it is uncertain as to whether this represents a familial form or whether it is due to some environmental factor, e.g. the cycad nut.

The mean survival in patients with MND is 3 years; however, those with bulbar onset have a shorter life expectancy because aspiration pneumonia is more common.

Men are more commonly affected than women, with a ratio of 1.5:1. However, the bulbar form is slightly more common in women.

DIFFERENTIAL DIAGNOSIS

The differential diagnosis depends on the mode of presentation:

Amyotrophic lateral sclerosis

Differential diagnoses for ALS include conditions that present with a mixture of UMN and LMN signs:

- Cervical spondylosis: combination of spinal cord compression (UMN), spinal root compression, and anterior horn cell loss (LMN).
- Spinal tumours: can cause LMN signs at the level of the pathology and also UMN signs below the level of the lesion.

- Hyperthyroidism: wasted, fasciculating muscles secondary to a myopathy with brisk reflexes.

Progressive muscular atrophy

Differential diagnoses for PMA include conditions with LMN signs only:

- Spinal muscular atrophy: a heterogeneous hereditary condition with anterior horn cell loss.
- Poliomyelitis (new onset is rare in the UK).
- Postpolio syndrome: progressive weakness and wasting 30–40 years after having had polio, which usually affects limbs involved in the initial disease. The exact cause is uncertain but it does not involve reactivation of the poliomyelitis virus.
- Multifocal motor neuropathy with conduction block: autoimmune condition with high levels of anti-GM1 antibody. This is treatable with intravenous immunoglobulin and immunosuppression.
- Lead neuropathy.

Pseudobulbar/bulbar palsy

Differential diagnoses for pseudobulbar palsy include conditions that cause bilateral UMN lesions:

- Cerebrovascular disease can cause a pseudobulbar palsy as well as UMN signs in the limbs.
- Multiple sclerosis usually gives a pseudobulbar picture in association with cerebellar features, optic atrophy, and other brainstem syndromes.

Differential diagnosis for bulbar palsy (i.e. a LMN syndrome with no UMN features), include:

- Myasthenia gravis.
- Multiple lower cranial nerve lesions caused by infiltrating tumours, e.g. nasopharyngeal carcinoma and glomus tumours.
- Rare neuropathies presenting with bulbar weakness, e.g. rare cases of Guillain–Barré or diphtheria.

DIAGNOSIS

The diagnosis is made clinically and this is supported by electromyography (EMG), which shows the presence of denervation in the muscles supplied by more than one spinal region (see Chapter 36, p. 251). The presence of EMG changes in the tongue in association with changes in the limbs is often helpful in confirming the diagnosis.

Other conditions must be excluded if suspected. This may require MRI of the brainstem and spinal cord in some cases.

TREATMENT

There is no cure for MND. The diagnosis should be carefully and fully discussed with the patient and carers. Ideally, counselling and multidisciplinary support should be available.

Drug treatment

The newly introduced drug riluzole has been shown to increase survival by 2–3 months but it has no effect on disability; it is now recommended by National Institute of Clinical Excellence (NICE). Many other drug trials are in progress, including the use of insulin-like growth factor-1 (Cephalon™).

Symptomatic treatment

Symptomatic treatment is of paramount importance in MND and includes:

- Speech therapy and communication aids.
- Altered food consistency for safe swallowing and, ultimately in some cases, a percutaneous endoscopic gastrostomy (PEG).
- baclofen or tizanidine for spasticity.
- Appropriate management of pain.
- Physiotherapy, splints, walking aids, and wheelchairs.
- Adaptations to allow patients to stay at home.
- Full palliative care in the terminal stages.
- Patients often have nocturnal hypoventilation due to neuromuscular respiratory weakness. This can often be helped with non-invasive respiratory support (NIPPV, CPAP).

Sensory signs do not occur in pure motor neuron disease and there is preservation of extraocular muscles and bladder function (Onuf's nucleus is unaffected by the disease process).

Radiculopathy and plexopathy

Objectives

- Understand the anatomy of the spinal nerve roots
- Describe the clinical features associated with radiculopathy
- Understand the difference in the clinical features between a central and lateral lumbar and cervical disc protrusion
- Describe the common causes of plexopathy

Anatomy

Thirty paired spinal nerve roots provide the means of entry and exit of information from the CNS. The dorsal root contains the sensory (afferent) fibres arising from sensory receptors in the periphery, as well as a collection of sensory cell bodies, termed the dorsal root ganglion (Fig. 22.1). The ventral (anterior) root contains the motor (efferent) fibres derived from the anterior horn cell bodies in the anterior horn of the spinal cord grey matter (see Fig. 22.1). The dorsal and ventral spinal roots lie within the spinal subarachnoid space and come together at the intervertebral foramen to become a mixed sensorimotor nerve called the spinal root.

The spinal roots are named by the vertebral level at which they emerge from the spinal cord. In the cervical region, the roots exit above each vertebral body and there are therefore eight cervical roots (C1–C8), even though there are only seven cervical vertebrae. By contrast, at all other levels the roots emerge below the respective vertebral body (i.e. T1–T12, L1–L5) (see Fig. 22.1).

After emerging from the intervertebral foraminae, the spinal roots pass into the brachial plexus to supply the upper limb or into the lumbosacral plexus to supply the lower limb. In the thoracic region, they form the intercostal nerves, which supply sensation and motor activity to the chest and upper abdominal wall.

The brachial plexus lies in the posterior triangle of the neck, between scalenius anterior and scalenius medius, and is derived from the C5–T1 spinal roots. At the root of the neck, the plexus lies behind the clavicle. The plexus gives off several motor branches before forming the 'cords' and ultimately becomes the median, ulnar, and radial nerves (see Fig. 12.5, p. 78).

The lumbosacral plexus is subdivided into the lumbar plexus (T12–L5) and the sacral plexus (L4–S3) (see Fig. 12.6, p. 78). The lumbar plexus is located in the psoas muscle and forms the femoral nerve (L2–L4). The sacral plexus is on the posterior wall of the pelvis and forms the sciatic nerve, which consists of two parts: those nerves that will form the common peroneal nerve (L4–L5, S1–S2 posterior divisions) and the tibial nerve (L4–L5, S1–S2 anterior divisions). The sciatic nerve divides into the tibial and common peroneal nerves in the popliteal fossa.

When a spinal nerve root is damaged then the patient is said to have a 'radiculopathy' and when a plexus is damaged the patient is said to have a 'plexopathy'.

RADICULOPATHY (SPINAL NERVE ROOT LESIONS)

Causes of radiculopathy include:

- Cervical and lumbar spondylosis (degenerative changes including disc prolapse, osteophytes).
- Trauma.
- Tumours, e.g. neurofibroma, metastases.
- Herpes zoster virus (shingles).
- Meningeal inflammation.
- Arachnoiditis.

The most common cause is degenerative changes affecting the cervical and lumbar regions.

Clinical features

- Pain: severe, sharp, shooting, and/or burning pain radiating into the cutaneous distribution

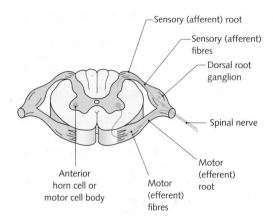

Fig. 22.1 Anatomy of spinal roots.

(dermatome) or muscle group (myotome) supplied by the root. It can be aggravated by movement, straining, or coughing.

- Neurological signs: lower motor neuron signs, i.e. wasting with or without fasciculations, flaccid weakness, and reduced/absent reflexes, in the affected myotome and sensory impairment in the affected dermatome.

Specific radiculopathies

Lateral cervical disc protrusion

Lateral disc protrusion in the cervical region often causes severe pain in the upper limb. A C6/C7 disc protrusion causing a C7 radiculopathy is the most common lesion followed by a C5/C6 disc lesion affecting C6. T1 radiculopathy is rarely caused by spondylotic disease and, if present, should be investigated promptly.

In cervical radiculopathies, there is root pain that radiates into the affected dermatome (into the middle finger with a C7 lesion). Subsequently, there is wasting and weakness of the muscles innervated by the root (triceps, and wrist and finger extensors in a C7 lesion), and the reflexes involved in this root will be lost (triceps jerk in a C7 lesion).

Lesions can be visualized on magnetic resonance imaging (MRI) or myelography with computed tomography (CT). Most cases in which pain is the only symptom recover with rest, the aid of a neck collar, and analgesia as the disc prolapse resolves spontaneously. When recovery is delayed, and especially if motor neurological signs exist or there is severe intractable pain, surgical spinal root decompression may be performed.

In some cases, the patient may have a central and a lateral disc protrusion, in which case the patient may have cervical cord compression with upper motor neuron signs in the legs and a sensory level as well as the radiculopathy at the level of the lesion.

Lateral lumbar disc protrusion

The most common lesion in the lumbar region causes compression of L5 and S1 roots due to lateral prolapse of L4/L5 and L5/S1 discs, respectively. (Fig. 22.2). This results in low back pain and 'sciatica' (pain radiating down the buttock and lower limb).

There is limitation of straight-leg-raising in the affected leg. There may be weakness of extension of the great toe (L5) or of plantar flexion (S1). The reflexes may be lost (ankle jerk in an S1 root lesion, or, rarely, the knee jerk in an L3/L4 lesion). Sensory loss may be found in the affected dermatome.

Investigations include MRI or myelography if MRI is not available. Most cases resolve with rest and analgesia but decompressive surgery may be required.

Central lumbar disc protrusion

The spinal cord ends at L1/L2. A central disc protrusion below this level will result in a polyradiculopathy and not a myelopathy. Multiple nerve roots (cauda equina) may be involved and will cause lower back pain with radiation down the legs, lower motor neuron weakness of the legs and feet, sacral numbness, retention of urine, bowel dysfunction, and impotence.

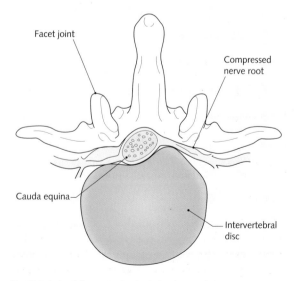

Fig. 22.2 Lateral disc protrusion in the lumbosacral region.

The onset may be acute, causing a flaccid paraparesis, or chronic, producing symptoms similar to intermittent claudication caused by vascular insufficiency; this is called 'neurogenic claudication'. A patient with back pain who develops retention of urine should be suspected of having a central lumbar disc protrusion. Urgent imaging and decompression should follow.

It is a common mistake to assume that a central lumbar disc protrusion causes spinal cord compression. The spinal cord ends at L1/2 and therefore the more common central disc protrusions (L4/5 or L5/S1) cause damage to the cauda equina, which is the loose bundle of nerve roots descending through the lumbosacral canal. The resulting syndrome is therefore a lumbosacral polyradiculopathy, i.e. pure LMN weakness with sensory loss in a dermatomal pattern (perineum and backs of legs) with severe sphincter dysfunction.

PLEXOPATHIES

Disease of the brachial and lumbosacral plexuses is relatively uncommon. Several specific conditions affect the plexuses.

Brachial plexopathies

Causes of brachial plexopathies include:

- Trauma.
- Neuralgic amyotrophy.
- Malignant infiltration.
- Radiotherapy.
- Compression, e.g. thoracic outlet syndrome (cervical rib or fibrous band).

Trauma

Trauma is the most common cause of a brachial plexus lesion (see Fig. 12.5, p. 78) and, in severe cases, early referral to a specialist unit with experience in the surgical repair of plexus injuries is advised as some recovery of function can be obtained even with complete disruption.

- Upper plexus lesion (C5, C6): upper plexus injury is usually caused by falling on the shoulder or traction on the neck and shoulder at birth ('Erb's palsy'). It is associated with the characteristic posture of a 'waiter's tip' with the arm internally rotated, extended, and slightly adducted with loss of shoulder abduction and elbow flexion. Sensory loss occurs in the outer aspect of the shoulder, arm, forearm and thumb in the C5, C6 dermatomes.
- Lower plexus lesion (C8, T1): lower plexus injury is usually caused by forced abduction of the arm, which may occur at birth ('Klumpke's palsy') and following trauma in later life, e.g. motorcycle accidents. There is characteristically a 'clawed hand' with loss of function of the intrinsic muscles of the hand and long flexors and extensors of the fingers as well as loss of sensation in C8 and T1 dermatomes and a Horner's syndrome.

Neuralgic amyotrophy (acute brachial neuropathy, brachial neuritis)

Neuralgic amyotrophy is a condition in which severe pain in the muscles of the shoulder is followed 2–7 days later, as the pain resolves, by rapid wasting and weakness in the proximal, more commonly than distal, muscles of the arm. It may occur bilaterally and tendon reflexes may be lost in the affected limb. Sensory findings are usually minor. It may follow an infection, inoculation, or surgery but most often a precipitating cause is not found. It is thought to be caused by an inflammatory process affecting the nerve roots and plexus. Recovery is gradual over many months but may not be complete. Recurrent episodes can occur. A very similar process can affect the lumbosacral plexus.

Episodic painful brachial neuropathy may be a presenting symptom of hereditary neropathy with liability to pressure palsies (HNPP). HNPP shows autosomal dominant inheritance and is characterized by episodes of mononeuropathy at vulnerable sites of nerve compression. A more generalized peripheral neuropathy may be evident upon clinical examination. Mildly reduced nerve conduction velocities are associated with a deletion of the PMP22 gene on chromosome 17. The same gene can be affected by different mutations and cause Charcot–Marie–Tooth disease type 1.

Malignant infiltration

Invasion of the brachial plexus usually occurs in association with metastatic or locally invasive breast carcinoma and can occur many years after the initial tumour was diagnosed and treated. There is usually severe and intractable pain in the arm.

Pancoast tumour

An apical lung tumour (usually squamous cell carcinoma) can involve the brachial plexus by affecting C8/T1-derived roots.

Clinically, the patient has:

- Severe pain in the arm.
- Ipsilateral weak and wasted hand.
- Sensory loss (C8, T1).
- Horner's syndrome.

Radiotherapy-induced plexopathy

Irradiation of the brachial plexus following breast carcinoma can lead to damage of the brachial plexus especially the lower parts. The onset is usually delayed between 5 and 30 months and can be difficult to differentiate from metastatic breast cancer.

Compression

Cervical rib (thoracic outlet syndrome)

A fibrous band or cervical rib extending from the tip of the transverse process of C7 to the first rib can stretch the lower part of the brachial plexus (C8, T1). There is pain along the ulnar border of the forearm and sensory loss initially in the distribution of T1, with wasting of the thenar muscles predominantly. There might also be a Horner's syndrome. Patients often complain of pain in the shoulder and numbness in the forearm especially on carrying heavy objects.

Some patients develop a vascular syndrome with compression of the subclavian artery or vein associated with unilateral Raynaud's phenomenon, pallor of the limb on elevation and loss of the radial pulse on abduction and external rotation of the shoulder. This is known as Adson's sign.

The vascular and neurological syndromes rarely coexist. Treatment is surgical decompression.

Lumbosacral plexus

Symptoms of a lumbosacral plexus lesion may be unilateral or bilateral. Diabetic 'amyotrophy' and malignant infiltration in the pelvis are the most common causes. Weakness, reflex change, and sensory loss depend on the location and extent of plexus damage. In general, the following features are found (see Fig. 12.6, p. 78):

- Upper plexus lesion: weakness of hip flexion and adduction, with anterior leg sensory loss.
- Lower plexus lesion: weakness of the posterior thigh (hamstrings) and foot muscles, with posterior leg sensory loss.

Diabetic amyotrophy

Diabetic amyotrophy is usually seen in older men with mild to moderate diabetes and may be associated with periods of poor glycaemic control. The site of the pathology may be in the lumbosacral plexus or in the roots and may have an inflammatory aetiology. Patients present with painful wasting – usually strikingly asymmetrical – of the quadriceps and psoas muscles. There is loss of the knee jerks and extreme tenderness in the affected area. There is usually minimal sensory loss. It resolves with careful control of blood glucose over many months.

Other causes of a lumbosacral plexopathy

- **Infiltration by neoplasia**, e.g. prostate, ovarian, and cervical, can infiltrate or metastasize to the lumbosacral plexus. This is usually associated with severe pain in the pelvis or/and legs.
- **Trauma** following abdominal or pelvic surgery, e.g. hysterectomy.
- **Compression** from an abdominal aortic aneurysm.

Disorders of the peripheral nerves

Anatomy

Peripheral nerves are made up of numerous axons bound together by three types of connective tissue – endoneurium, perineurium, and epineurium (Fig. 23.1). The vasa nervorum located in the epineurium provides the blood supply.

Peripheral nerve trunks contain myelinated and unmyelinated fibres. Myelin is a protein–lipid complex that forms an insulating layer around some axons, resulting in increased rates of conduction in these fibres.

All peripheral nerves have a cellular sheath, the Schwann cell, but only in some does the membrane of the cell 'spiral' around the axon, forming the multilayered myelin sheath.

Schwann cells of myelinated nerves are separated by nodes of Ranvier. At these points, the axons are not surrounded by myelin. During conduction, impulses jump from one node to the next, which is called saltatory conduction. Conduction in unmyelinated nerves is slower and dependent on the diameter of the axon.

Within the peripheral nerve, the axons vary structurally and this is related to function. Three distinct types of fibre can be distinguished (Fig. 23.2). All are myelinated apart from the C fibres, which carry impulses from painful stimuli.

The function of peripheral nerves can be disrupted by damage to the cell body, the axon, the myelin sheath, the connective tissue, or the blood supply.

Two basic pathological processes occur:

1. **Wallerian degeneration:** the axon and myelin sheath degenerates distal to injury to the axon. The process occurs within 7–10 days of the injury and the degenerating portion of the nerve is electrically inexcitable. Regeneration can occur because the basement membrane of the Schwann cell survives and acts as a skeleton along which the axon regrows up to a rate of about 1mm per day.

2. **Demyelination:** segmental destruction of the myelin sheath occurs mostly without axonal damage although prolonged demyelination may cause secondary axonal damage. The primary lesion affects the Schwann cell and causes marked slowing of conduction or conduction block. Local demyelination is caused by pressure, e.g. entrapment neuropathies or by inflammation, e.g. Guillain–Barré syndrome.

DEFINITIONS OF NEUROPATHIES

- **Neuropathy:** a pathological process that affects a peripheral nerve or nerves and may involve axonal degeneration (Wallerian degeneration) or demyelination, as discussed above.
- **Mononeuropathy:** when a single nerve is affected, e.g. the median nerve in carpal tunnel syndrome. If multiple single nerves are affected in an asymmetrical pattern, it is termed **multifocal neuropathy** or mononeuritis multiplex.
- **Polyneuropathy:** a diffuse, symmetrical disease process that is usually distal with some proximal progression. It affects the longest axons first, i.e. to the feet, and gradually involves shorter axons in the legs and hands. It can be acute, subacute, or chronic. It may be progressive, relapsing, or transient, and can be motor, sensory, autonomic, or mixed (sensorimotor ± autonomic).

Fig. 23.1 Transverse section of a peripheral nerve.

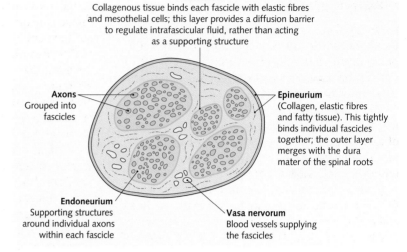

Perineurium
Collagenous tissue binds each fascicle with elastic fibres and mesothelial cells; this layer provides a diffusion barrier to regulate intrafascicular fluid, rather than acting as a supporting structure

Axons
Grouped into fascicles

Epineurium
(Collagen, elastic fibres and fatty tissue). This tightly binds individual fascicles together; the outer layer merges with the dura mater of the spinal roots

Endoneurium
Supporting structures around individual axons within each fascicle

Vasa nervorum
Blood vessels supplying the fascicles

Fig. 23.2 Fibre types in peripheral nerve

Fibre type	Fibre diameter (μm)	Velocity (m/s)	Function/nerve type
Type A (myelinated); Group I	12–20	90	Vibration and position sense alpha motor neurons
Group II	6–12	50	Touch and pressure afferents
Group III	1–6	30	Gamma afferents
Type B (myelinated)	2–6	10	Autonomic preganglionic
Type C (unmyelinated)	<1	2	Pain and temperature afferents autonomic postganglionic

SYMPTOMS OF NEUROPATHY

Sensory symptoms

Negative symptoms (loss of sensation)

Large myelinated fibre disease causes loss of touch, vibration, and joint-position sense (proprioception), leading to:

- Difficulty discriminating textures.
- Feet and hands feeling like 'cotton wool'.

- Gait unsteady through loss of position sense, especially at night when vision cannot compensate.

Small unmyelinated fibre disease causes loss of pain and temperature appreciation, leading to:

- Painless burns and trauma.
- Damage to joints (Charcot's joint), resulting in painless deformity.

Positive symptoms

Large myelinated fibre disease can cause paraesthesiae ('pins and needles'). Small unmyelinated fibre disease produce painful positive symptoms:

- Burning sensations.
- Dysaesthesia: pain on gentle touch.
- Hyperalgesia: lowered threshold to pain.
- Hyperpathia: pain threshold is elevated, but pain is excessively felt.
- Lightning pains: sudden, very severe, shooting pains, which usually suggest a diagnosis of tabes dorsalis (tertiary syphilis).
- Allodynia: when non-painful stimuli are perceived as painful.

Sensory examination
Functions of large myelinated sensory fibres include:

- Light touch.
- Two-point discrimination.
- Vibration sense.
- Joint-position sense.

Functions of small unmyelinated and thinly myelinated sensory fibres include:

- Temperature perception.
- Pain perception.

A classic polyneuropathy will produce sensory loss in the characteristic 'glove-and-sock' distribution. This phenomenon is usually length related and therefore signs in the hands will not develop until there is sensory loss up to at least mid-shin level.

When joint-position sense is lost, gait may be abnormal due to sensory ataxia. Romberg's test is positive (loss of joint-position sense is compensated for by vision, therefore when the eyes are closed, the stance becomes unsteady, whereas it is steady when the eyes are open).

Sensory examination should include the search for neuropathic burns, trauma, ulcers on the heels and between the toes and Charcot joints. There might also be trophic changes within the skin due to loss of sensory and autonomic fibres. These changes include loss of hairs, oedema, purple discoloration, and shiny featureless skin (see also p. 244, sensory testing).

Motor symptoms

Weakness is usually the main presenting feature. This is usually distal (e.g. difficulty clearing the kerb when walking or unable to open jars) but some neuropathies can be proximal (e.g. difficulty climbing stairs or combing hair).

Patients may also complain of cramps and twitching of muscles (fasciculations), although these symptoms are more commonly due to diseases affecting the anterior horn cell (e.g. motor neuron disease).

Motor examination

The classic features of a lower motor neuron abnormality include:

- Distal wasting of muscles: Distal wasting can also occur with generalized weight loss but weakness is rare, although the muscles may fatigue easily in this context.
- Fasciculations.
- Flaccid weakness of muscles.
- Depressed or absent tendon reflexes.

INVESTIGATION OF PERIPHERAL NEUROPATHY

In up to 30% of cases, the cause of a neuropathy may not be identified. The following investigations may be helpful in the diagnosis:

- **Blood tests:** routine blood tests to exclude certain causes of peripheral neuropathy should include full blood count (FBC), erythrocyte sedimentation rate (ESR), C-reactive protein (CRP), urea and electrolytes (U&E, especially renal function tests), liver function tests, glucose, vitamin B_{12}, and protein electrophoresis.
- **Nerve conduction studies:** these can differentiate axonal degeneration (reduced amplitude of electrical impulse) from demyelination (reduced conduction velocity) and can characterize whether sensory and/or motor fibres are involved. They can also localize the sites of abnormality, e.g. in entrapment neuropathies.
- **Electromyography (EMG):** use of a fine needle inserted into the muscle can discern whether complete or partial denervation is present and whether reinnervation is occurring. This can help in localization depending on the distribution of muscles affected.
- **Nerve biopsy:** the sural nerve is the most commonly biopsied because it is purely sensory and the small resulting clinical deficit is therefore trivial. Pathological information can be gained from light and electron microscopy.
- **Cerebrospinal fluid (CSF) examination:** this may be helpful, for example, in inflammatory demyelinating neuropathies (Guillain–Barré syndrome or chronic inflammatory demyelinating polyradiculoneuropathy; see p. 154), when the protein content is usually raised, without inflammatory cells.

SPECIFIC NEUROPATHIES

Mononeuropathies

Peripheral nerve compression and entrapment neuropathies

Nerves can be damaged by compression either acutely (e.g. by a tourniquet or a tight-fitting cast over the leg) or chronically (e.g. carpal tunnel syndrome). This usually causes localized demyelination although, if prolonged, it may lead to axonal degeneration.

Acute compression tends to affect nerves that lie superficially to the skin (e.g. the common peroneal nerve at the fibular head by prolonged knee crossing or a tight-fitting plaster cast, or the radial nerve as it passes around the humerus, causing 'Saturday-night palsy').

Chronic compression causes 'entrapment neuropathies', which occur when the nerve passes through tight anatomical spaces (e.g. the median nerve in the carpal tunnel).

The most common nerves to be involved by compression are described below.

Carpal tunnel syndrome (median nerve compression at the wrist)

Carpal tunnel syndrome is usually idiopathic but can be associated with:

- Hypothyroidism.
- Pregnancy.
- Diabetes mellitus.
- Rheumatoid arthritis.
- Acromegaly.

It presents with tingling, pain, and numbness in the hand, which tends to wake the patient from sleep or in the morning. The pain may extend up the arm to the shoulder and be relieved by shaking of the arm and hand. In some cases there is weakness of the thenar muscles especially abductor pollicis brevis. Sensory loss affects the palm and the lateral three- and-a-half digits. If it is longstanding and severe then there may be wasting of abductor pollicis brevis. Tinel's sign may be present – tapping on the carpal tunnel reproduces tingling and pain.

Diagnosis is clinical and by electrophysiology confirming slowing of the impulse across the wrist with a reduced amplitude in some cases. Surgical decompression is the definitive procedure, although splints and steroid injections into the carpal tunnel may provide temporary relief (Fig. 23.3).

Ulnar nerve compression

Ulnar nerve compression is less common than carpal tunnel syndrome. Entrapment typically occurs at the elbow, where the nerve is compressed within the olecranon groove within the cubital tunnel, which lies behind the medial epicondyle. It can follow fracture of the ulna or prolonged/recurrent pressure at this site. The ulnar nerve may be compressed at other sites within the cubital tunnel such as between the two heads of flexor carpi ulnaris.

Ulnar neuropathy causes wasting and weakness of ulnar-innervated muscles of the forearm and hand and sensory loss in the ulnar one-and-a-half fingers. The patient characteristically develops an 'ulnar claw hand', especially when the nerve is affected at the wrist leaving the long ulnar flexors unopposed.

Electrophysiology localizes the lesion. Surgical decompression or anterior transposition can be performed but results from the latter procedure are generally poor and it is seldom performed in modern practice.

A more distal ulnar compression neuropathy can occur in the deep motor branch as it passes across the palm. This is due to regular pressure from tools, e.g. screwdrivers, crutches, or cycle handlebars (Fig. 23.4).

Radial nerve compression

Radial nerve compression occurs when the radial nerve is compressed against the humerus, e.g. when the arm is draped over the back of a chair for several hours ('Saturday-night palsy'), and results in wrist drop and weakness of finger extension and brachioradialis. Sensation is lost in the region of the 'anatomical snuffbox' on the dorsum of the hand over the base and shafts of the first two metacarpals. Recovery is usually spontaneous, but may take up to 3 months (Fig. 23.5).

Fig. 23.3 Carpal tunnel syndrome.

Motor loss	Reflex loss	Sensory loss
Abductor pollicic brevis	None	

Nerve sensitivity
Sometimes at the level of the carpal tunnel

Fig. 23.4 Ulnar nerve compression.

Motor loss	Reflex loss	Sensory loss
Flexor carpi ulnaris	None	
Flexor digitorum profundus to little and ring fingers		
All the small muscles of the hand except abductor pollicis brevis, opponens pollicis, lateral two lumbricals and part of flexor pollicis brevis		

Nerve sensitivity

Often quite marked on the medial side of the elbow

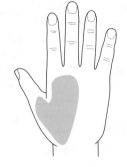

Fig. 23.5 Radial nerve compression.

Motor loss	Reflex loss	Sensory loss
Brachioradialis	Absent brachioradialis (supinator) jerk	
All extensors of wrist, fingers and thumb except extensor carpi ulnaris		

Nerve sensitivity

Usually none

Common peroneal nerve palsy

Common peroneal nerve palsy occurs when the nerve is compressed at the fibular head and can result from prolonged squatting or leg crossing, wearing a tight plaster cast, prolonged bed rest, or coma. It results in a foot drop and weakness of eversion and dorsiflexion, with sensory loss on the anterolateral border of the shin and dorsum of the foot. Recovery is usual, but not invariable, within a few months (Fig. 23.6).

Meralgia paraesthetica

This is the syndrome caused by the entrapment of the lateral cutaneous nerve of the thigh, beneath the inguinal ligament, which causes burning, tingling, and numbness on the anterolateral surface of the thigh. It usually occurs in overweight patients and weight loss may help (Fig. 23.7).

Multifocal neuropathy (mononeuritis multiplex)

Certain systemic illnesses are associated with multiple mononeuropathies. They can be caused by preferential sites of entrapment but also by a focal pathological process in a nerve(s) (e.g. infarction in diabetes). These include:

- Diabetes mellitus.
- Connective tissue disease, e.g. polyarteritis nodosa, systemic lupus erythematosus (SLE), rheumatoid arthritis – the pathology is usually a small vessel vasculitis.
- Sarcoidosis.
- Amyloidosis.
- Neurofibromatosis.
- AIDS.
- Leprosy.

Fig. 23.6 Common peroneal nerve palsy.

Motor loss	Reflex loss	Sensory loss
Foot evertors	None	
Foot dorsiflexors		
Toe dorsiflexors		

Nerve sensitivity

Sometimes, at the neck of the fibula

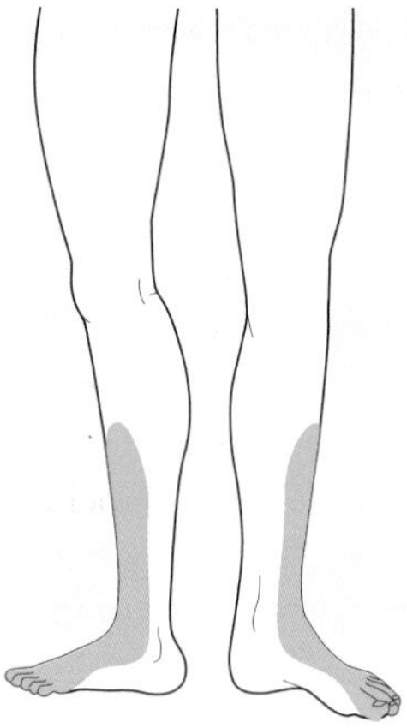

Fig. 23.7 Meralgia paraesthetica.

Motor loss	Reflex loss	Sensory loss
None	None	

Nerve sensitivity

Usually none

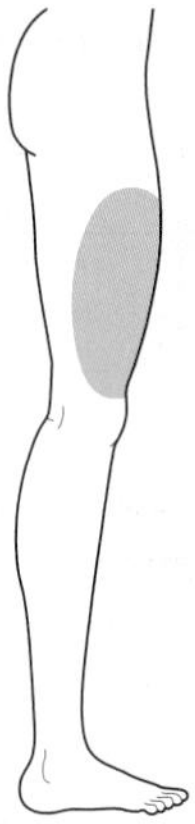

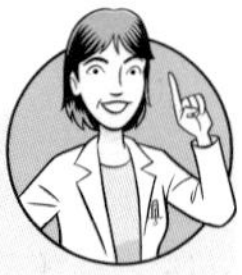

Small vessel vasculitic neuropathy can occur in isolation or in association with other connective tissue diseases, e.g. SLE, rheumatoid arthritis. Characteristically, it is associated with severe pain in the affected nerves and multiple mononeuropathy. It often affects muscle as well and therefore a combined biopsy of both muscle and nerve is often performed if the diagnosis is suspected. It is an important cause not to miss as a delay in diagnosis and treatment can lead to severe neurological deficits.

Polyneuropathies

Polyneuropathies can be classified according to their mode of onset, functional or pathological type, distribution, or causation. The classification used below is based on causation.

Polyneuropathies associated with systemic disease

A wide range of systemic diseases can affect the peripheral nerve. The following represent a small selection of the most common conditions.

Diabetic neuropathy

The neuropathies found in diabetes mellitus are often related to poor glycaemic control. The exact cause of the nerve damage is uncertain but may relate to sorbitol accumulation or to vascular disease in both large and small vessels.

A number of different types of neuropathy complicate diabetes:

- Distal symmetrical polyneuropathy: most commonly sensory but may be motor or autonomic. Improving glycaemic control has been demonstrated to reduce the risk of developing peripheral neuropathy.
- Proximal asymmetrical motor neuropathy: known as 'diabetic amyotrophy', acutely painful and occurs in older men.
- Autonomic neuropathy: with gastroparesis and resultant diarrhoea, arrhythmias, and postural hypotension.
- Mononeuropathies can be single or multiple, especially entrapment.
- Cranial nerve lesions: especially isolated third and sixth nerve palsies.
- Mononeuritis multiplex.

Renal disease

Chronic renal failure produces a progressive sensorimotor neuropathy. The response to dialysis is variable but the neuropathy usually improves after renal transplantation.

Paraneoplastic polyneuropathy

Malignant disease, especially small-cell carcinoma of the bronchus, can produce a sensory neuropathy affecting the large fibres leading to a sensory ataxic neuropathy. This is often associated with 'anti Hu' antineuronal antibodies. The neuropathy may predate the appearance of the malignancy by months or years.

Haematological malignancies such as multiple myeloma and other monoclonal gammopathies characteristically produce peripheral neuropathies that resemble chronic inflammatory demyelinating polyradiculoneuropathy (CIDP).

Connective tissue diseases and vasculitides

Connective tissue diseases and vasculitides classically produce a very painful mononeuritis multiplex, although individual diseases may produce a symmetrical sensorimotor neuropathy (especially SLE), entrapment neuropathy (rheumatoid arthritis), or trigeminal neuropathy (Sjögren's syndrome).

Porphyria

Acute intermittent porphyria produces a predominantly motor neuropathy in addition to abdominal pain, psychosis, and seizures. The onset is usually acute or subacute, similar to Guillain–Barré.

Amyloidosis

Amyloid is deposited around the vessels in the nerve, causing distortion. The neuropathy is characterized by predominantly sensory, painful, dysaesthetic features. Autonomic features are common.

Neuropathies caused by drugs and toxins

Drugs

A wide variety of drugs are known to cause a peripheral neuropathy. Most produce a chronic, progressive, sensorimotor polyneuropathy and are generally reversible. Examples of the most common include:

- Sensory axonal neuropathy: chloramphenicol, isoniazid (by affecting pyridoxine metabolism), phenytoin, Taxol.
- Motor axonal neuropathy: amphotericin, dapsone, gold.
- Sensorimotor axonal neuropathy: chlorambucil, cisplatin, disulfiram, nitrofurantoin, vincristine.
- Sensorimotor demyelinating neuropathy: amiodarone.

Toxins

A wide variety of metals and industrial toxins have been shown to cause polyneuropathy. Peripheral nerve involvement is often accompanied by other systemic features. For example:

- Lead causes a motor neuropathy.
- Arsenic and thallium cause a painful peripheral sensory neuropathy.
- Acrylamide, trichloroethylene, and fat-soluble hydrocarbons, e.g. as in glue sniffing, cause a progressive polyneuropathy.

Alcoholic neuropathy

Alcohol is the most common toxin associated with peripheral neuropathy. Alcoholic neuropathy is one of the most common forms of peripheral neuropathy (up to 30% of all cases of neuropathy).

It progresses slowly, with distal sensory loss, paraesthesiae, and burning pains. Distal muscle weakness may occur and spread proximally, with muscle cramps and gait disturbance.

The cause may be primarily due to alcohol toxicity but also due to a secondary deficiency of vitamins, particularly in thiamine and other B vitamins, as well as often having an inadequate general dietary intake.

Abstinence from alcohol, supplementation of thiamine, and a balanced diet constitute the principal therapy. The painful symptoms may be eased with the use of tricyclic agents (e.g. amitriptyline) or gabapentin.

Inflammatory demyelinating neuropathies

The group 'inflammatory demyelinating neuropathies' includes an acute neuropathy (Guillain–Barré syndrome) and CIDP.

Guillain–Barré syndrome (postinfective polyneuropathy)

Guillain–Barré syndrome (GBS) is an inflammatory, demyelinating polyradiculoneuropathy. It occurs world wide with an annual rate of 1.5 cases per 100 000 persons.

It often follows 1–3 weeks after a respiratory infection or diarrhoea, which may have been mild. *Campylobacter jejuni* has been particularly implicated as a cause of the diarrhoea and is associated with a more severe form. It may follow other infections such as HIV seroconversion or following vaccines.

The classic presentation is with distal paraesthesiae, often with little sensory loss, and weakness tends to occur proximally, distally spreading proximally or generalized. The symptoms ascend up the lower limbs and body over days to weeks. Facial weakness is present in 50% of cases. In severe cases, respiratory and bulbar involvement occurs, and ventilation may be required. If the vital capacity drops to 1 litre or below, artificial ventilation is often necessary. Autonomic dysfunction may also occur and cause arrhythmias.

A proximal variant of GBS exists, involving ocular muscles and associated with areflexia and ataxia (Miller–Fisher syndrome).

Diagnosis is usually clinical, supported by slowed conduction velocities on nerve conduction studies and a raised CSF protein. Both these investigations may be normal early in the disease.

Differential diagnoses include other paralytic illnesses such as poliomyelitis, myasthenia gravis, botulism, and primary muscle disease.

The use of intravenous immunoglobulin has been shown to produce significant improvement in the course of the disease and is equivalent to the more invasive plasmapheresis. Corticosteroids and immunosuppressive agents have not been successful in acute GBS. Careful management of the paralysed patient, and ventilation as indicated, are also essential. Recovery, although gradual over many months, is usual, but may be incomplete. Approximately 5% of patients develop a relapsing and remitting disease. A mortality rate of 10% is associated with inadequate ventilatory support, complications of immobility (aspiration, pulmonary embolism) and arrhythmias. By definition, the symptoms and signs cease to progress after 6 weeks or the disease becomes termed CIDP.

Chronic inflammatory demyelinating polyradiculoneuropathy (CIDP)

CIDP represents an often milder syndrome that is related to GBS but has a more protracted clinical course. The clinical, diagnostic features and pathology are similar to those of GBS. It is rarely associated with preceding infection.

Drug treatment includes corticosteroids, with or without other immunosuppressive agents such as azathioprine or cyclophosphamide, or recurrent intravenous immunoglobulin infusions/plasmapheresis.

Neuropathies caused by nutritional deficiencies

Thiamine (vitamin B_1) deficiency (beriberi)

Thiamine deficiency is strongly implicated in the causation of alcoholic neuropathy. In addition to the peripheral neuropathy, deficiency can cause Wernicke–Korsakoff syndrome (see Chapter 31, p. 211).

Pyridoxine (vitamin B_6) deficiency

Pyridoxine deficiency causes a mainly sensory neuropathy. It may be precipitated by isoniazid therapy for tuberculosis, and pyridoxine is therefore given in association with this drug.

Vitamin B_{12} deficiency

Peripheral neuropathy can occur in association with subacute combined degeneration of the cord (spastic paraparesis, loss of proprioception, paraesthesiae); B_{12} deficiency is also linked to optic neuropathies and dementia. Treatment involves intramuscular replacement injections (see Chapter 20, p. 136).

Vitamin E deficiency

Vitamin E deficiency occurs in the context of fat malabsorption. The onset of neurological symptoms takes many years. It involves a large-fibre sensory neuropathy with spinocerebellar degeneration.

Hereditary neuropathies

This section will consider the group of conditions known as the hereditary motor sensory neuropathies

(HMSN). These are also termed peroneal muscular atrophy or Charcot–Marie–Tooth (CMT) disease. Other types of hereditary neuropathy will be considered in Chapter 32.

With the advent of molecular genetic studies, the original classification system for HMSN is undergoing modification. Categories are as follows:

- CMT type I: most common form, autosomal dominant demyelinating neuropathy with hypertrophy of nerves ('onion-bulb' formation on electron microscopy); onset at age between 5 and 15 years.
- CMT type II: autosomal dominant axonal neuropathy; onset 10 and 20 years.

- CMT type III (Dejerine–Sottas disease): autosomal dominant or recessive demyelinating neuropathy with gross hypertrophy of peripheral nerves and often the CSF protein is raised due to hypertrophied nerve roots.
- Complex forms of HMSN: additional features such as optic atrophy, retinitis pigmentosa, deafness, and spastic paraparesis can coexist.

General characteristics of hereditary motor sensory neuropathies

All forms of HMSN are characterized by distal wasting of the lower limbs, which progresses, often over many years, and may involve the upper limbs.

When the wasting in the legs is severe they resemble 'inverted champagne bottles' (Fig. 23.8). The wasting is accompanied by reduced or absent reflexes and a variable loss of sensation.

Pes cavus (loss of lateral arch) with clawing of the toes is almost invariable. These features may be the only signs in mild cases. Clawing of the hands may also be seen.

The age of onset varies from childhood to middle age. There is variability within subgroups and within families.

The causes of peripheral neuropathies are summarized in Fig. 23.9.

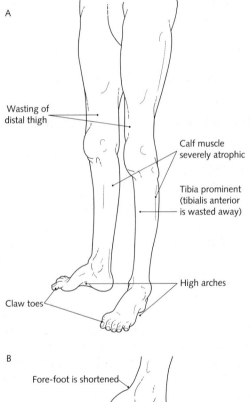

A

Wasting of distal thigh

Calf muscle severely atrophic

Tibia prominent (tibialis anterior is wasted away)

High arches

Claw toes

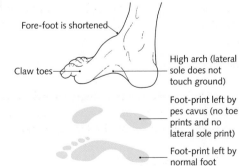

B

Fore-foot is shortened

Claw toes

High arch (lateral sole does not touch ground)

Foot-print left by pes cavus (no toe prints and no lateral sole print)

Foot-print left by normal foot

Fig. 23.8 'Inverted-champagne-bottle' legs of hereditary motor sensory neuropathy.

Fig. 23.9 Summary of causes of peripheral neuropathies	
Inflammatory	Guillain–Barré syndrome Chronic inflammatory demyelinating polyradiculoneuropathy
Metabolic	Diabetes Renal disease Porphyria
Nutritional deficiencies	Vitamin B_1 Vitamin B_6 Vitamin B_{12} Vitamin E
Toxic	Drugs: isoniazid, vincristine, nitrofurantoin Alcohol Lead
Connective tissue disease	Systemic lupus erythematosus Rheumatoid arthritis Polyarteritis nodosa
Malignancy (paraneoplastic)	Bronchus Breast, ovarian, uterus
Hereditary	HMSN syndromes
Trauma	Entrapment mononeuropathies Limb injuries

Disorders of the neuromuscular junction

Objectives

- Understand the anatomy and neurophysiology of the neuromuscular junction
- Describe the clinical features of myasthenia gravis
- Understand the investigations and management of myasthenia gravis

The normal anatomy and physiology of the neuromuscular junction are outlined in Fig. 24.1. A normal electrical impulse passes down motor nerves towards skeletal muscle. Each motor axon divides up into a number of terminal branches just before it reaches the muscle. Each one of these branches ends at the presynaptic nerve terminal. The electrical impulse causes calcium to flood into the terminal and acetylcholine-containing vesicles to fuse with the nerve membrane, thereby releasing acetylcholine into the synaptic cleft. The acetylcholine crosses the synaptic cleft and binds to acetylcholine receptors on the postsynaptic muscle end-plate membrane. This results in depolarization of the muscle fibre and subsequent contraction of the muscle. The acetylcholine is then broken down by acetylcholinesterase, which is bound to the basement membrane in the synaptic folds.

Two main diseases of neuromuscular transmission will be discussed in this chapter – myasthenia gravis and Lambert–Eaton myasthenic syndrome (LEMS).

MYASTHENIA GRAVIS

Myasthenia gravis is an acquired, organ-specific autoimmune disorder, of unknown cause, in which antibodies are directed against the postsynaptic acetylcholine receptor. This results in weakness and fatigability of skeletal muscle groups. The most commonly affected muscles are the proximal limbs, the ocular and bulbar muscles.

There is often an associated abnormality of the thymus in patients with myasthenia gravis. Thymic hyperplasia is found in 70% of patients below the age of 40 years. In 10% of all patients with myasthenia gravis, a benign thymic tumour (thymoma) is found. The incidence of thymomas increases with age. In patients with thymoma, antibodies to striated muscle may also be found.

There appear to be two distinct groups of patients who develop myasthenia gravis, split by age and sex:

- Young women (20–35 years), who tend to have an acute, severely fluctuating, more generalized condition, with increased association with HLA-B8 and HLA-DR3.
- Older men (60–75 years), who tend to have a more oculobulbar presentation.

There is some crossover between the groups, and myasthenia gravis is seen in young men and older women, but much less frequently.

Clinical features

The clinical features of myasthenia gravis are listed in Fig. 24.2. The most important of these is fatiguability of power. This causes fluctuating weakness, which is worse after exercise and at the end of the day.

Fatiguability can be demonstrated by exercising affected muscles (e.g. making a patient in whom ptosis is sometimes apparent, look upwards for 1–2 minutes). The ptosis will become more severe and the eyes may drift to the primary position. Similar manoeuvres can be carried out for the proximal limb muscles.

Limb reflexes are normal or hyperactive but fatigue on repeated testing. Muscle wasting is rare, occurring at a late stage in only a minority of more severe cases. It is rarely as severe as in disorders affecting the motor cell body or nerve. Sensory examination is normal.

Fig. 24.1 The neuromuscular junction. Antibodies directed against acetylcholine receptors cause myasthenia gravis, whereas antibodies against the presynaptic voltage-gated calcium channels cause Lambert–Eaton myasthenic syndrome.

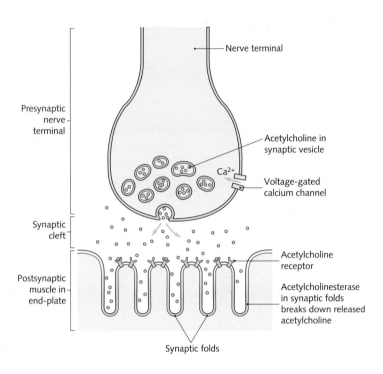

Presynaptic nerve terminal

Synaptic cleft

Postsynaptic muscle in end-plate

Nerve terminal

Acetylcholine in synaptic vesicle

Ca^{2+}

Voltage-gated calcium channel

Acetylcholine receptor

Acetylcholinesterase in synaptic folds breaks down released acetylcholine

Synaptic folds

Fig. 24.2 Symptoms of myasthenia gravis

Ocular	Ptosis
	Diplopia
Other cranial muscles	Weak face and jaw
	Dysarthria
	Dysphonia
	Dysphagia
Limb weakness	Usually proximal-shoulder and hips
Axial weakness	Neck and trunk
	Respiratory muscle

Any young woman with a complex ophthalmoplegia is likely to have myasthenia, MS or thyroid eye disease. With bilateral ptosis in addition to ophthalmoplegia, myasthenia is probable and, very rarely, ocular myopathies. In thyroid eye disease there will typically be proptosis, not ptosis, and in MS usually other brainstem symptoms or signs.

Investigations

Tensilon (edrophonium) test

Edrophonium is a fast-acting anticholinesterase (i.e. it antagonizes the action of acetylcholinesterase and thus prevents the breakdown of acetylcholine). This enables more acetylcholine to stimulate the reduced numbers of acetylcholine receptors. When edrophonium is given as an intravenous bolus, usually with atropine to prevent cardiac side effects, weakness improves within seconds and for only 2–3 minutes. This can be used as a diagnostic test for myasthenia gravis, although many neurologists are now relying on the other tests available and reserving this test if the others are negative and the clinical suspicion is high.

Serum acetylcholine receptor antibody

The highly specific acetylcholine receptor antibody is present in the serum of up to 85% of patients with generalized myasthenia gravis.

Electromyography

There are two classic electromyographic findings in myasthenia gravis:

- A decrement in amplitude (progressive 'fatigue') of the compound muscle action potential following repetitive stimulation.
- Increased jitter using a single-fibre electrode.

Thymus imaging

It is essential to image the chest with computed tomography or magnetic resonance imaging for the presence of thymic hyperplasia or tumour, as removal of a hyperplastic thymus may improve the condition in some patients and removal of thymomas prevents malignant transformation.

Autoantibodies

Other autoantibodies may be present, especially those against striated muscle and thyroid.

Spirometry

The patient's vital capacity (VC) needs to be checked. A VC falling below 1.5 L requires transfer of the patient to ITU/HDU before frank ventilatory failure occurs.

Any known myasthenic with new onset bulbar dysfunction should have their VC carefully monitored. There can often be very few other features of myasthenia at the start of a relapse and neuromuscular respiratory weakness can be missed. Patients may complain that their breathing is difficult lying flat but this is not invariable.

Management

The illness may have a protracted and fluctuating course. Acute exacerbations may be unpredictable or may follow infections or treatment with certain drugs. It is important to recognize respiratory involvement, as assisted ventilation may be required. Patients may remit permanently, however, especially after thymectomy or with immunosuppressive treatment.

Oral acetylcholinesterases

Pyridostigmine is the most widely used drug; it has a duration of action of about 3–5 hours. The patient's response will determine the dosage required.

Overdosage causes a cholinergic crisis with severe weakness, which may be difficult to differentiate from the myasthenic weakness. Colic and diarrhoea may also occur.

Acetylcholinesterases are excellent symptomatic drugs but do not alter the natural history of the disease.

Thymectomy

In patients with thymic hyperplasia, thymectomy, for unknown reasons, improves the prognosis of the disease, especially in those under 40 years of age and in those who have had the disease for less than 10 years.

In patients with a thymoma, surgery is essential to remove a potentially malignant tumour but this rarely results in improvement of the myasthenia.

Immunosuppression

Corticosteroids provide the mainstay of immunosuppressive treatment. An excellent response is seen in 70% of patients but the dose must be increased slowly, preferably in hospital, as there is often a temporary exacerbation of symptoms before the therapeutic effect.

Plasmapheresis is sometimes used, especially during an acute exacerbation or when there is respiratory involvement. The effects only last a few days and therefore must be repeated if required.

Intravenous immunoglobulin may be used in the acute setting to control severe myasthenia especially if the respiratory muscles are involved.

Azathioprine is used as a steroid-sparing agent.

Myasthenia gravis mainly affects younger woman who can find the disfigurement of ptosis, facial weakness and ophthalmoplegia distressing at diagnosis. The patient should be reassured that the disease is highly treatable with a good prognosis.

LAMBERT–EATON MYASTHENIC SYNDROME

Lambert–Eaton myasthenic syndrome (LEMS) is a rare condition associated with antibodies that are directed against the presynaptic voltage-gated calcium channels at the neuromuscular junction. This results in a failure of acetylcholine release from the presynaptic nerve terminal. In many cases, it is a non-metastatic manifestation of malignancy, especially small-cell carcinoma of the lung.

LEMS is characterized by weakness of the proximal limb muscles, especially in the lower limbs. Ocular and other cranial muscles are typically spared. There may be fatiguability but, characteristically, there is a paradoxical initial improvement in power after exercise, followed by sustained weakness. Reflexes are usually absent, but then return following use of the muscle ('post-tetanic potentiation'). Autonomic involvement is especially common in cases associated with an underlying malignancy.

The diagnosis can be confirmed electromyographically by an 'incremental' increase of the compound muscle action potential after repetitive stimulation (the opposite to myasthenia gravis). A search should be made for malignancy, especially bronchial, although the tumour may not be found initially, only to appear several years later.

Guanethidine hydrochloride and 4-aminopyridine may enhance acetylcholine release. Steroids and plasmapheresis may also help. The prognosis for those with a primary lung tumour is usually poor.

OTHER MYASTHENIC SYNDROMES

Even rarer myasthenic syndromes include:

- Congenital myasthenia gravis: patients develop weakness as newborns often due to mutations within the apparatus that allows release of acetylcholine from the presynaptic terminal.
- Neonatal myasthenia gravis: this is caused by transfer of antibodies to the acetylcholine receptor across the placenta to the baby and usually resolves after delivery.
- Penicillamine-induced myasthenia.

BOTULINUM TOXIN

Clostridium botulinum is a bacterium that can make a preformed toxin which, when ingested, can cause food poisoning. It is a very rare condition and the toxin can damage the neuromuscular junction, resulting in a condition resembling severe, acute myasthenia gravis. However, this very powerful neuromuscular-blocking toxin is used routinely in neurological practice, in small doses, to treat unwanted muscular activity. The indications include cervical dystonia, blepharospasm, and severe limb spasticity following stroke or multiple sclerosis.

Disorders of skeletal muscle

- Understand the basic anatomy of skeletal muscle
- Describe the features in the history which help diagnose a muscle disorder
- Understand the tests used to investigate muscle disease
- Understand the main clinical features of hereditary and inflammatory myopathies
- Describe the myopthies associated with systemic disease

Anatomy

Skeletal muscle is made up of large numbers of multinucleated muscle fibres, which have an outer membrane (sarcolemma) and cytoplasm (sarcoplasm) and in which lie the contractile components of the muscle (myofibrils). The fibres are separated by connective tissue (endomysium) and arranged in bundles (fasciculi). Each fasciculus has a connective tissue sheath (perimysium). The muscle is made up of a number of fasciculi bound together and surrounded by a connective tissue sheath (epimysium) (Fig. 25.1).

There are two broad types of muscle fibre, which are functionally different:

1. Type I: rich in myoglobulin, with low metabolism (aerobic) and rich in sarcoplasm.
2. Type II: low in myoglobin, with high metabolism (aerobic or anaerobic) and little sarcoplasm.

CLINICAL FEATURES OF MUSCLE DISEASE (MYOPATHY)

Muscle has rather uniform structure and function and thus diseases of muscles from a variety of causes can produce similar clinical features. The general features of muscle disease will therefore be summarized prior to discussion of the most common and important specific diseases.

Weakness

Myopathies are characterized by weakness of muscles and the distribution is usually proximal, involving shoulders, hips, trunk, neck and sometimes face.

Each muscle disease exhibits a particular pattern of involvement (e.g. proximal limb, facial, and proximal upper arm), which is an important diagnostic clue. Careful examination of all muscle groups is important to classify a myopathy, and to differentiate it from a lower motor neuron (LMN) disorder or CNS disorder.

Changes in muscle tone

There may be a loss of tone (hypotonia) secondary to disease of muscle, although this sign can be difficult to differentiate from normal tone.

Changes in muscle bulk

Wasting of the affected (proximal) muscles is distinctive, in contrast to the distal wasting of most neuropathies.

Enlargement of muscle may be the result of overactivity or an early sign in certain dystrophies, caused by infiltration of fat, exacerbating the weakness (pseudohypertrophy).

Changes in reflexes

These are usually preserved in muscle disorders, at least until wasting and weakness is severe, which helps to distinguish myopathies from LMN syndromes.

Changes in muscle contractility

Myotonia – persistence of contraction, often for several seconds, during attempted relaxation – is found in myotonic dystrophy, paramyotonia congenita, hyperkalaemic periodic paralysis, and congenital myotonia. On electromyography (EMG), the characteristic findings consist of rhythmic discharges. This phenomenon may also be elicited by a sharp tap on

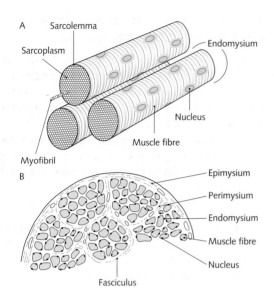

Fig. 25.1 Normal skeletal muscle morphology: (A) longitudinal muscle fibres; (B) cross-section of muscle.

the muscle belly (percussion myotonia). Myotonia must be differentiated from neuromyotonia, which is derived from nerve abnormalities.

In McArdle's syndrome, there is a characteristic fixed shortening of the muscle that follows a series of strong contractions. This needs to be differentiated from cramp.

Pain

Pain is a rare complaint in primary muscle disease except in deficiencies of certain enzymes of the carbohydrate or lipid pathways or in severe inflammatory myopathy (e.g. polymyositis, vasculitis).

FAMILY HISTORY

Many muscle diseases are inherited and therefore a full family history is essential. Inherited muscles diseases include:

- X-linked: Duchenne muscular dystrophy, Becker's muscular dystrophy, Emery–Dreifuss dystrophy.
- Autosomal dominant: facio-scapulo-humeral dystrophy, scapuloperoneal dystrophy, myotonic dystrophy.
- Autosomal recessive: limb-girdle dystrophy, all deficiencies of enzymes of glycolytic and lipid metabolism.

- Mitochondrial: sometimes maternal inheritance. Chronic progressive external ophthalmoplegia, Kearns–Sayre syndrome.

INVESTIGATION OF MUSCLE DISEASE

The diagnosis may be possible from the clinical features in some causes of muscle disease. Other helpful tests include:

- **Serum creatine phosphokinase (CPK; creatine kinase, CK):** this is often significantly raised in many dystrophies and in inflammatory muscle disorders, e.g. polymyositis.
- **EMG:** needle examination will reveal 'myopathic units' (small, short-duration, spiky polyphasic units). There may be evidence of myotonic discharges in myotonias.
- **Muscle biopsy:** this can yield information about fibre type (type I or II), inflammation, and dystrophic and histochemical changes. Electron microscopy is sometimes required.

SPECIFIC DISEASES

Myopathies can be subdivided as in Fig. 25.2. Important examples are discussed below.

Hereditary myopathies

Muscular dystrophies

Duchenne muscular dystrophy

Duchenne muscular dystrophy is an X-linked recessive condition caused by an absence of dystrophin, a protein that is vital for connecting the cytoskeleton of muscle cells to the extracellular matrix through the membrane. It occurs in 20–30/100 000 liveborn males. It also affects skeletal and cardiac muscle.

Clinical features Patients with Duchenne muscular dystrophy display no abnormality at birth but the condition is apparent by the fourth year. The child is usually wheelchair-bound by 10 years old and death is usual by the age of 20, from respiratory failure or cardiomyopathy.

There is initially proximal muscle weakness with pseudohypertrophy of the calves. The weakness then spreads. When rising to an erect position, there is a

Fig. 25.2 Hereditary and acquired myopathies

Hereditary myopathies	Muscular dystrophies	Duchenne Becker's Facio-scapulo-humeral Limb-girdle
	Myotonic disorders	Myotonic dystrophy Myotonia congenita
	Metabolic myopathies	Myophosphorylase deficiency (McArdle's disease) Phosphofructokinase deficiency Lactate dehydrogenase deficiency Carnitine palmityl transferase deficiency
	Periodic paralyses	Hypokalaemic Hyperkalaemic
	Mitochondrial myopathies	Kearn Sayres
Acquired myopathies	Inflammatory	Polymyositis Dermatomyositis Inclusion body myositis
	Metabolic or endocrine myopathies	Cushing's syndrome Hyper- or hypothyroidism Hypokalaemia
	Drug-induced	Zidovudine (AZT), steroids, statins, amiodarone, alcohol
	Paraneoplastic	Often necrotising
	Critical Illness	Probably multifactorial

characteristic manoeuvre in which the patient has to 'climb' his legs with his hands (Gower's sign) (Fig. 25.3).

Diagnosis The diagnosis of Duchenne muscular dystrophy is often made clinically. The CK is grossly elevated (often 10 000 U/L). The EMG is myopathic

and muscle biopsy shows fatty infiltration and absence of staining for dystrophin.

Management There is no cure for Duchenne muscular dystrophy so the management is supportive. Steroids may provide short-term improvement. Genetic counselling is important. Carrier females may have a raised CK and mildly myopathic EMG but without any clinical symptoms or signs. An accurate and rapid DNA diagnosis is now available, allowing reliable identification of carrier status and prenatal diagnosis if required.

Becker's muscular dystrophy
Becker's muscular dystrophy is also an X-linked recessive condition, with similar characteristics to Duchenne muscular dystrophy, but it has a much milder course. Dystrophin is altered rather than absent.

Clinical features The symptoms of Becker's muscular dystrophy begin in the first decade, although often are not noticed until later. Children continue to walk into their teens and early adult life. Cramps associated with exercise are common. The effects of the cardiomyopathy can be worse than the skeletal weakness and patients are predisposed to developing arrhythmias. These patients often succumb to the cardiac effects before the skeletal muscle problems.

Other muscular dystrophies
Other muscular dystrophies include facio-scapulo-humeral dystrophy (autosomal dominant), scapuloperoneal dystrophy (autosomal dominant), and limb-girdle dystrophy (can be autosomal recessive or dominant). The clinical presentations vary from mild and slowly progressive to rapidly fatal.

Myotonic disorders

Myotonic dystrophy (dystrophia myotonica)
Myotonic dystrophy is an inherited condition caused by an expanded trinucleotide repeat (CTG) on

Fig. 25.3 Gower's sign. This involves having to climb up the legs with the hands to overcome pelvic muscle weakness. It is found in any condition with pelvic muscle weakness.

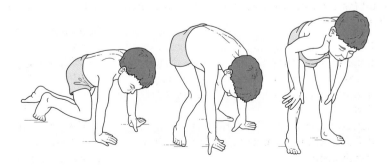

chromosome 19 and thus causes 'anticipation', whereby successive generations are more severely affected. Myotonic dystrophy is unusual in that it is female transmission that results in more severely affected offspring rather than paternal transmission which is seen in other forms of anticipation. The features may be very mild in some cases if the length of the expanded repeat is only just above normal.

It is a multisystem disease resulting in (Fig. 25.4):

- Progressive proximal and distal muscle weakness especially in the upper limbs.
- Myotonia (worse in the cold).
- Myopathic facies (weakness and thinning of the face and sternomastoids).
- Ptosis.
- Cataracts.
- Frontal balding.
- Mild intellectual impairment and sleep disturbance.
- Cardiomyopathy and conduction defects.
- Gynaecomastia and testicular atrophy.
- Bronchiectasis.
- Glucose intolerance/diabetes mellitus

The features develop between the ages of 20 and 50 years, and progress gradually.

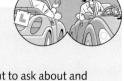

Patients with myotonic dystrophy are often polysymptomatic and hypersomnolent. It is important to ask about and investigate for nocturnal hypoventilation and test for diabetes as these are two common causes of fatigue and sleepiness. Patients are also prone to cardiac conduction deficits and therefore require regular ECGs (at least yearly or when symptomatic).

Metabolic myopathies

Any disturbance of the biochemical pathways that support ATP levels in muscle will cause exercise intolerance, with pain during exercise and extreme fatigue. Continued exercise will lead to destruction of muscle (rhabdomyolysis) and the release of myoglobin, which may cause the patient's urine to turn red-orange and renal failure can ensue.

There are a large number of specific enzyme deficiencies with autosomal recessive inheritance where the gene has been described. Only one will be discussed here.

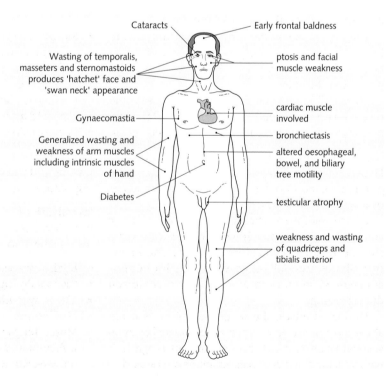

Fig. 25.4 Clinical features of myotonic dystrophy.

Cataracts

Early frontal baldness

Wasting of temporalis, masseters and sternomastoids produces 'hatchet' face and 'swan neck' appearance

ptosis and facial muscle weakness

Gynaecomastia

cardiac muscle involved

bronchiectasis

Generalized wasting and weakness of arm muscles including intrinsic muscles of hand

altered oesophageal, bowel, and biliary tree motility

Diabetes

testicular atrophy

weakness and wasting of quadriceps and tibialis anterior

Myophosphorylase deficiency (McArdle's syndrome)

McArdle's syndrome is an autosomal recessive condition with deficiency of myophosphorylase in skeletal muscle. Symptoms begin during teenage years, with fatigue and severe pain during exercise. Continued exercise cause true contractures, which are silent on EMG (as opposed to cramp), and there is a risk of developing myoglobinuria.

A diagnostic sign is the absence of a rise in venous lactate during an ischaemic forearm exercise test (using a blood-pressure cuff).

Periodic paralyses

The periodic paralyses are rare membrane disorders that are now recognized to be among a group of disorders known as channelopathies. They are characterized by episodes of sudden weakness with alterations in serum potassium levels.

Hypokalaemic periodic paralysis

Hypokalaemic periodic paralysis is an autosomal dominant condition that is caused by abnormalities in L-type calcium channels.

Patients present between 10 and 20 years of age and may remit after 35 years of age. Attacks of generalized weakness develop after a heavy carbohydrate meal or after a period of rest following strenuous exertion (e.g. the following morning).

During an attack, the serum potassium falls to below 3.0 mmol/L. Attacks may last from 4 to 24 hours. The weakness responds to treatment with potassium chloride.

The condition is rarely fatal, as the diaphragm and respiratory muscles tend to be spared. Similar weakness with hypokalaemia may occur in thyrotoxicosis.

Hyperkalaemic periodic paralysis

Hyperkalaemic periodic paralysis is an autosomal dominant condition that is caused by abnormalities of voltage-gated sodium channels.

It becomes apparent between 5 and 15 years of age and tends to remit after 20 years of age; however, a chronic proximal myopathy may persist. The attacks of weakness, especially of proximal muscles, become apparent 30 minutes to 2 hours after exercise and during fasting.

During an attack, the serum potassium is raised above 5.0 mmol/L. Attacks may be terminated by intravenous calcium gluconate or by salbutamol. Prophylaxis with thiazide diuretics or acetazolamide can be used.

Mitochondrial myopathies

The final oxidative pathway involves the respiratory chain in mitochondria, which have their own DNA. Abnormalities of mitochondrial DNA (maternally inherited) cause a wide range of different conditions affecting muscle, the CNS, and other systems within the body. Mutations in nuclear genes encoding mitochondrial proteins are now being described and may also present with a muscle disorder.

Inflammatory myopathies

Polymyositis and dermatomyositis

Polymyositis and dermatomyositis are conditions in which there is inflammation within the muscle. There may be associated connective tissue disease (25%) or underlying carcinoma (10%), especially if skin changes are present (dermatomyositis).

Clinical features

Polymyositis and dermatomyositis usually present in the fourth to fifth decade, with women more commonly affected than men. Proximal muscle weakness is the cardinal symptom (difficulty rising from a chair or climbing stairs). Pain and tenderness of the muscles occurs in less than half the patients.

The associated skin changes (dermatomyositis) include:

- Macular erythema on the face-especially in the periorbital area, where it is heliotrope (blue-violet) in colour.
- Erythematous plaques over the dorsal aspects of the fingers (Gottron's papules).
- Nail-fold haemorrhages.
- Photosensitivity.

As the disease progresses, there may be widespread wasting and weakness, with bulbar dysfunction and respiratory muscle weakness.

Investigations

Investigations for polymyositis and dermatomyositis include the following:

- Erythrocyte sedimentation rate (ESR): raised.
- CK: usually highly raised.
- EMG: myopathic picture but may include fibrillations.
- Muscle biopsy: muscle fibre necrosis with an inflammatory infiltrate which is distinct for polymyositis and dermatomyositis

- Autoantibodies (anti-Jo, antinuclear antibodies, rheumatoid factor, ENAs): present in up to 25% of patients.
- Investigation for underlying carcinoma (chest X-ray as a minimum).

Treatment

Corticosteroids and other immunosuppressive drugs (e.g. azathioprine, cyclophosphamide) reduce the symptoms in about 75% of cases of polymyositis and dermatomyositis that are not associated with malignancy. Removal of an associated tumour may cause complete remission.

There is full recovery in about 10% of patients. The remainder of patients have varying degrees of disability and the disease may become inactive or 'burnt out' after a few years. When associated with connective tissue disease, the prognosis is linked to the course of this disease.

Patients with an inflammatory myopathy often have neck weakness and this is one cause of presentation with a 'dropped head', i.e. forward flexion of the neck. Others are motor neuron disease and myasthenia gravis.

Inclusion body myositis

This degenerative disease of muscle is becoming more widely recognized. It is the most common cause of muscle disease in people aged over 50 years, occurs more frequently in men, and often presents with weakness and wasting of the flexor muscles of the forearm and hand. The proximal muscles can also become involved, particularly the quadriceps, and the oesophagus may be affected as the disease progresses.

The investigation of choice is the muscle biopsy as characteristic inclusions are seen in muscle fibres. Occasionally, there may be inflammation on the biopsy and some patients have a limited response to steroids. The underlying cause is not known but the association of other autoimmune diseases with inclusion body myositis suggests that it may have an immunological basis, although other evidence suggests it is a degenerative disease of age.

The prognosis is progressive disability and death from the consequences of immobility.

Acquired electrolyte and endocrine myopathies

A wide range of diseases (especially endocrinological), acquired biochemical abnormalities, and drugs can result in myopathy (Fig. 25.5). The weakness tends to be proximal. Most cases are reversible with treatment of the primary condition or removal of the drug.

Thyrotoxicosis

Patients often have greater shoulder than pelvic girdle involvement. Reflexes are brisk. Fasciculations and atrophy may be present.

Cushing's syndrome

A proximal myopathy can be seen in patients who are taking long-term steroids or who have an underlying steroid-secreting neoplasm.

Fig. 25.5 Common investigations and causes of aquired myopathies

Investigation	Cause of myopathy
Full blood count and ESR	Polymyositis systemic connective tissue disease Carcinoma
Electrolytes and renal function tests	Hypokalaemia (diuretics or laxatives) Renal disease Cushing's syndrome
Liver function tests	Alcohol abuse chronic liver disease
Calcium; phosphate; alkaline phosphatase	Vitamin D deficiency
Thyroid function tests	Thyrotoxicosis Hypothyroidism
Cortisol studies	Cushing's disease
Creatine kinase	Raised in many myopathies
CXR; abdominal Ultrasound; mammogram	Underlying carcinoma
History of drugs or toxins	Alcohol Steroids Statins Clofibrate Chloroquine Zidovudine (AZT)

Hypokalaemia

Hypokalaemia can be associated with a painless proximal myopathy. This is often caused by potassium-losing drugs, including liquorice.

Vitamin D deficiency

Proximal muscle pain and wasting can occur in the context of vitamin D deficiency. The weakness often improves over several weeks with vitamin replacement.

Drug-induced myopathies

Statins are increasingly recognized to be associated with a variety of muscle disorders, ranging from asymptomatic raised creatine kinase through to muscle pain and overt myopathy. The causative statin should be stopped in all but the mildest cases and a different statin commenced and monitored. Steroids are a common cause of drug-induced myopathy. Chloroquine, amiodarone and doxorubicin can all cause a dose-related vacuolar myopathy associated with proximal weakness. The causative drug should be stopped.

Zidovudine (AZT) is used in the treatment of HIV infection and can cause a dose-related proximal myopathy associated with mitochondrial dysfunction. Recovery usually occurs after the drug is stopped.

Paraneoplastic myopathy

A necrotizing myopathy can occur with malignancies, especially colorectal, lung, and breast, independent of either polymyositis or dermatomyositis.

Critical Illness myopathy

Patients who are ventilated can sometimes develop a severe myopathy. It can present as an inability to wean off the ventilator and may be associated with prolonged use of paralysing agents (e.g. vecuronium). It is a symmetric proximal myopathy but the neck flexors may be involved and respiratory failure occurs in 80% of cases. Patients often show a slow improvement but associated illness leads to a mortality of up to 50%. Muscle biopsy shows myosin loss in muscle fibres and the cause of this remains uncertain.

Vascular diseases of the nervous system

- Define: stroke and TIA
- Understand the vascular supply to the brain and spinal cord
- Describe the main stroke syndromes
- Understand the management of stroke and TIA – what risk factors are treatable?
- Understand the presentation and management of subarachnoid haemorrhage

CEREBROVASCULAR DISEASE

Cerebrovascular disease is a principal cause of mortality and morbidity in the developed world. Strokes of all types rank third as a cause of death and are surpassed only by heart disease and cancer.

Definitions

Stroke

Stroke is a focal, non-convulsive, neurological deficit caused by a vascular lesion. The onset is sudden and the symptoms last longer than 24 hours, if the patient survives.

Thromboembolic vascular occlusion accounts for 85% of strokes and the most common presentation is hemiplegia caused by occlusion of the contralateral middle cerebral artery. These are called 'ischaemic' strokes because they cause ischaemia and infarction distal to vessel occlusion. This is in contrast to strokes due to intracerebral haemorrhage, which are usually caused by rupture of microaneurysms (Charcot–Bouchard aneurysms), secondary to chronic hypertension. These are less common but it is often difficult to distinguish them clinically from thromboembolic strokes. Ischaemic and infarcted brain can occasionally become haemorrhagic; this is called 'haemorrhagic transformation' and is important to recognize because it is a cause of later deterioration in a patient with an ischaemic stroke.

Transient ischaemic attack (TIA)

A TIA is a focal, non-convulsive, neurological deficit lasting less than 24 hours, with complete clinical recovery, caused by focal hypoperfusion within the brain. Examples of the types of deficits that can occur as listed in Fig. 26.1. The symptoms are often recurrent and repeated episodes are often stereotypical. The onset of symptoms is usually sudden.

Almost a third of patients who have a TIA will develop a disabling stroke within 5 years; the majority of strokes will occur within 18 months and the risk is highest during the days and weeks after a TIA. Prompt investigation and preventive strategies are therefore essential.

Incidence of stroke

The incidence of stroke is 150–200 cases per 100 000 persons per annum (this varies regionally around the UK).

The incidence of TIA is 30 cases per 100 000 persons per annum, although many probably go unreported.

The rates increase markedly with advancing age.

Aetiology of stroke

The causes of stroke are as follows (the first five are responsible for the majority of cases):

- **Atherosclerosis:** this causes thrombotic stroke in large extracranial arteries, most commonly the carotid arteries, or intracranial arteries arising from the Circle of Willis.
- **Cardiac or carotid embolism:** embolic stroke usually arises from pieces of ruptured atherosclerotic plaques or cardiac thrombus lodging in distal narrow sites. The bifurcation of the common carotid and akinetic segments of myocardium, e.g. after a heart attack or in atrial fibrillation, are the most common sources of emboli.

Fig. 26.1 Clinical features of transient ischaemic attacks (TIAs)

Anterior circulation (carotid arteries)	Posterior circulation (vertebrobasilar arteries)
Amaurosis fugax	Diplopia, vertigo
Dysphasia	Dysarthria/dysphagia
Contralateral hemiparesis	Unilateral/bilateral or alternating paresis or sensory loss
Contralateral homonymous visual field loss	Binocular visual loss
Any combination of the above	Ataxia
	Loss of consciousness (rare)
	Any combination of the above

- **Arterial dissection:** in the younger population, dissection of either the carotid or vertebral arteries is being acknowledged as a relatively common cause of stroke. There may be no antecedent history of injury to the neck, but sudden twisting movements or flexion/extension injuries, e.g. 'whiplash' are associated. Emboli from mural thrombosis associated with the dissection is a common mechanism of stroke in this setting.
- **Intracerebral haemorrhage:** this is most often secondary to chronic untreated hypertension but can be caused by other factors, e.g. trauma, anticoagulant therapy, neoplasia, and coagulation disorders, such as haemophilia, or abnormalities of platelet number or function.
- **Lipohyalinosis of small arteries:** this degenerative process especially affects small perforating arteries that supply structures deep to the cortex, e.g. basal ganglia, internal capsule and pons. It usually occurs in patients with chronic untreated hypertension. Occlusion of these penetrating arteries causes subcortical infarcts, less than 1.5 cm in diameter, which are called 'lacunes'. Occasionally, their rupture can lead to a small, but clinically devastating, haemorrhage.
- **Diseases of the vessel wall:** these are rarer than the above causes but should always be considered, especially in young patients who present with stroke. Causes include rheumatoid vasculitis, systemic lupus erythematosus, polyarteritis nodosa, and temporal arteritis (in the elderly). Infections involving the base of the brain, e.g. tertiary syphilis and TB meningitis, can also block large blood vessels.

Risk factors

- **Hypertension:** this is a major factor in the development of ischaemic and haemorrhagic stroke.
- **Diabetes mellitus:** this increases the risk of cerebral infarction twofold and should be treated aggressively because it is a recognized risk factor for atherosclerosis.
- **Cardiac disease:** in addition to cardiac causes of embolic strokes, e.g. atrial fibrillation, cardiomyopathy, arrhythmias, and valve disease; the presence of coronary artery disease is a marker for atherosclerosis elsewhere and is therefore a marker for stroke.
- **Hyperlipidaemia:** this is less significant for stroke than for coronary artery disease.
- **Smoking:** cessation of smoking lowers the risk of ischaemic stroke.
- **Family history:** close relatives are at slightly greater risk than non-genetically related family members of a stroke patient. Diabetes and hypertension show familial propensity, thus clouding the significance of pure hereditary factors.
- **Obesity and diet:** these are probably less significant for stroke than for coronary artery disease.
- **Oral contraceptive:** this may increase risk of thromboembolic stroke, cerebral venous thrombosis, and subarachnoid haemorrhage in vulnerable individuals.

Vascular anatomy

A knowledge of the arterial blood supply to the brain and of the common sites for atheromatous plaque formation is important for an appreciation of the various presentations and significance of cerebrovascular disease.

The circle of Willis (Fig. 26.2) is supplied anteriorly by the two carotid arteries and posteriorly by the basilar artery, which is formed by the union of the two vertebral arteries (Fig. 26.3). It is therefore common to classify strokes into those affecting the anterior (carotid) and posterior (vertebrobasilar) circulations.

The most common sites for atheromatous plaques are:

- The origin of the internal carotid arteries.
- Within the carotid syphon.
- The origin of the vertebral arteries.

The anterior, middle, and posterior cerebral arteries arise from the circle of Willis. These supply specific

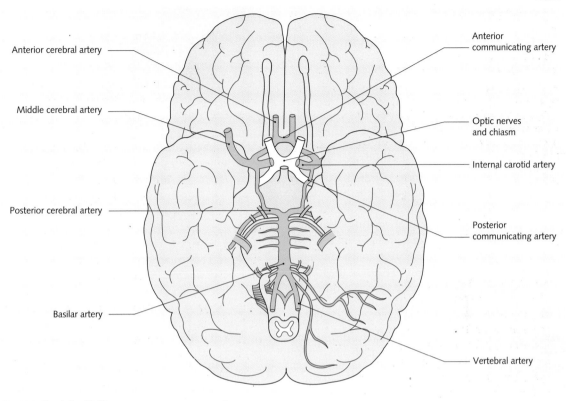

Anterior cerebral artery

Middle cerebral artery

Posterior cerebral artery

Basilar artery

Anterior communicating artery

Optic nerves and chiasm

Internal carotid artery

Posterior communicating artery

Vertebral artery

Fig. 26.2 The circle of Willis.

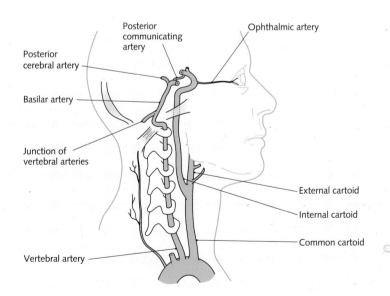

Posterior cerebral artery

Basilar artery

Junction of vertebral arteries

Vertebral artery

Posterior communicating artery

Ophthalmic artery

External cartoid

Internal cartoid

Common cartoid

Fig. 26.3 The vertebrobasilar and carotid arteries.

portions of the cerebral hemispheres (Figs 26.4, 26.5 and 26.6); thus, reduction in perfusion in each territory will cause different and specific deficits.

Clinical syndromes

Middle cerebral artery occlusion

The middle cerebral artery is the largest branch of the internal carotid artery and supplies the largest area of the cerebral cortex (see Fig. 26.4 and Fig. 1.1, p. 4). It is the most commonly involved artery in stroke. As well as supplying the motor and sensory cortices, the middle cerebral artery supplies the areas of the cortex pertaining to the comprehension (Wernicke's area) and expression (Broca's area) of speech (see Fig. 26.4 and Fig. 26.5). These areas are found in the dominant hemisphere only, and thus, in the majority of right-handed individuals, speech production will be affected only when there is occlusion of the left middle cerebral artery. Non-dominant lesions often cause visuospatial problems, e.g. inattention. Lesions of either side can be associated with hemianopia.

The signs of a middle cerebral artery occlusion are listed in Fig. 26.7. Initially, the limbs are flaccid and areflexic. After a variable period, the reflexes recover and become exaggerated, and the plantar responses become extensor, with spastic limb tone. There is variable recovery of weakness over the course of days, weeks, or months.

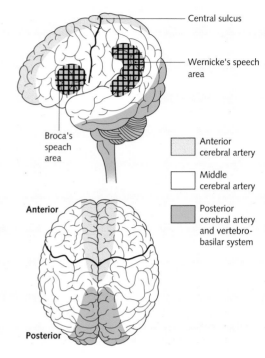

Fig. 26.4 The distribution of the three major cerebral arteries (lateral and tomographic views).

Anterior cerebral artery occlusion

The anterior cerebral artery is a branch of the internal carotid artery and runs above the optic nerve to follow the curve of the corpus callosum. The two arteries are linked by the anterior communicating artery and thus

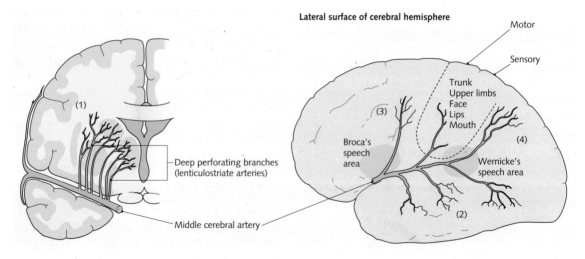

Fig. 26.5 The middle cerebral artery is the largest branch of the internal carotid artery. It gives off (1) deep branches (perforating vessels – lenticulostriate), which supply the anterior limb of the internal capsule and part of the basal nuclei. It then passes out to the lateral surface of the cerebral hemisphere at the insula of the lateral sulcus. Here it gives off cortical brances: (2) temporal, (3) frontal, and (4) parietal.

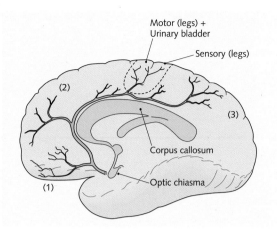

Motor (legs) +
Urinary bladder

Sensory (legs)

(2)

(3)

Corpus callosum

Optic chiasma

(1)

Fig. 26.6 Medial surface of the right cerebral hemisphere. The anterior cerebral artery is a branch of the internal carotid and runs above the optic nerve to follow the curve of the corpus callosum. Soon after its origin, the vessel is joined by the anterior communicating artery. Deep branches pass to the anterior part of the internal capsule and basal nuclei. Cortical branches supply the medial surface of the hemisphere: (1) orbital; (2) frontal, and (3) parietal.

Fig. 26.7 Signs of middle cerebral artery occlusion

Contralateral hemiplegia (including the lower part of the face and relative sparing of the leg)
Contralateral cortical hemisensory loss
Dominant hemisphere (usually left): aphasia
Non-dominant hemisphere: neglect of contralateral limb and dressing apraxia
Contralateral homonymous hemianopia

---

the effect of occlusion depends on the relation with respect to the anterior communicating artery (see Fig. 26.2 and Fig. 26.6). Occlusion proximal to the anterior communicating artery is normally well tolerated because of adequate cross-flow, and thus few symptoms result. Occlusion distal to the anterior communicating artery causes contralateral weakness and cortical sensory loss in the leg (see Fig. 12.1, p. 72 and Fig. 13.1, p. 82). Incontinence is often present, and occasionally a contralateral grasp and other primitive reflexes. It is relatively uncommon for the anterior cerebral to be purely involved in stroke; it is often involved secondary to occlusion more proximally in the internal carotid.

Posterior cerebral artery occlusion

The posterior cerebral arteries are the terminal branches of the basilar artery. In addition to cortical branches to the temporal lobe and occipital and visual cortices, there are perforating branches that supply the midbrain and thalamus.

The effect of occlusion depends on the site:

- Proximal occlusion: midbrain syndrome (Weber's syndrome), third nerve palsy and contralateral hemiplegia, thalamic syndrome, chorea or hemiballismus, hemisensory disturbance.

- Cortical vessel occlusion: homonymous hemianopia with macular sparing (the macular area is additionally supplied by the middle cerebral artery).
- Bilateral occlusion: Anton's syndrome (cortical blindness). The patient is blind but lacks insight into the degree of visual loss and often denies it.

Lacunar infarction

Approximately 25% of ischaemic strokes are due to infarction of the internal capsule subsequent to occlusion of small perforating vessels. These originate from the origin of the middle cerebral artery and dive deep within the brain to supply parts of the internal capsule, basal ganglia, and thalamus. Although these vessels supply a very small area, a number of extremely important structures pass through this space. A very small lesion can cause a marked neurological deficit. Lacunes also occur in the brainstem, especially the pons. These are usually associated with lipohyalinosis and chronic hypertension affecting the small perforating vessels. Chronic hypertension can be associated with very small Charcot–Bouchard aneurysms within the internal capsule and basal ganglia. These structures can rupture and cause up to 70% of primary intracerebral haemorrhages in hypertensive patients.

Primary intracerebral haemorrhage

The most common non-traumatic causes include chronic hypertension, aneurysms, and vascular malformations. When in conjunction with chronic hypertension, primary intracerebral haemorrhage often occurs in the internal capsule and/or basal ganglia, but it can occur in any part of the cortex, as well as in the pons and cerebellum. The clinical signs depend on the location but are often associated with mass effect and therefore reduced conscious level. It is otherwise very difficult to clinically differentiate a haemorrhage from an infarct.

Brainstem stroke

Multiple patterns of deficit can arise depending on the exact location of the lesion with respect to the long tracts (i.e. corticospinal, medial and lateral lemnisci, brainstem connections to the cerebellum, and cranial nerve nuclei). Possible clinical features are summarized in Fig. 26.8.

Specific brainstem syndromes

Lateral medullary syndrome (posterior inferior cerebellar artery syndrome; Wallenberg's syndrome) Lateral medullary syndrome (Fig. 26.9) is the most widely recognized brainstem syndrome. Clinical features

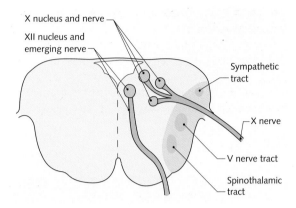

Fig. 26.9 Posterior inferior cerebellar artery syndrome (lateral medullary syndrome).

comprise sudden onset vertigo, vomiting, nystagmus, ipsilateral ataxia (cerebellar connections), ipsilateral facial numbness (fifth cranial nerve descending tract), ipsilateral Horner's syndrome (sympathetic tract), contralateral loss of pain and temperature sensation in the limbs (ascending spinothalamic tract) and dysarthria and dysphagia (tenth nerve). See also Fig. 13.4, p. 85.

'Locked-in syndrome' This distressing state is caused by a bilateral infarction in the ventral pons, with or without medullary involvement. The patient is conscious (intact brainstem reticular formation) but is mute and paralysed. Patients can often move their eyes because of sparing of the third and fourth cranial nuclei in the midbrain.

Weber's syndrome Weber's syndrome is caused by a lesion in one half of the midbrain, resulting in an ipsilateral third nerve palsy (III nucleus) and contralateral hemiplegia (descending pyramidal tract above the decussation).

Clinical evaluation of strokes

History

It is essential to take a good history from the patient, if possible, or from a relative or friend. The onset is usually acute, over several minutes to hours, with the development of a fixed neurological deficit (e.g. hemiplegia). The course may be slightly stuttering over hours or there may have been a 'warning TIA' in the previous hours or days. The presence of a severe progressive headache may indicate haemorrhage, although ischaemic infarcts can also present with headache. A slowly progressive course may indicate

Fig. 26.8 Features of brainstem infarction

Clinical features	Structures involved
Upper motor neuron Hemiparesis or tetraparesis	Corticospinal tracts (pyramidal tracts)
Hemisensory or bilateral sensory impairment	Medial lemniscus or Spinothalamic tracts
Diplopia	3rd, 4th (midbrain), and/or 6th (pons) cranial nerves or nuclei or their connections, e.g. median longitudinal fasciculus
Facial sensory loss	5th cranial nerve nucleus (midbrain, pons, medulla)
Lower motor neuron facial weakness (upper and lower face)	7th nerve nucleus (pons)
Nystagmus, vertigo	Vestibular nuclei (pons and medulla) and connections
Dysphagia, dysarthria	9th and 10th cranial nerve nuclei (medulla)
Dysarthria, ataxia, vomiting, hiccoughs	Cerebellum and cerebellar brainstem connection
Horner's syndrome (meiosis, ptosis, enophathalmos, and disturbed sweating)	Sympathetic fibres in lateral brainstem
Altered consciousness	Reticular formation

an alternative diagnosis such as tumour with progressing oedema.

Progressive impairment of consciousness may indicate raised intracranial pressure secondary to a large cerebral haemorrhage, a large complete anterior circulation infarct or coning caused by a cerebellar haemorrhage, and must be acted upon urgently.

> The clinical picture of 'stroke' may also be caused by other conditions such as tumour, abscess, subdural haematoma, and subarachnoid haemorrhage. Any unusual features in the history and examination must be further investigated.

Risk factors

Risk factors should be elucidated and a drug history taken, especially for use of anticoagulants.

Past medical history

A history of TIAs point towards a thromboembolic stroke. A history of connective tissue disease, neoplasia, bleeding disorders, arrhythmias, and other cardiological diseases should be sought.

Examination

In the examination, particular care should be taken to find possible causes of embolus (atrial fibrillation, carotid bruit, valve lesion, or evidence for endocarditis), and to ascertain whether the patient is or has been hypertensive and whether there is asymmetry between the two brachial pressures (evidence for subclavian stenosis).

Initial investigations

The following routine investigations should be performed:

- Full blood count (FBC): polycythaemia; infection.
- Erythrocyte sedimentation rate (ESR); C-reactive protein (CRP): inflammatory disease.
- Urinalysis and blood sugar: diabetes mellitus.
- Fasting lipids.
- Blood culture: if endocarditis or a superadded infection is suspected.
- Autoantibodies and coagulation studies in young patients: connective tissue disease or prothrombotic disorder.

- Electrocardiography (ECG): arrhythmia or myocardial ischaemia/infarction.
- Chest X-ray: neoplasia/heart failure.

Special investigations

Imaging

Current guidelines suggest that patients should have a computed tomography (CT) scan within 24 hours of a stroke. This is mainly to differentiate between an ischaemic and a haemorrhagic stroke, which determines how soon the patient is commenced on antiplatelet agents. In elderly patients, in whom strokes are most common, information gained by CT scanning rarely changes the management. However, if there is any doubt about the aetiology of the stroke, or there is the possibility of surgical intervention (e.g. cerebellar haemorrhage), a CT scan should be undertaken.

Magnetic resonance imaging (MRI) should be considered if the lesion is clinically located in the posterior fossa (i.e. brainstem and cerebellum) as these regions are poorly visualized by CT because of artefacts caused by the surrounding bone. MRI should also be considered in patients who may have had a small stroke, which may not be visible on CT and so the diagnosis is uncertain. Vascular reconstructive imaging using CT angiography (CTA) and MR angiography (MRA) is helpful in visualizing the intra- and extracranial carotids and the posterior circulation to look for atheromatous disease, dissections, and aneurysms.

Carotid Doppler

Carotid Doppler is an extremely effective, non-invasive means of demonstrating internal carotid artery stenosis when carotid thromboembolism is suspected or a carotid bruit is heard. Progress to carotid endarterectomy is considered if there is greater than 70% stenosis in a vessel, which corresponds to contralateral symptoms within the last 6 months. If the patient is left with a very dense hemiplegia and other cortical problems (e.g. dysphasia) then there is little value in performing carotid Doppler. If the patient makes a partial or full recovery then there is brain left to protect and the patient might benefit from carotid investigation and intervention.

Angiography

The advent of carotid Doppler and MRA has meant that conventional cerebral angiography is now used less in stroke patients; however, it is used for location of intracerebral aneurysms and for diagnosis of cerebral vasculitides, which are both still poorly detected with MRA. In patients with a recent completed stroke, angiography should not be considered until 1–2 weeks have elapsed.

Management of transient ischaemic attacks

- Confirm the diagnosis from history and examination.
- Investigate possible sites of the primary lesion, e.g. carotid stenosis, cardiac embolus secondary to atrial fibrillation.
- Identify and treat risk factors, e.g. hypertension.
- Aspirin: this reduces platelet aggregation and should be routinely used unless any contraindications exist to reduce the risk of further events.
- Dipyridamole: the concomitant use of this antiplatelet drug with aspirin has been shown in one trial to reduce the incidence of completed stroke by almost half that of aspirin alone.
- Anticoagulation (heparin and warfarin): this is not to be encouraged routinely because anticoagulants can precipitate haemorrhagic stroke and cause haemorrhage into an infarct. However, they are indicated in patients with a known cardiac source of embolus and atrial fibrillation, once a scan has excluded haemorrhage.

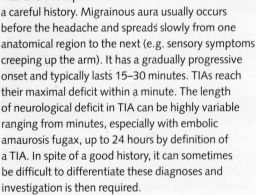

Distinguishing between TIAs and migrainous aura is vital and this is possible with a careful history. Migrainous aura usually occurs before the headache and spreads slowly from one anatomical region to the next (e.g. sensory symptoms creeping up the arm). It has a gradually progressive onset and typically lasts 15–30 minutes. TIAs reach their maximal deficit within a minute. The length of neurological deficit in TIA can be highly variable ranging from minutes, especially with embolic amaurosis fugax, up to 24 hours by definition of a TIA. In spite of a good history, it can sometimes be difficult to differentiate these diagnoses and investigation is then required.

- Clopidogrel: this may be used if aspirin is ineffective or poorly tolerated. There is growing evidence that it prevents reocclusion of vascular stents.

Management of a completed stroke

The management of a completed stroke is mainly supportive at present, although trials of thrombolytic agents over the past few years have demonstrated that tissue plasminogen activator (tPA) – a thrombolytic agent – reduces mortality and morbidity from ischaemic infarcts if given within 3 hours of the onset of the stroke; in selected cases it may be beneficial up to 6 hours. The logistics of transferring patients to hospital and performing a CT head scan has precluded this treatment from all but the most dedicated and specialized centres in the UK.

The management aims are as follows:

- Confirm diagnosis (history, examination, and investigations).
- Prevent progression of present event.
- Prevent development of complications, e.g. aspiration pneumonia, pressure sores, dislocated shoulders.
- Rehabilitate the patient, e.g. physiotherapy, occupational therapy, and speech therapy.
- Control hypertension only if it is severely elevated, i.e. systolic >220 mmHg and diastolic >120 mmHg. An acute drop in blood pressure can reduce perfusion to an already ischaemic brain.
- Encourage the patient to stop smoking and initiate the patient into a formal programme. This measure improves the longevity of the patient by reduction of coincidental ischaemic heart disease as well as stroke.
- Correct lipid abnormalities.
- Good glycaemic control in diabetic patients.
- Give aspirin (300 mg o.d.) and dipyridamole.
- Remove or treat embolic source, e.g. anticoagulation, antibiotics for endocarditis, or endarterectomy. Note: anticoagulation is indicated for cardiac embolus but only once haemorrhage has been excluded and not for at least 7 days after an acute event, to prevent a haemorrhagic infarct.
- Treat inflammatory or connective tissue diseases.
- Stop thrombogenic drugs, e.g. oral contraceptives.

Prevention of cerebrovascular disease by identifying and controlling risk factors has a greater effect in the reduction of death and disability than any medical or surgical intervention once a stroke has occurred.

Prognosis

The mortality of stroke is 10% in the first week, 20% in the first month and 30% within one year. The mortality is greater in patients with intracerebral haemorrhage, although these patients can recover well from acutely severe deficits because of the gradual reduction of the effects of associated oedema.

A worse prognosis is indicated by coma (suggesting raised intracranial pressure and 'coning'), defects in conjugate gaze with hemiplegia (suggesting involvement of the total anterior circulation), and severe hemiplegia.

There is a 10% recurrence of stroke within the first year.

There is a further 60–70% mortality rate within 3 years resulting from complications (e.g. chest infection, pulmonary embolus) and from other atherosclerotic disease (e.g. myocardial infarction).

Among the survivors, gradual improvement usually occurs but many are left with severe residual deficits. About a third of patients return to independent mobility but even these patients often have subtle to overt cognitive deficits (e.g. poor memory or concentration). Depression is very common in patients after a stroke and it should be treated aggressively because it can limit rehabilitation. The cardiac side-effects limit the use of the older tricyclic antidepressants.

INTRACRANIAL HAEMORRHAGE

Intracranial haemorrhage can be subdivided by site:

- Primary intracerebral haemorrhage (considered in the section on cerebrovascular disease).
- Subarachnoid haemorrhage.
- Subdural and extradural haemorrhage.

Subarachnoid haemorrhage

Subarachnoid haemorrhage is caused by spontaneous (rather than traumatic) arterial bleeding into the subarachnoid space.

Incidence

The incidence of subarachnoid haemorrhage is 10–15 cases per 100 000 persons per year.

Causes

- Saccular ('berry') aneurysms: 70%.
- Arteriovenous malformations (AVMs): 10%.
- Not defined: 20%.

Clinical features

- Patients complain of a severe headache of instantaneous onset (like a sudden 'blow to the head'). The patient often describes it as the worst headache they have ever had.
- Transient or prolonged loss of consciousness or seizure may follow immediately.
- Nausea and vomiting often occur due to raised intracranial pressure.
- Drowsiness or coma may continue for hours to days.
- Signs of meningism occur after 3–12 hours: neck stiffness on passive flexion; positive Kernig's sign (lifting the leg and extending the knee with the patient lying supine, stretches the nerve roots and causes meningeal pain).
- Focal signs from a haematoma may be present, e.g. limb weakness, dysphasia.
- Papilloedema may be present and may be accompanied by subhyaloid and vitreous haemorrhage.

Investigation

CT scanning is the investigation of choice and shows subarachnoid or intraventricular blood in 90% of patients.

Lumbar puncture should only be carried out if a CT scan is not available or if the scan is inconclusive, and then only if the patient is alert and orientated without focal signs, i.e. no evidence of raised intracranial pressure. In a patient with a mass lesion, lumbar puncture can precipitate transtentorial herniation or 'coning'. The diagnosis of subarachnoid haemorrhage can be made when the cerebrospinal fluid (CSF) is uniformly bloodstained or xanthochromic (straw-coloured supernatant), due to breakdown products of haemoglobin accumulating over a period of six hours or more. An extra 5% of cases of subarachnoid haemorrhage can be diagnosed after lumbar puncture. Therefore, 95% of cases can be diagnosed following CT head and CSF analysis but, in the remaining 5% of cases, these tests are normal and if the clinical history is suggestive of subarachnoid haemorrhage, formal angiography will need to be performed to exclude the diagnosis.

Angiography is carried out at the earliest convenience in most patients, but is delayed in patients with a poor clinical condition. Angiograms are required to localize aneurysms and arteriovenous malformations prior to intervention and to confirm the cause of the diagnosis.

Immediate management

- Regular neurological observations.
- Bed rest and fluid replacement.
- Analgesia for headache: codeine or dihydrocodeine (stronger analgesics may depress conscious level and mask deterioration).
- Nimodipine (a calcium-channel blocker): reduces vasospasm and morbidity/mortality.
- Control of hypertension (but care should be taken to avoid hypotension, which can cause deterioration).
- The routine use of prophylactic anticonvulsants is controversial, but if seizures occur anticonvulsants should be commenced.
- Transfer to neurosurgical unit.

Subsequent management

Berry aneurysms are the most common finding at angiography. There is growing evidence that the majority of aneurysms are best treated endovascularly by placing platinum coils in the aneurysm if the anatomy is suitable. In selected cases, surgery to clip the neck of the aneurysm still provides excellent results and is most appropriate when the neck of the aneurysm is very wide or the aneurysm itself is very large. The timing of surgery is up to the individual surgeon; however, some believe that early surgical intervention may be harmful, because of retraction of a swollen non-compliant brain, and the usual wait is between 3 and 14 days from the haemorrhage, depending on the patient's condition and the grade of the haemorrhage. Current trials are elucidating which approach is best in different clinical scenarios.

Arteriovenous malformations can be treated conservatively, or with direct surgery, radiosurgery, endovascular embolization, or a combination of these.

Prognosis

There is a mortality rate of almost 50% prior to admission to hospital. Of patients surviving the initial bleed, 30% die within 3 months; of these, 10–20% die from further bleeding within the first month. Almost half the survivors make a good functional recovery.

Operative mortality ranges from 5 to 50%, depending on the patient's clinical condition and the timing of embolization or surgery.

Prognostic guides include age, quantity of subarachnoid blood on CT scan, loss of consciousness at ictus, clinical condition on admission, and presence of pre-existing hypertension or arterial disease.

Subdural and extradural haemorrhage

Both subdural and extradural haemorrhage can be fatal unless treated promptly.

Subdural haematoma

Subdural haematoma occurs as a result of rupture of cortical veins bridging the dura and brain. It is almost invariably caused by trauma to the head in a patient with a shrunken brain (e.g. elderly and alcoholics).

In an acute subdural haemorrhage, there can be rapid accumulation of blood with a space-occupying effect, leading to rapid transtentorial 'coning'.

With a chronic subdural haematoma, the initial injury may be minor and there may be a latent interval, from days to months, between injury and symptoms. Chronic subdural haematoma is common in the elderly and in alcoholics. Symptoms can be indolent and fluctuate and include headache, drowsiness (a key feature), and confusion. However, focal deficits (usually hemiparesis), seizures, stupor, and coma can occur.

Extradural haemorrhage

Extradural haemorrhage is caused by a traumatic tear in the middle meningeal artery, usually associated with a temporal or parietal skull fracture.

Blood accumulates rapidly in the extradural spaces, over minutes to hours. After a lucid period, the patient may then develop focal signs, coma, and transtentorial coning, leading to death.

Management

Diagnosis is by CT scan (Fig. 26.10).

Urgent surgical drainage is undertaken for acute subdural or extradural haematoma. Chronic subdural haematoma is often evacuated through burr holes as an elective procedure.

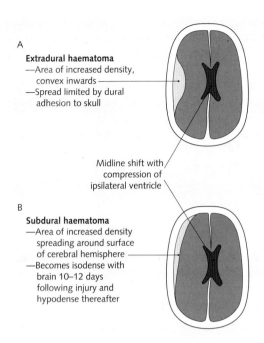

A

Extradural haematoma
—Area of increased density,
 convex inwards
—Spread limited by dural
 adhesion to skull

Midline shift with
compression of
ipsilateral ventricle

B

Subdural haematoma
—Area of increased density
 spreading around surface
 of cerebral hemisphere
—Becomes isodense with
 brain 10–12 days
 following injury and
 hypodense thereafter

Fig. 26.10 (A) Extradural haematoma: biconvex, high-density lesion abutting the inner margin of the skull. Midline ventricular shift and sulcal effacement can occur in both subdural and extradural haematomas if they are sufficiently large. (B) Subdural haematoma: crescent-shaped, high-density lesion lying adjacent to the inner margin of skull. As the haematoma ages, it can become isodense with the brain substance.

CEREBROVASCULAR INVOLVEMENT IN VASCULITIS AND CONNECTIVE TISSUE DISEASE

The vasculitides and connective tissue diseases cause inflammation and necrosis of blood vessels. Cerebral involvement can be part of a generalized systemic disease or isolated to the cranial vessels (Fig. 26.11).

All these conditions can cause stroke (ischaemic or haemorrhage) and should be considered in any young patient with stroke or any patient with unusual or systemic features. Seizures are relatively common and the history is often one of step-wise progression.

Many of the conditions can present with other signs of neurological involvement of either the central or peripheral nervous system (e.g. a painful neuropathy).

Investigations

Investigations should include ESR, CRP, autoantibodies, imaging (MRI), angiography, CSF, and, if appropriate, biopsy of the skin, muscle, kidney, or other affected organ. If there is a strong suspicion of vasculitis confined to the CNS and angiography shows no diagnostic features, then biopsy of the brain and meninges may be necessary to make the diagnosis.

Fig. 26.11 Connective tissue diseases and vascultides that can present with stroke

Connective tissue diseases	Vasculitides
• Systemic lupus erythematosus • Rheumatoid arthritis • Sjögren's syndrome	• Polyarteritis nodosa • Wegener's granulomatosis • Giant-cell arteritis – temporal arteritis • Takayasu's arteritis • Behçet's disease • Granulomatous angilitis

Treatment

Treatment is with steroids and other immuno-suppressive drugs such as cyclophosphamide.

CEREBRAL VENOUS THROMBOSIS

Blood from the brain is drained by cerebral veins, which empty into dural sinuses, which subsequently drain into the internal jugular veins.

Venous sinus thrombosis is associated with:

- Pregnancy, puerperium, oral contraception.
- Haematological diseases, e.g. polycythaemia.
- Dehydration, e.g. prolonged vomiting.
- Infection: the middle ear, paranasal sinuses and face all drain into the dural sinuses.

- Inflammatory disorders, e.g. Behçet's disease, sarcoidosis, systemic lupus erythematosus.
- Head injury.
- Malignant meningitis.

The superior sagittal sinus is most commonly involved, followed by the lateral sinus and cavernous sinus, although all are uncommon.

Clinical features

The clinical features of thrombosis in the major sinuses and cerebral veins are variable. The most common presentations are headache, motor and sensory deficit, seizures, altered consciousness, and papilloedema. The thrombosis within the sinus may lead to venous infarction in the territory draining into the affected sinus.

Cavernous sinus thrombosis

Cavernous sinus thrombosis warrants a special mention because it has a distinctive clinical picture. The cavernous sinus drains venous blood from the eye and many important structures run by or through it, including the carotid artery and the third, fourth, fifth (ophthalmic division), and sixth cranial nerves. In classic, acute cases of cavernous sinus thrombosis, there is proptosis, chemosis, and painful ophthalmoplegia.

Diagnosis

MRI is now a key procedure for diagnosis of cerebral venous thrombosis.

Treatment

Treatment regimens for cerebral venous thrombosis remain controversial and vary in different centres. Symptomatic treatments include anticonvulsants, antibiotics (if associated with infection) and methods to reduce intracranial pressure. Anticoagulation with heparin is controversial but most clinicians would commence anticoagulation if the degree of venous infarction is not too severe.

SPINAL CORD VASCULAR DISEASE

The blood supply to the spinal cord is complex. The main vessels are the paired posterior spinal arteries, which run down the posterior surface of the cord, and the single anterior spinal artery, which runs down the median fissure anteriorly (Fig. 26.12).

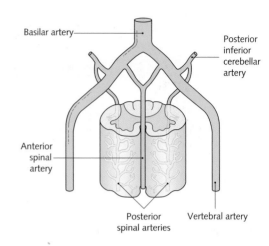

Fig. 26.12 Vascular supply of the spinal cord.

During development, five to eight radicular arteries become predominant and provide most of the flow to the spinal cord through the anterior spinal artery. The largest is the artery of Adamkiewicz, which enters at the T9–T11 level and supplies the major portion of blood to the lower thoracic cord and lumbar enlargement.

The midthoracic region is most vulnerable because the supply to the anterior spinal artery often consists of only one significant radicular artery and because there is a poor anastomotic network at this level.

The posterior spinal arteries have a rich collateral supply and therefore the posterior part of the cord is relatively protected from the effects of vascular disease, including the dorsal columns.

Figure 26.13 shows the vascular supply of the cord in cross-section and indicates the supply of the major pathways.

Anterior spinal artery syndrome

If the anterior spinal artery becomes occluded, the supply to the anterior two-thirds of the cord is disrupted causing anterior spinal artery syndrome, resulting in disruption of the corticospinal and spinothalamic tracts bilaterally (see Fig. 26.13).

Causes

- Small-vessel disease, e.g. diabetes, polyarteritis, systemic lupus erythematosus.
- Arterial compression or occlusion, e.g. disc fragments, extradural mass, dissecting aortic aneurysm, aortic surgery.

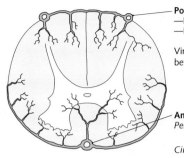

Posterior spinal artery territory
—Posterior one-third of spinal cord
—Dorsal columns

Virtually no anastomotic communication
between anterior and posterior territories

Anterior spinal artery territory
Penetrating braches   —Anterior and part of
                                posterior grey matter
Circumferential branches—Anterior white matter
                                —Anterior two-thirds
                                of spinal cord

Fig. 26.13 Cross-sectional view of the vascular supply of the spinal cord.

- Embolism, e.g. aortic angiography, decompression sickness.
- Hypotension: the arterial watershed at the midthoracic region is especially susceptible to hypoperfusion, e.g. pericardiac arrest.

Clinical features

The clinical features of anterior spinal artery syndrome are dependent on the level of the lesion and include:

- Segmental pain at onset: usually in the back and around the trunk.
- Sphincter disturbance: usually urinary retention but incontinence of bladder and bowel can occur.
- Flaccid paraparesis, which progresses to spasticity over days (corticospinal tracts). Tetraparesis is

less common because the thoracic cord is most vulnerable.

- Areflexia below the level of the lesion, which progresses to hyperreflexia and extensor plantar responses over days.
- Loss of pain and temperature sensation up to the dermatome level at which the lesion occurred (spinothalamic tracts).

Note: vibration and joint-position sense are not affected as the dorsal columns are supplied by the posterior spinal artery.

Management

Treatment is symptomatic. The prognosis for recovery is variable but usually poor.

Intracranial tumours can be defined as benign or malignant lesions within the cranial cavity. They can be:

- **Primary:** primary intracranial tumours account for approximately 10% of all neoplasms and represent 60% of all intracranial neoplasms. They can be derived from neuroepithelial cells (gliomas), the meninges (meningiomas), nerve sheath cells (Schwannomas), the anterior pituitary (adenomas), or blood vessels (haemangiomas).
- **Secondary:** metastatic carcinoma (e.g. lung, breast) or lymphoma.

The relative frequencies of the most common intracranial tumours are shown in Fig. 27.1.

TYPES OF INTRACRANIAL TUMOUR

Gliomas

Gliomas are malignant, intrinsic brain tumours originating from astrocytes and oligodendrocytes. They usually occur within the cerebral hemispheres. They virtually never metastasize outside the CNS and spread only by direct extension.

There are many different types. The most common are presented below.

Astrocytoma

Astrocytomas arise from astrocytes and are the most common primary brain tumour. They can be separated histologically into four grades dependent on the degree of malignancy (grade I: slow-growing over years; grade IV: death within months).

Glioblastoma multiforme

A glioblastoma multiforme is a highly malignant tumour with no cell differentiation, preventing identification of its tissue of origin.

Oligodendroglioma

Oligodendrogliomas arise from oligodendrocytes and form slow-growing, sharply defined tumours that may become calcified. Variants include an anaplastic form and a mixed astrocytoma/oligodendroglioma.

Ependymoma

Derived from ependymal cells and choroid plexus, ependymomas can arise anywhere throughout the ventricular system or spinal canal but usually in the fourth ventricle or cauda equina. They spread through cerebrospinal pathways and infiltrate surrounding tissue.

Meningiomas

Meningiomas are benign tumours that arise from the arachnoid membrane and granulations and may grow to a large size, usually over many years. They tend to compress adjacent brain structures rather than infiltrate. Calcification is common and they may erode adjacent bone. They are rare below the tentorium cerebelli.

Pituitary tumours

Pituitary tumours may cause endocrine dysfunction that is not always apparent to the patient. They may also present with visual symptoms due to chiasmal compression and can result in bitemporal hemianopia

Fig. 27.1 Relative frequencies (RF) of the most commonest intracranial tumours

Tumour	RF %
Metastases	40
Gliomas	33
Meningiomas	8
Pituitary adenomas	8
Schwannomas	3
Haemangioblastomas	3
Others	5

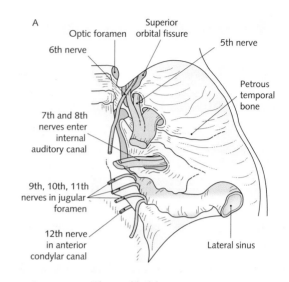

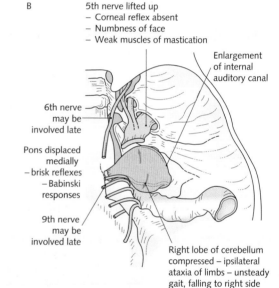

Fig. 27.2 Acoustic neuroma. Vestibular Schwannoma. (A) is a view from above of an opened skull with the brain removed showing the middle cranial fossa and its relation to the cranial nerves and lateral sinus. (B) demonstrates the spatial effect of a neuroma on the surrounding cranial nerves.

(see Fig. 5.2 and Fig. 5.3, p. 28). The visual failure may progress and become irreversible if the tumour is left untreated.

The most common types of pituitary tumour include:

- Prolactinomas: usually microadenomas.
- Non-functioning adenomas.
- Growth-hormone-secreting adenomas (causing acromegaly and usually macroadenomas).
- ACTH-secreting adenomas or hyperplasia: Cushing's disease.

Neurofibromas and schwannomas

Schwannomas arise from Schwann cells; neurofibromas arise from Schwann cells and other cells in the peripheral nerves such as fibroblasts. The principal intracranial site of schwannomas is in the cerebellopontine angle, where they arise from the vestibular portion of the eighth cranial nerve sheath (Fig. 27.2). They are a common finding in neurofibromatosis type 2, when they can be bilateral, although they are usually sporadic and unilateral. Clinical features of a vestibular schwannoma include ipsilateral sensorineural deafness and fifth nerve involvement (sometimes only loss of the corneal reflex, with no sensory symptoms), then later facial weakness (seventh nerve) and ipsilateral cerebellar signs. Ultimately, contralateral pyramidal signs and hydrocephalus may develop.

Haemangioblastomas

Haemangioblastomas are derived from blood vessels and occur within the cerebellar parenchyma or spinal cord. They are found in von Hippel–Lindau disease in association with similar tumours in the retina and cystic lesions in the pancreas and kidney.

Metastases

Metastases are the most common intracranial tumour, especially in the elderly. The most common primaries are from the lung, breast, and melanomas. More than half are solitary lesions at presentation but there are usually many micrometastases that cannot be resolved with magnetic resonance imaging (MRI) or computed tomography (CT) scanning.

CLINICAL FEATURES OF INTRACRANIAL TUMOURS

Mass lesions or space-occupying lesions within the cranium may present with one or more of the following features:

- Effects of raised intracranial pressure: headache, vomiting, papilloedema.
- Focal neurological signs occurring singly or in various combinations, caused by the direct effects of the tumour (compression, infiltration, or oedema).
- Diffuse cerebral symptoms: seizures, cognitive impairment.

Primary and secondary intracranial tumours are the most common cause of these symptoms, but any space-occupying lesion can present similarly, e.g. cerebral abscess, tuberculoma, subdural or intracerebral haematoma.

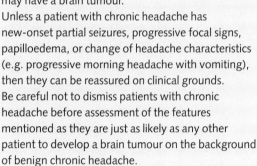

Many patients with chronic headache are afraid that they may have a brain tumour.
Unless a patient with chronic headache has new-onset partial seizures, progressive focal signs, papilloedema, or change of headache characteristics (e.g. progressive morning headache with vomiting), then they can be reassured on clinical grounds.
Be careful not to dismiss patients with chronic headache before assessment of the features mentioned as they are just as likely as any other patient to develop a brain tumour on the background of benign chronic headache.

Raised intracranial pressure

Raised intracranial pressure produces the classic triad of headache, vomiting, and papilloedema. However, these features, especially papilloedema, are relatively infrequent early presentations, as the symptoms usually imply obstruction to the cerebrospinal fluid pathways. The full picture is more common early in posterior fossa tumours, when the flow of cerebrospinal fluid is disrupted and lesions are usually within a very confined space. Progressive early morning or nocturnal headache is a common first symptom of intracranial tumours although focal neurological signs and symptoms often occur without headache.

The raised pressure caused by an expanding mass and the associated oedema can cause symptoms and signs distant to the tumour, including:

- Herniation.
- False localizing signs.

Herniation

There may be compression of the medulla by herniation of the cerebellar tonsils through the foramen magnum ('coning'), which leads to impairment of consciousness, respiratory depression, bradycardia, decerebrate posturing, and death (Fig. 27.3). This is called 'tonsillar herniation'. Similarly, the uncus of the temporal lobe may herniate through the tentorial opening (see Fig. 27.3). This is called 'uncal herniation' and the resulting compression of the third nerve is the cause of the dilating pupil on the side of the tumour, then later bilaterally. There may also be ipsilateral hemiparesis (see below).

False localizing signs

These are 'false' in that they are distant to the site of the mass and caused by the raised pressure. They include:

- Sixth nerve palsy: this is caused by compression of the nerve during its long intracranial course. It is often unilateral initially, then bilateral.
- Third nerve palsy: caudal herniation of the uncus of the temporal lobe causes pupillary dilatation and then later ophthalmoplegia.
- Hemiparesis on the same side as the tumour: this is caused by compression of the brainstem on the free edge of the tentorium in uncal herniation.

False localizing signs are very important because they indicate an increase in pressure with brain shift and require urgent investigation and treatment, which may include surgery.

Focal neurological signs

Focal neurological signs may be caused by direct effects of the tumour (compression, infiltration, or oedema) or be false localizing signs (as discussed above). The direct effects will depend on the site of the tumour (Fig. 27.4).

Fig. 27.3 Herniation of (A) the temporal lobe (supratentorial tumours) and (B) the cerebellar tonsils (infratentorial tumours; coning).

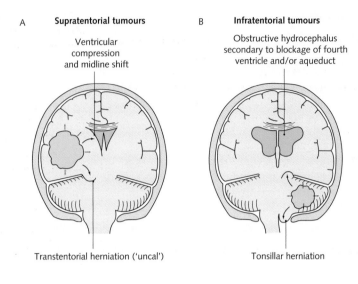

A **Supratentorial tumours**

Ventricular compression and midline shift

Transtentorial herniation ('uncal')

B **Infratentorial tumours**

Obstructive hydrocephalus secondary to blockage of fourth ventricle and/or aqueduct

Tonsillar herniation

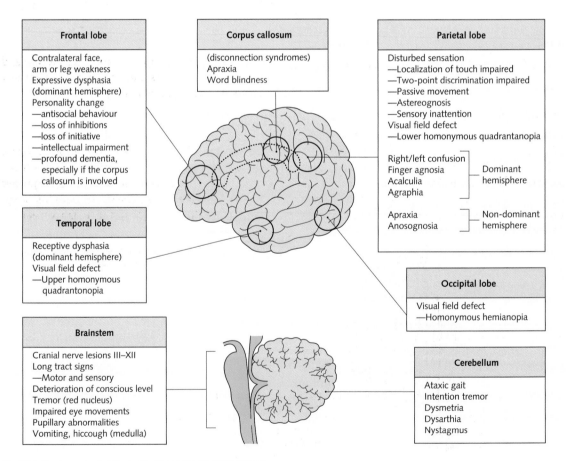

Frontal lobe

Contralateral face, arm or leg weakness
Expressive dysphasia (dominant hemisphere)
Personality change
—antisocial behaviour
—loss of inhibitions
—loss of initiative
—intellectual impairment
—profound dementia, especially if the corpus callosum is involved

Corpus callosum

(disconnection syndromes)
Apraxia
Word blindness

Parietal lobe

Disturbed sensation
—Localization of touch impaired
—Two-point discrimination impaired
—Passive movement
—Astereognosis
—Sensory inattention
Visual field defect
—Lower homonymous quadrantanopia

Right/left confusion
Finger agnosia   Dominant
Acalculia   hemisphere
Agraphia

Apraxia   Non-dominant
Anosognosia   hemisphere

Temporal lobe

Receptive dysphasia (dominant hemisphere)
Visual field defect
—Upper homonymous quadrantonopia

Occipital lobe

Visual field defect
—Homonymous hemianopia

Brainstem

Cranial nerve lesions III–XII
Long tract signs
—Motor and sensory
Deterioration of conscious level
Tremor (red nucleus)
Impaired eye movements
Pupillary abnormalities
Vomiting, hiccough (medulla)

Cerebellum

Ataxic gait
Intention tremor
Dysmetria
Dysarthia
Nystagmus

Fig. 27.4 Focal neurological signs according to the site of the tumour.

Seizures

Partial seizures, whether simple or complex, are characteristic of many focal hemispheric lesions. They may then secondarily generalize to a tonic–clonic seizure. The seizures caused by tumours are often difficult to control with drugs but are often helped by steroids in the acute setting.

INVESTIGATIONS

Lumbar puncture is contraindicated in any case of suspected or definite intracranial mass because it can lead to herniation ('coning') and prove fatal.

Imaging of the head is essential if an intracranial tumour is suspected. However, as many intracranial tumours are metastatic, more systemic investigations may also be necessary (e.g. chest X-ray, abdominal imaging, and mammography).

Computed tomography

CT scans should be carried out with contrast, as enhancement of a lesion (which may not be visible precontrast) adds to the discriminating ability.

However, CT scans show only the presence and site of a mass, and whether there is oedema, shift, or hydrocephalus; they do not provide much information about the type of tumour. Different intracranial masses, i.e. tumours (benign and malignant), cerebral abscesses, and tuberculomas, all have characteristic, but not entirely diagnostic, appearances (Fig. 27.5).

Magnetic resonance imaging

MRI usually provides more anatomical information than CT scanning and is always the investigation of choice for suspected posterior fossa mass lesions and pituitary tumours. Small metastases and meningeal lesions may also be missed by CT scans.

Electroencephalography (EEG)

EEG is rarely indicated or helpful in the investigation of tumours. There may be abnormal electrical activity in the region of the mass, but the EEG may be normal.

Skull X-ray

Skull X-ray is rarely indicated except to define bony landmarks or pathology in selected cases prior to surgery.

Specialized neuroradiology

Angiograms may be required to define the site and blood supply of a mass and ensure it is not entirely vascular in nature (i.e. an aneurysm).

Stereotactic brain biopsy

A frame is positioned on the head with identifiable external reference (fiducial) markers. CT or MRI can then be used to place a biopsy needle into the precise coordinates of the lesion. The subsequent histological findings help determine further management.

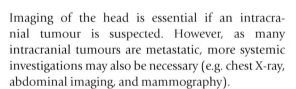

Fig. 27.5 CT scan features of various intracranial tumours.

Extra-axial
e.g. meningioma

Intra-axial
e.g. glioma

Single or multiple lesions
(if multiple more likely to be
metastases or infective)

Mass effect
• Midline shift
• Ventricular compression
• Hydrocephalus (secondary to 3rd
  ventricular or posterior fossa lesion)

Effect of contrast enhancement
• None – low-grade glioma
• Ring enhancing or irregular
  – malignant glioma
  (or could be an abscess)
• Homogeneous – meningioma

TREATMENT

Cerebral oedema

The oedema round the tumour can be rapidly reduced with the use of corticosteroids (dexamethasone) or intravenous mannitol in a neurosurgical emergency setting.

Seizures

Seizures are treated with anticonvulsants but are often difficult to control and the patient may be left with mild ongoing partial seizures.

Surgery

Benign tumours (e.g. meningiomas) can often be removed entirely. The location of benign tumours is critical and sometimes not all of the tumour can be removed, especially if it is in a difficult anatomical postion (e.g. sphenoid wing). Malignant tumours cannot be totally removed and therefore they are usually debulked for palliation.

Radiotherapy

Radiotherapy is usually recommended for gliomas and radiosensitive metastases to provide palliation.

Chemotherapy

Chemotherapy is sometimes given as adjunctive treatment (e.g. PCV regimen or temozolomide) but unfortunately the response is often poor with primary brain tumours.

PROGNOSIS

The prognosis for malignant brain tumours is poor. There is an overall 1-year survival of less than 50%. Benign tumours, especially meningiomas and neurofibromas, can often be removed entirely and therefore cured.

- Describe the presentation, bacterial differential diagnosis and management of meningitis
- Describe the clinical presentation and management of encephalitis
- Consider the predisposing causes for cerebral abscess
- Understand how HIV may affect the nervous system
- Be aware of the manifestations of TB within the nervous system

This chapter will consider only the most common and important infections of the nervous system. General conditions will be considered first, followed by diseases caused by individual organisms.

GENERAL CONDITIONS

Meningitis

Definition

Meningitis is inflammation of the meninges: the pia and arachnoid maters and the cerebrospinal fluid (CSF) that they enclose.

The term 'meningitis' typically refers to inflammation caused by an infective agent; however, it can also be applied to inflammation of the meninges caused by malignant cells, inflammatory disease (e.g. sarcoidosis), drugs, contrast media, and blood following subarachnoid haemorrhage. All of these causes can have a similar presentation to infective causes of meningitis.

Infective agents can reach the meninges from direct spread (e.g. from sinuses, the nasopharynx or the inner ear), through fractures of the skull, or, more commonly, from the bloodstream (haematogenous).

Causative agents

Infective meningitis can be caused by a variety of organisms, including bacteria, viruses, and fungi.

Bacteria

Among Gram-staining bacteria, the most likely causative organisms vary with age and predisposing factors.

In the neonate, they include:

- Gram-negative bacilli, e.g. *Escherichia coli, Klebsiella* species.
- *Haemophilus influenzae* type B.

In children, they include:

- *Haemophilus influenzae* type B.
- *Streptococcus pneumoniae* (pneumococcus).
- *Neisseria meningitidis* (meningococcus).

In adults, they include:

- *Neisseria meningitidis*.
- *Streptococcus pneumoniae*.

In immunodeficiency, trauma, or neurosurgery (e.g. ventricular shunts), they include:

- *Staphylococcus aureus*.
- *Listeria monocytogenes*.
- *Proteus* species.
- group A streptococci.

Tuberculous meningitis

Acid-fast bacilli that can cause meningitis include *Mycobacterium tuberculosis*. Tuberculous meningitis is generally considered separately from the other bacterial meningitides because the presentation is somewhat different in that it is a subacute meningitis that particularly affects the base of the brain.

Spirochaetes

Spirochaetes causing meningitis include:

- *Treponema pallidum* (syphilis).
- *Borrelia burgdorferi* (Lyme disease).

These are also often subacute/chronic meningitides rather than acute.

Viruses

Viruses that can cause meningitis include:

- Enteroviruses: echovirus, coxsackie virus, and polio virus.
- Mumps.
- Herpes simplex type 2 (rarely type 1) and Epstein–Barr virus (EBV).
- HIV: due to the primary infection.

Fungi

Fungi that cause meningitis include:

- *Cryptococcus neoformans*: a common opportunistic organism in HIV-positive and other immunocompromised patients.
- *Histoplasma capsulatum*.

Clinical features

The classic clinical triad of 'meningism' is:

- Headache.
- Photophobia.
- Neck stiffness.

There is often a fever, with or without rigors, although with 'aseptic' meningitis (i.e. not bacterial) this may be variable.

There may be a prodromal infection with myalgia and lethargy, or a likely source of infection may be evident (e.g. otitis media, pneumonia).

Bacterial meningitis

Bacterial meningitis is characterized by a sudden onset, with high fevers and rigors accompanying the classical triad. A non-blanching petechial rash, which may not be very obvious, indicates meningococcaemia and may be associated with meningitis. The patient may also present with septicaemic shock. Meningococcal septicaemia can occur without the meningitis and is often as life threatening as the meningitis itself because it is associated with thrombosis within arteries (e.g. to limbs).

Bacterial meningitis is a medical emergency with a high mortality rate. Meningococcal meningitis, in particular, can progress extremely rapidly. If there is a high index of suspicion of bacterial meningitis, and especially if a petechial rash develops (meningococcaemia), treatment should be started immediately, prior to confirmation of the diagnosis with lumbar puncture.

Viral meningitis

Viral meningitis is acute or subacute. It is usually self-limiting and lasts 4–10 days. Headaches may last for some weeks but serious sequelae are rare. If the virus then proceeds to affect the brain substance (encephalitis) then the patient can become very unwell.

Tuberculous meningitis

Tuberculosis meningitis (TBM) typically causes a chronic meningitis, but it may present more acutely. TBM may occur years after the primary infection and in many cases there is no history of prior tuberculosis (TB). Meningitic signs may take many weeks to develop, having been preceded by non-specific symptoms such as a vague headache, malaise, anorexia, and vomiting. The infection often affects the base of the brain where it can damage the brainstem, arteries to the brain and block the flow of CSF causing hydrocephalus.

Fungal meningitis

Cryptococcal meningitis is the most common fungal meningitis in Europe and is especially associated with immunocompromised patients. The presentation is similar to TBM.

Diagnosis

Diagnosis is made by lumbar puncture. This should be carried out immediately to prevent delay in treatment. However, if there are any signs of raised intracranial pressure, a computed tomography (CT) scan should be carried out first to look for radiological signs of raised intracranial pressure so that the risk of coning can be assessed.

Typical CSF findings are listed in Fig. 28.1. Other investigations include the following:

CSF pressure

This is characteristically elevated ($>200\,mmH_2O$) especially in cryptococcal and tuberculous meningitis.

Staining of CSF

- Gram stain: to diagnose bacterial meningitis. Gram-positive diplococci: pneumococcus. Gram-negative intracellular diplococci: meningococcus.
- Ziehl–Neelson stain: demonstrates acid-fast bacilli of tuberculosis (acid-fast bacilli visualized in only 20% of cases of TBM).
- Indian-ink stain: for fungi.

Blood cultures and CSF culture

Including culture in Lowenstein–Jensen medium for TB (results take 6 weeks for TB).

Fig. 28.1 CSF findings in meningitis

	Normal	Bacterial	Viral	Tuberculous
Appearance	Clear	Turbid/pus	Clear/turbid	Turbid/viscous
Neutrophils	Nil	200–10 000/mm³	Nil/few	0–200/mm³
Lymphocytes	<5 mm³	<50/mm³	10–100/mm³	100–300/mm³
Protein	0.2–0.4 g/L	0.5–2.0 g/L	0.4–0.8 g/L	0.5–3.0 g/L
Glucose	>1/2 blood glucose	<1/3 blood glucose	<1/2 blood glucose	<1/3 blood glucose

Blood glucose

This is compared with CSF glucose taken at the same time.

Blood and CSF serology

These are carried out for likely viral causes.

CSF polymerase chain reaction (CSF PCR)

This is being increasingly performed to look for TB and viruses in the CSF. The sensitivities and specificities of the tests vary and false positives can be common.

Chest/skull X-rays/CT with bone windows

These are carried out if there is a possibility that infection has spread from the chest or via a fracture, following head trauma.

Complications

Consciousness is not severely impaired in uncomplicated meningitis, although a high fever may cause delirium. Marked changes in conscious level, focal neurological signs, seizures, and papilloedema indicate that complications may be developing or that an alternative diagnosis should be considered (e.g. cerebral abscess or encephalitis). Complications include:

- Hydrocephalus due to obstruction of CSF outflow, leading to raised intracranial pressure: this is especially common in TB meningitis.
- Cerebral oedema.
- Venous sinus thrombosis.
- Subdural empyema.
- Cerebral abscess.
- Arteritis and endarteritis: TB can often inflame the origin of the cerebral vasculature as it rises from the base of the brain. In severe cases, this can lead to occlusion of the artery causing a large vessel stroke. Meningitis can also inflame the smaller arteries within the meninges causing further damage from ischaemia.

Treatment

Bacterial meningitis is a medical emergency. Each hour of delay increases the likelihood of a fatal outcome or permanent neurological deficit.

It is usually possible to distinguish between bacterial meningitis and meningitis caused by other organisms in the clinical setting and with initial visualization of the CSF.

If there is any suspicion that a patient may have bacterial meningitis, treatment with intravenous broad-spectrum antibiotics should be started immediately: cefotaxime or ceftriaxone (depending on local sensitivities) for meningococcus and pneumococcus, and chloramphenicol for *Haemophilus*. High-dose ampicillin is used to treat *Listeria* meningitis; vancomycin or rifampicin can be used in drug-resistant pneumococcus.

Tuberculous meningitis is treated for at least 9 months with a combination of isoniazid, rifampicin, and pyrazinamide, with the peripheral nerve side effects of isoniazid protected by pyridoxine. Other possible agents include ethambutol, streptomycin, and ciprofloxacin.

Steroids are known to improve prognosis and reduce the complication rate in childhood meningitis and there is now evidence of similar benefit in adults, particularly in patients with TB or pneumococcal meningitis, when given early and in high dosages.

Viral meningitis is usually benign and self-limiting and the treatment is symptomatic.

Prophylaxis

Contacts of patients with bacterial meningitis, including family, school, and work contacts, should be considered for prophylactic treatment with oral rifampicin.

Encephalitis

Definition

Encephalitis is inflammation of the brain parenchyma, usually caused by viruses, but occasionally due to bacteria or other organisms (e.g. *Mycoplasma*, *Rickettsia*, and *Histoplasma*).

The temporal course of encephalitis can differ depending on the virus. Three main forms of viral encephalitis exist:

- Direct: when the infective organism directly causes the encephalitis at the time of infection (acute viral meningoencephalitis or encephalitis).
- Immune-mediated: causing an allergic or postinfectious encephalomyelitis, which can also follow after vaccination.

Causative organisms

The causative organisms are often not identified and the viral aetiology is presumed.

The most common organisms identified in cases of adult encephalitis in the UK are:

- Echovirus.
- Coxsackie virus.
- Mumps virus.
- Herpes simplex: causes the most severe viral encephalitis in the UK and is often associated with haemorrhagic changes within the temporal lobes and progressive personality changes and memory loss.

Slightly rarer causes include adenovirus, varicella-zoster, measles, and influenza.

In the Far East, the most common cause is Japanese B arbovirus, which causes epidemic encephalitis with a high mortality.

Clinical features

Many of the causative organisms will cause a mild self-limiting illness with headache and drowsiness, but some cases will present with a severe illness with depressed conscious level, focal signs, and seizures.

Herpes simplex type 1 accounts for most of the severe cases.

Clinical features can be categorized as follows:

- Non-specific features: headache, pyrexia, myalgia, malaise.
- Meningism (from meningeal involvement): headache, photophobia, neck stiffness, and lymphocytic pleocytosis in the CSF.
- Parenchymal involvement: depends whether the inflammation is diffuse or focal, e.g. confusion, dysphasia, hemiparesis, seizures, ataxia, cranial nerve palsies, autonomic dysfunction.
- Virus-specific features, e.g. parotid swelling in mumps.

Diagnosis

Definitive diagnosis is often difficult in viral encephalitis. Herpes simplex type 1 is the commonest identified cause of encephalitis in the UK and there is a specific treatment for this agent. There are probably many viruses which are never detected or isolated.

Investigations

- CT scanning: often shows cerebral oedema, which is non-specific.
- Magnetic resonance imaging (MRI): is preferable if the patient can tolerate it. Subtle inflammatory changes are much more apparent and the appearances of herpes simplex encephalitis in one or both temporal lobes are very distinctive.
- Electroencephalogram (EEG): may show non-specific slow-wave changes and/or periodic complexes; however, if these findings are restricted to temporofrontal regions, a diagnosis of herpes simplex is suggested.
- Viral serology/PCR of blood and CSF.
- Brain biopsy: seldom performed since the advent of MRI and PCR for herpes simplex but can provide more definitive information in difficult cases.

Treatment

Any case of suspected herpes simplex encephalitis should be treated immediately with intravenous acyclovir. Otherwise, treatment of encephalitis is supportive and symptomatic, including:

- Supportive treatment for comatose patients.
- Anticonvulsants for seizures.

- Control of cerebral oedema.
- Corticosteroids in the first week of illness is controversial.

Prognosis

The prognosis is very variable and depends on the causative organism.

In the UK, herpes simplex carries the highest mortality. There is 80% mortality for untreated herpes simplex encephalitis; this falls to 30% with treatment. By contrast, the mortality for mumps encephalitis is 2%, even though there is no specific treatment.

The likelihood of neurological sequelae is also variable and depends on the severity of the encephalitis. Memory impairment is a common sequel to herpes simplex encephalitis.

Cerebral abscess

Definition

A cerebral abscess is a focal encapsulated area of infection within the cerebrum or cerebellum.

The abscess passes through several stages, over about 2 weeks, from localized suppurative cerebritis to complete encapsulation. There may be a solitary abscess or multiple abscesses.

The brain is relatively resistant to abscess formation but abscesses can occur under conditions that cause necrosis of tissue with simultaneous infection by an appropriate organism.

The infection can reach the brain by local spread or via the bloodstream. Disease states that predispose to cerebral abscess formation include:

- Chronic lung infections, e.g. bronchiectasis, chronic sinusitis, otitis, or mastoiditis.
- Congenital heart disease, especially those with 'right to left' shunts.
- Bacterial endocarditis.
- Infections in immunocompromised patients.

Causative organisms

Bacteria are the usual causative organisms; however, in immunocompromised patients, other organisms (e.g. fungi and protozoa) are more common.

Anaerobic and microaerophylic organisms are the main pathogens:

- *Streptococcus* species, especially *S. viridans* and *S. milleri*.
- *Bacteroides* species.

- Enterobacteria, e.g. *Escherichia coli* and *Proteus* species.
- *Staphylococcus aureus*.

The following organisms are important in immuno-compromised patients:

- *Toxoplasma*.
- *Aspergillus*.
- *Candida*.
- *Listeria*.
- *Strongyloides*.

Clinical features

The history in patients with cerebral abscess is usually short (less than 1 month) and progressive.

Brain abscesses present as space-occupying lesions with features of raised intracranial pressure:

- Headache.
- Vomiting.
- Deterioration in conscious level.
- Papilloedema.

There may also be focal features associated with the space occupation:

- Seizures (occur in 30% of cases).
- Hemiparesis.
- Dysphasia.
- Visual field defects.
- Ataxia.

There may also be symptoms of systemic infection (e.g. pyrexia, malaise) or of focal infection (e.g. cough, earache) but these may not be present, particularly in immunocompromised patients.

Diagnosis

CT scanning or, if available, MRI, is the investigation of choice. Lumbar puncture is contraindicated in the presence of a mass lesion because of the risk of herniation. Other investigations include X-rays/CT of the chest, sinuses, and middle ear, which may reveal the primary source of the infection, and blood cultures.

The classic appearance seen on a CT scan with contrast (Fig. 28.2) comprises:

- 'Ring enhancement' of the lesion, which is usually spherical.
- Central area of low density.
- Surrounding area of oedema.

In addition, there may be ventricular compression and midline shift due to a mass effect.

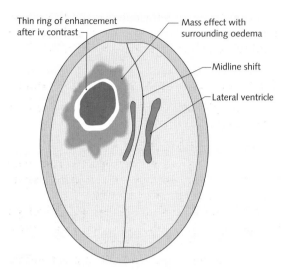

Thin ring of enhancement after iv contrast

Mass effect with surrounding oedema

Midline shift

Lateral ventricle

Fig. 28.2 CT appearance of a cerebral abscess (similar appearances may be produced by an intracranial tumour).

Treatment

Treatment consists of four parts:

- Treatment of the brain abscess with appropriate antibiotics or organism-specific drugs: a combination of drugs is often used to target all likely pathogens until the organism has been isolated. For example, penicillin, chloramphenicol, and metronidazole may be used for non-immunocompromised patients, and pyrimethamine (toxoplasma), amphotericin (fungi), and ampicillin (listeria) for immunocompromised patients.
- Surgical drainage or excision of the brain abscess in association with medical treatment.
- Treatment of raised intracranial pressure and seizures.
- Treatment of the source of infection, e.g. drainage of chronic sinus infection.

Prognosis

The mortality rate since the advent of CT scanning and better bacteriological techniques for anaerobic organisms has fallen to 5–15% (it was 30–50% prior to CT).

Poor prognostic indicators are:

- Reduced preoperative level of consciousness.
- Brain herniation.
- Rupture of the abscess into the ventricles or subarachnoid space.
- Immunocompromised patient.
- Poor general medical condition, e.g. severe pulmonary disease.

Of survivors, 25–50% have neurological sequelae, 30–50% have persistent seizures, 15–30% have a persistent hemiparesis, and 10–20% have disorders of speech and language.

SPECIFIC ORGANISMS AND THEIR ASSOCIATED DISEASES

Tuberculosis

TB is an infection that, in humans, is most commonly caused by *Mycobacterium tuberculosis*. It can also be caused by *M. bovis*, and now, with immunosuppression secondary to HIV infection, there is an increasing incidence of cases due to *M. avium-intracellulare*. TB meningitis is described above.

Diagnosis

The diagnosis of neurological TB involves chest X-ray (for evidence of pulmonary TB, although this is often normal), tuberculin testing, CSF (as long as no space-occupying lesion exists), CT scanning and MRI, and biopsy. CSF PCR for TB is increasingly being used but care in interpretation is needed because false positives may be high.

Conditions associated with TB

- Tuberculous meningitis complicated by hydrocephalus, cranial nerve palsies and cerebral infacts (see p. 190).
- Tuberculoma (brain and spine).
- Pott's disease of the spine (vertebrae).
- Spinal arachnoiditis causing myelopathy and radiculopathy.

Tuberculoma

Tuberculoma presents as a cerebral abscess and may produce a space-occupying effect. Most cases resolve with antituberculous therapy.

Pott's disease

Tuberculous osteomyelitis of the vertebral bodies can cause chronic epidural infection. The lower thoracic region is usually involved, with pain over the affected area (which is only relieved by rest) and features of cord compression (20% of cases). Occasionally, there may be vertebral collapse or spread of infection into the pleura, peritoneum, or psoas muscle.

A needle biopsy is usually sufficient to establish the diagnosis, but occasionally exploratory surgery is required.

Treatment comprises long-term antituberculous therapy and, if signs of cord compression develop, surgical decompression.

Spinal arachnoiditis

Spinal arachnoiditis may result from downwards spread of intracranial infection or from direct spread from epidural infection.

The presentation is of spreading myelitis with root involvement:

- Weakness: pyramidal and radicular.
- Root pain.
- Sensory loss.
- Sphincter disturbance.

Treatment

Antituberculous therapy for neurological TB should be continued for at least 12–18 months and involves a combination of isoniazid, rifampicin, pyrazinamide, and ethambutol, with pyridoxine to cover the peripheral nerve side effects of isoniazid.

Syphilis

Syphilis is caused by the motile spirochaete *Treponema pallidum* and transmission is almost invariably through sexual contact.

The natural history of untreated infection is divided into three stages. Neurological involvement occurs in the third stage, which is typically many years after the initial infection. Neurosyphilis occurs in less than 10% of all untreated cases. Penicillins are widely used for the treatment of other infections and thus many unsuspected cases of syphilis are treated without progressing to stages two and three.

Diagnosis

The combined use of the serological tests veneral disease reference laboratory (VDRL), *T. pallidum* haemagglutination assay (TPHA), and fluourescent treponema antibodies absorbed (FTA-Abs), provides specific results. For practical purposes, negative serology excludes the diagnosis, although these tests can be negative on the sera but positive on the CSF in neurosyphilis.

Treatment

Parenteral penicillin is given for all forms of neurosyphilis for 2–3 weeks. Established neurological disease can be arrested but may not be reversed.

Jarisch–Herxheimer reactions (severe allergic reactions) may occur following treatment and high-dose steroid cover is often given with the penicillin.

Conditions associated with neurosyphilis

The main syphilitic syndromes that affect the nervous system are described below.

Asymptomatic neurosyphilis

During the long interval between the secondary and tertiary stages of the disease, neurosyphilis may actively persist but be asymptomatic.

CSF examination reveals positive syphilis serology, lymphocytosis ($100–1000/mm^3$), elevated protein (0.5–2.0 g/L), and reduced glucose.

Treatment with penicillin will prevent further progression.

Meningitis

Approximately 25% of untreated patients will develop an acute symptomatic meningitis within 2 years of infection. This may present in three ways:

- Acute basal meningitis: with hydrocephalus, cranial nerve palsies, and papilloedema.
- Focal meningitis: when a gumma presents as an expanding intracranial mass, favouring the meninges rather than parenchyma, and presenting with seizures, raised intracranial pressure, and focal signs.
- Meningovascular meningitis (5–10 years after primary infection): causing an obliterative endarteritis and periarteritis and presenting as a 'stroke', most often in a young person.

Treatment with penicillin will prevent progression.

Tabes dorsalis

Tabes dorsalis is a late presentation of syphilis (15–20 years after primary infection), causing a meningoradiculitis with degeneration of the dorsal columns and pupillary involvement.

The classic features include:

- Lightning pains: irregular, severe, sharp stabbing pains, usually in the lower limb, chest, or abdomen, caused by dorsal root involvement.
- Visceral crises: abdominal pain, diarrhoea, and tenesmus.
- Argyll Robertson pupils: small, irregularly shaped pupils that do not react to light but do accommodate.

- Ptosis: with compensatory over activity of the frontalis muscle.
- Optic atrophy.
- Impaired vibration and joint-position sense, and reduced deep pain.
- Patchy loss of pin-prick and temperature sensation.
- Trophic skin lesions and Charcot joints (painless joint damage).
- Sensory ataxia: positive Romberg's test and stamping gait.
- Hypotonia and reduced reflexes.
- Extensor plantar responses in spite of absent ankle jerks: caused by the combination of radiculopathy and upper motor neuron involvement.

General paralysis of the insane

General paralysis of the insane develops 10–25 years after primary infection and, as its historical name indicates, involves psychiatric abnormality and weakness.

There are two phases:

- Preparalytic: with progressive dementia.
- Paralytic: with involvement of the corticospinal tracts and extrapyramidal system.

Clinical features include:

- Dementia: usually similar to that associated with Alzheimer's disease but occasionally involves manic behaviour or delusions of grandeur.
- Seizures and incontinence.
- Pupil abnormalities: pupils are large, unequal, and unreactive in 75% of cases; the remainder have Argyll Robertson pupils.
- Tremor of tongue ('trombone' tongue).
- Dysarthria.
- Hypertonia with brisk reflexes and extensor plantar responses.

Human immunodeficiency virus

Infection with the retrovirus HIV can cause neurological involvement either directly or via opportunistic infections. Neurological involvement develops in 80% of patients.

Both the central and peripheral nervous system can be affected.

Central nervous system involvement

Primary HIV infection

The direct effects of the virus can cause:

- HIV encephalopathy ('AIDS dementia'): subacute or chronic onset.

- HIV myelopathy: a reversible form can occur during seroconversion, but a later form (when not caused by an opportunistic organism) is irreversible.
- Acute atypical meningitis: self-limiting and occurs at seroconversion, with cranial neuropathies and pyramidal signs.

Opportunistic infection

A wide variety of organisms may be responsible. The most common conditions include:

- CNS toxoplasmosis: the most commonly encountered neurological opportunistic infection (occurs in 28% of patients with AIDS). It usually presents as a focal cerebral abscess.
- Cryptococcal meningitis: *Cryptococcus neoformans* is the third most common infectious agent causing neurological disease in AIDS. Classic clinical markers of meningitis may be absent. Pyrexia and headache, or even purely non-specific symptoms, may be the only sign.
- Progressive multifocal leucoencephalopathy (PML): caused by JC papovavirus and resulting in a relentlessly progressive central demyelination with a poor prognosis.
- Cytomegalovirus (CMV): can cause a retinitis, myelitis, sacral radiculitis, and encephalitis.
- Herpes simplex type 2: myelitis.
- Varicella-zoster: radiculitis and encephalitis.
- Other infections: *Candida*, *Aspergillus*, and *Coccidioides* may affect the CNS.

Neoplasia

HIV infection may cause:

- Primary CNS lymphoma: presents as mass lesions (occurs in 1.5% of AIDS patients as compared with 0.2% of other immunocompromised patients).
- Other malignancies, e.g. spread from systemic non-Hodgkin's lymphoma or, rarely, metastases from Kaposi's sarcoma.

Peripheral nervous system involvement

Peripheral neuropathy

HIV may be associated with the following peripheral neuropathies:

- Distal symmetrical polyneuropathy: the most common type of neuropathy (10–30% of patients). It is usually a late feature, with pain and paraesthesiae of the feet. Treatment is symptomatic.

- Chronic inflammatory demyelinating polyradiculoneuropathy (CIDP): an early feature. It comprises a subacute, predominantly motor polyneuropathy, affecting proximal muscles more than distal, without painful dysaesthesia. Plasmapheresis may help unlike in forms of CIDP in non-HIV positive patients.
- Guillain–Barré syndrome (GBS): the acute counterpart of CIDP. This is an early feature that can occur at seroconversion. It has the same clinical features as seronegative GBS but with a high CSF lymphocyte count. Plasmapheresis may help.
- Multifocal neuropathy: nerve infarction leads to sudden-onset sensory and motor deficits. Herpes zoster radiculitis must be excluded.

Myopathy

Myopathies caused by HIV include:

- Polymyositis: indistinguishable from seronegative polymyositis. Immunosuppressive treatment results in improvement.
- Type-2 fibre muscle atrophy: frequent finding on biopsy in patients with proximal weakness and normal creatine kinase (CK) levels.
- Drug-induced myopathy, especially from zidovudine.

Poliomyelitis

Polio virus is one of the enteroviruses; it is a picorna-virus (pico, small; rna, RNA).

The incidence of primary infection has been extremely low in the UK since immunization began in 1957 but many patients have residual disability following infection before the 1950s.

Poliomyelitis remains endemic in the tropics, occurring especially in late summer and autumn.

Mode of spread

Poliomyelitis is spread by the faeco–oral route and then enters the bloodstream, causing a viraemia. Neurological involvement occurs only in some patients and targets the anterior horn cells of the spinal cord and the motor nuclei of the brainstem.

Clinical features

The incubation period is 10–14 days. There is considerable variation in symptoms:

- Asymptomatic (95%): with resultant immunity.

- Abortive poliomyelitis (4–5%): a self-limiting illness with gastrointestinal and mild upper respiratory symptoms and pyrexia.
- Non-paralytic poliomyelitis (0.5%): features of abortive poliomyelitis with meningism. Recovery is complete.
- Paralytic poliomyelitis (0.1%): initially there are features of abortive poliomyelitis, which subside and then recur with meningism and myalgia. There is subsequent asymmetrical paralysis with no sensory involvement. Respiratory failure is due to paralysis of the respiratory muscles. The lower limb or limbs are most commonly affected, especially in children. Bulbar symptoms can occur with cranial nerve involvement. When paralytic poliomyelitis occurs before puberty, the patient is often left with a wasted, shortened limb.

Diagnosis of paralytic poliomyelitis

Paralytic poliomyelitis is distinguished clinically from GBS by the lack of sensory signs and the asymmetry.

CSF findings are similar to those in other viral meningitides (raised protein, increased number of lymphocytes, and normal glucose), but there are usually increased numbers of polymorphs initially.

The virus may be grown from throat swabs, stool, and CSF, and paired serology will show a rising titre.

Treatment of paralytic poliomyelitis

Patients with paralytic poliomyelitis should be isolated and contacts immunized.

Other measures include:

- Careful nursing, as for all paralysed patients, to prevent pressure ulcers.
- Physiotherapy, to avoid deformities.
- Fluid and electrolyte replacement.

Respiratory failure requires artificial ventilation.

Prognosis

Lack of ventilatory support for respiratory paralysis is the usual cause of death, but otherwise mortality rates are very low. Improvement in muscle power can commence a week after paralysis and continue for up to a year. Bulbar palsies recover usually well. Some muscles may remain permanently paralysed and fasciculations may persist.

In affected limbs in children, bone growth is retarded, resulting in a wasted, shortened limb.

Vaccination

Routine immunization from 2 months of age occurs in the UK.

Up to 1962, Salk (inactivated) vaccine was used. Since then, the Sabin (live, attenuated) vaccine has been used. It is given orally in three doses, 1 month apart, starting at the age of 2 months, and then a reinforcing dose is given at school-entry age.

Note: live virus will be excreted in the stool after immunization and therefore great care must be taken to avoid transmission of infection to immunocompromised and non-vaccinated individuals.

Post-polio syndrome

A deterioration in function with atrophy in the affected as well as unaffected limbs can occur many years after the primary infection (usually between 20 and 40 years). The cause is uncertain but it may represent the normal ageing process (i.e. loss of anterior horn cells) with the symptoms accentuated by the prior reduction in anterior horn cell number caused by the original infection.

Lyme disease

The causative agent in Lyme disease is the spirochaete *Borrelia burgdorferi*, which is transmitted by the tick *Ixodes dammini*. The organism is prevalent throughout Europe and North America (e.g. Lyme, Connecticut, where the disease was first recognized).

Clinical features

The clinical course of Lyme disease can be divided into three stages.

Stage 1 begins 3–30 days after the tick bite and consists of a relapsing remitting pyrexia and arthralgia, with a characteristic skin lesion (erythema chronicum migrans) developing at the site of the bite. This stage resolves after about 4 weeks.

Stage 2 occurs a few weeks or months after stage 1 and consists of neurological (15%) or cardiac symptoms (10%), which can last up to 8 weeks. Neurological manifestations include:

- Subacute lymphocytic meningitis: often mild and self-limiting but can recur if not treated.
- Subacute encephalitis: often mild and self-limiting.
- Cranial nerve involvement.
- Peripheral neuropathy with painful radiculitis.

Stage 3 occurs several months or years later and consists of recurrent and often erosive arthritis. Signs of diffuse CNS involvement may also develop, with focal encephalitis, seizures, behavioural disorders, and a multiple-sclerosis-like illness.

Diagnosis

Clinical features and epidemiological considerations are indicative. Serological and PCR techniques give the best probability of making the diagnosis. Cultures often give a low yield.

Treatment

Treatment comprises:

- Stage 1: oral antibiotics (penicillin or tetracycline).
- Stages 2 and 3: high-dose intravenous penicillin or ceftriaxone for 14 days. This shortens the course of neurological illness and prevents further parenchymal damage.

Prognosis

Focal deficits that do not improve after treatment and normalization of the CSF indicate fixed parenchymal damage and are hence unlikely ever to improve.

A patient that presents with a unilateral or bilateral Bell's palsy, a rash and a systemic upset, e.g. fever, should always be considered to have possible Lyme disease.

Creutzfeldt–Jakob disease

Creutzfeldt–Jakob disease (CJD) is an extremely rare disease that has received public awareness recently because of the possibility that the equivalent disease in cattle, bovine spongiform encephalitis (BSE), may be transmissible to humans.

Transmission

CJD, BSE, and similar diseases (scrapie in sheep, and kuru, which is found in Papua New Guinea) are transmitted by a protein (the prion protein) that is found within the nervous and in variant CJD within the lymphatic systems of affected humans or animals.

The transformed, pathogenic prion protein is resistant to formalin, heat, irradiation, and procedures that modify nucleic acids.

CJD is not contagious but is infectious. It can be transmitted experimentally and there are a number of examples of iatrogenic transfer (e.g. human pituitary-derived growth hormone given to growth-retarded children and transfer via corneal grafts).

There is no evidence so far of transmission via whole organ transplantation, or across the placenta.

Incidence

The UK annual incidence remains within the worldwide range: 0.5–0.9 per million.

However, from 1994 to 2006, there have been reports of 159 cases of definite or probable variant CJD; these have occurred in persons between the ages of 12 and 74 years (median 28 years). The peak annual incidence occurred in 2000 and is subsequently dropping, although surveillance continues because of concerns regarding a late epidemic.

Features of classical CJD

Classical CJD has a long incubation period, up to several years, and usually presents in the sixth decade of life. It is characterized by the triad of:

- Dementia: rapid onset and progressive, with ultimate loss of language function.
- Myoclonus: brief, shock-like involuntary movements, often exaggerated on being startled.
- A characteristic but non-specific EEG abnormality: generalized slowing or pseudoperiodic sharp waves.

An MRI scan can often show a high signal in the caudate and putamen and a protein called 14–3-3 is almost always elevated in the CSF, although this can also be elevated in other diseases where neurons die rapidly (e.g. cerebral infarction).

The disease is rapidly progressive and invariably fatal, often within 6 months from the onset of symptoms. Brain pathology shows characteristic spongiform (vacuolated) changes in the brain.

Features of new variant CJD (vCJD)

New variant CJD is a young-onset form that was not seen in the UK before 1994. Clinical features include behavioural change, ataxia, cognitive impairment,

and a tendency to a more prolonged duration of illness (up to 40 months, median 14 months).

The EEG is not typical as in classical sporadic CJD. Brain pathology shows marked spongiform change and extensive amyloid plaques.

The diagnosis of vCJD

- Clinical picture.
- Brain biopsy and tonsil biopsy.
- MRI scans may demonstrate high signal in the back of the thalamus or 'pulvinar'.
- Elevated protein 14-3-3 in the CSF is not as sensitive as in classical CJD but is helpful if raised.
- Autopsy: unfortunately, the definitive diagnosis is often made this way.

Treatment

There is no treatment for CJD or other prion diseases at the current time, although several potential drugs are under trial.

Comment

The current opinion from the Spongiform Encephalopathy Advisory Committee (SEAC) concerning the young cases of new variant CJD is that 'in the absence of any credible alternative, the most likely explanation at present is that these cases are linked to exposure to BSE before the Specified Bovine Offal (SBO) ban was introduced in 1989'.

The SBO ban prohibits the use of the tissues most likely to contain the infective agent of BSE in products for human consumption. These tissues include brain, spinal cord, thymus, tonsils, spleen, intestines, and, more recently, bones. As of May 2007 there have also been four cases linked to contaminated blood products in the UK.

A rapidly progressive dementia (over weeks or months), especially with myoclonus, should always be considered to be prion disease unless an alternative diagnosis can be made. This has implications for how all samples from the patient, including blood and CSF, are handled by medical and laboratory staff.

Multiple sclerosis

Objectives

- Understand the epidemiology and possible pathogenic mechanism of MS
- Describe the neurological systems typically affected by MS
- Understand the investigations needed to make a firm diagnosis of MS
- What are the differential diagnoses of white matter disease?
- Understand the pharmaceutical and non-pharmaceutical management of patients with MS

Multiple sclerosis (MS) is a common disease in Europe and North America. There are multiple areas of demyelination affecting white matter tracts within the CNS. The episodes of demyelination are separated in time and place within the CNS, and, classically, the disease runs a relapsing-remitting course initially and then becomes progressive.

EPIDEMIOLOGY

MS occurs worldwide but is far more common in temperate climates. The prevalence increases in proportion to the distance from the equator. This applies in the northern and southern hemispheres. In England, at between 50° and 65° latitude, the prevalence is 60–100 cases per 100 000 inhabitants, whereas in southern Italy (40° latitude), the prevalence is about 15 per 100 000; at the equator.

Interestingly, on moving from a high-prevalence area to a low-prevalence area prior to puberty, the risk of developing the disease takes on the rate of the low-prevalence area; however, if such a move is made following puberty, the risk of the high-prevalence area is retained.

The disease usually occurs in young adults, the peak age of onset being between 20 and 30 years. More females than males are affected.

PATHOGENESIS

A large number of hypotheses exist regarding the pathogenesis of MS and the exact cause remains uncertain. Immunological mechanisms undoubtedly play a role, although the causation is probably multifactorial.

Immunological mechanisms

Evidence points towards the presence of immunoregulatory defects in MS. Recent research has suggested that cytokines may play a critical role in the pathophysiology, both by regulating aberrant autoimmune responses and by mediating myelin damage.

Genetic factors

There is an increased familial incidence of MS, with a relative of an affected individual having a 20-fold increased risk of developing the disease. There is not a clear-cut pattern of inheritance but there is a positive association with HLA-A3, B7, B18, DR2, and DW2.

Infection

The defective immunological response in patients with MS suggests a viral aetiology. Raised titres to many common viruses have been found in the serum and cerebrospinal fluid (CSF) of MS patients, but attempts to induce MS experimentally with viruses have been unsuccessful.

Biochemical mechanisms

No biochemical effect has been demonstrated. Myelin is normal prior to breakdown. Reports that excess dietary fats or fat malabsorption are important have not been substantiated.

PATHOLOGY

Areas of demyelination are found in the white matter of the brain and spinal cord. These areas are called plaques. The lesions lie in close relationship to post-capillary venules (perivenular).

- There is a particular predilection for certain sites within the CNS:
- Periventricular region of the cerebral hemispheres.
- Corpus callosum.
- Brainstem, (including medial longitudinal fasciculus), cerebellum and cerebellar peduncles.
- Cervical cord.
- Optic nerves.

There is myelin destruction with relative preservation of axons. An inflammatory infiltrate containing mononuclear cells and lymphocytes is found. Interstitial oedema occurs in acute lesions. Remyelination is rare and the mechanism of functional recovery is uncertain. It is postulated that chronic demyelination may account for the loss of axons and subsequently the cell bodies. This may explain the clinical irreversibility of some of the relapses.

CLINICAL FEATURES

MS can present in a multitude of ways and no single presentation is diagnostic. For instance, a young woman with a history of two or more episodes of CNS dysfunction that have remitted would be highly suggestive but not diagnostic.

Three main patterns of disease progression are recognized:

- Relapsing and remitting: with lesions often occurring in different parts of the CNS at different times. This makes up 90% of cases initially.
- Secondary progressive: when the disease starts with a relapsing–remitting picture but eventually recovery from each successive relapse becomes less complete, causing residual progressive disability. Over half of the patients presenting with relapsing-remitting disease eventually develop secondary progressive disease.
- Primary progressive: in which there is little or no recovery from relapses, with a cumulative disability from the onset. Only 10% of patients present with this form of disease.

There is a marked variability in the disease progression, but, by 15 years after the onset of symptoms, 30% of patients are still working and 40% still walking.

The most common presentations are discussed below.

Optic and retrobulbar neuritis

Optic neuritis presents as subacute visual loss, usually unilateral, associated with a central scotoma and pain on ocular movement. Recovery is usual over a few weeks. The ophthalmological findings depend on whether the lesion is in the optic nerve head (papillitis) or in the optic nerve behind the eye (retrobulbar neuritis). In the former, a pink swollen disc is seen, whereas in the latter, the disc looks normal.

There are usually no residual symptoms following optic neuritis, although a relative afferent pupillary defect (Fig. 29.1), small central scotomata, and defects in colour vision may be demonstrated. Following an attack, optic atrophy (pale disc) often develops several weeks later.

Optic neuritis may be an isolated event, it may occur simultaneously with a transverse myelitis (Devic's syndrome), or it may be a forerunner for

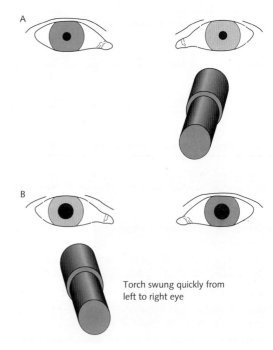

Torch swung quickly from left to right eye

Fig. 29.1 Afferent pupillary defect in right eye: light shone into the normal left eye (A) causes consensual constriction of both pupils. (B) Both pupils consensually dilate when the torch swings to the abnormal right eye because less light reaches the afferent arc of the reflex, due to the right optic nerve lesion.

further episodes of CNS demyelination, i.e. MS. Up to 70% of cases fall into the last category.

In some patients, optic nerve demyelination may be asymptomatic and only discovered clinically by the presence of optic atrophy or by the use of visual evoked potentials (see Chapter 36, p. 251).

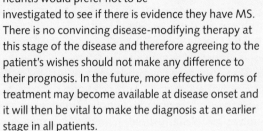

Some patients who have an isolated episode of optic neuritis would prefer not to be investigated to see if there is evidence they have MS. There is no convincing disease-modifying therapy at this stage of the disease and therefore agreeing to the patient's wishes should not make any difference to their prognosis. In the future, more effective forms of treatment may become available at disease onset and it will then be vital to make the diagnosis at an earlier stage in all patients.

Papillitis can look similar to papilloedema through an ophthalmoscope. Papillitis causes early and profound loss in vision, with a central scotoma, impaired colour vision and pain on eye movement. In papilloedema, visual deterioration occurs only at a late stage, when there is enlargement of the blind spot and sometimes constriction of the fields.

Brainstem presentation

Demyelination may initially affect the brainstem including the cerebellar connections and medial longitudinal fasciculus (see Fig. 19.3, p. 125) in the brainstem.

Classical presentations include:

- Diplopia: often due to internuclear ophthalmoplegia (failure of adduction of one eye, sometimes with coarse nystagmus of the other abducting eye on lateral gaze), caused by a lesion of the medial longitudinal fasciculus. This may be unilateral or, more commonly, bilateral.
- Nystagmus (due to cerebellar disease).
- Vertigo.
- Dysarthria (often cerebellar).
- Facial numbness and even trigeminal neuralgia as it affects the exiting fifth nerve and nucleus.
- Dysphagia.

- Ataxia (trunk and limbs).
- Pyramidal signs: with involvement of the corticospinal tracts.
- Hemisensory or patchy sensory changes in the limbs

Spinal cord lesion (myelopathy)

A spinal cord lesion is a common presentation and results in a spastic paraparesis (thoracic cord) or tetraparesis (cervical cord), often with tonic spasms of the limbs. There is associated difficulty walking and sensory loss. Bladder symptoms are extremely common.

Lhermitte's symptom, in which there is a brief, electric-shock-like sensation down the limbs on flexion of the neck, may be present. It is often indicative of lesions within the spinal cord, which can occur with processes other than demyelination, e.g. vitamin B_{12} deficiency before treatment.

The symptoms and signs of MS tend to get worse with heat, e.g. in the bath or during hot weather (Uthoff's phenomenon).

DIFFERENTIAL DIAGNOSIS

Initial presentation may cause diagnostic difficulty but few other conditions follow a similar subsequent pattern of relapsing and remitting CNS disease. The exceptions are Behçet's disease, CNS sarcoidosis, and systemic lupus erythematosus.

There are multiple causes of optic neuritis, brainstem syndromes, and myelopathy, and these must be excluded on initial presentation.

INVESTIGATIONS

There is no diagnostic test for MS, but the clinical suspicion is supported by the following three tests.

Magnetic resonance imaging (MRI)

Computed tomography scans do not accurately pick up areas of demyelination, whereas MRI is far more sensitive at showing the white-matter disease. Hyperintense lesions are seen on T2-weighted images. Widespread MRI abnormalities are often seen at presentation, in spite of the symptoms being isolated to one or two sites. Similar hyperintense lesions may be seen in multi-focal vascular and granulomatous disorders. Contrast enhancement of some lesions on the MRI and not of others suggests that the lesions are separated in time as well as space, which is an important criterion for making the diagnosis of MS.

Cerebrospinal fluid examination

A mild lymphocyte pleocytosis may be present, especially during relapses. The protein may be slightly elevated. However, the presence of 'oligoclonal bands' (several intense bands of staining for IgG on Western blotting) in the CSF but not in the serum is highly suggestive of MS.

Oligoclonal bands in the CSF and often the serum may also be found in many chronic infective or inflammatory conditions involving the CNS.

Evoked potentials

Visual evoked potentials (VEPs)

If there has been demyelination at any time along the optic nerve (i.e. optic neuritis), whether symptomatic or asymptomatic, the conduction of visual images (usually a changing checkerboard) to the occipital cortex will be delayed. The normal response takes about 100 milliseconds.

Somatosensory evoked potentials (SSEPs)

Measurement of SSEPs may detect a delay in central sensory pathways.

Brainstem auditory evoked potentials (BAEPs)

Measurement of BAEPs during auditory testing, may detect brainstem lesions.

MANAGEMENT

Treatments for the disease process

Anti-inflammatory treatment

Steroid therapy, usually given intravenously as methylprednisolone (high dose, 1 gramme, for 3 days), is the mainstay treatment used for severe acute relapses. This may shorten the duration of the relapse but does not affect eventual clinical outcome.

Suppression or modulation of the immune system

Interferon-β1a and 1b and glutiramer acetate are currently being used in selected patients, especially those with relapsing and remitting disease. Current guidelines suggest that a patient must have had at least two significant relapses within the past 2 years to qualify for treatment. The clinical relapse rate is modestly reduced by 30%. National Institute for Clinical Excellence (NICE) guidelines currently suggest that these treatments are not cost-effective when cost is compared to improvement in 'quality of life years' (QALYs) but it is still prescribed to selected individuals who appear to benefit. These drugs also demonstrate a slight effect on secondary progressive disease, although they are less widely used for this and the benefit is less convincingly supported by evidence from clinical trials.

Symptomatic treatment

Spasticity

Spasticity can be a considerable problem, especially if painful spasms develop. Drugs such as baclofen, dantrolene, diazepam, and tizanidine can be helpful. Care must be taken not to reduce the tone too far, as some patients require the increased tone to walk as they use their spastic leg as a 'stick'.

Contractures may be prevented with physiotherapy but sometimes require injections of botulinum toxin to reduce the tone in the muscle.

Bladder dysfunction

Anticholinergic drugs may help if incontinence is a problem (e.g. oxybutynin, tolterodine). Intermittent self-catheterization or a permanent urinary catheter may be required. Intravesical capsaicin has also been shown to help in some cases.

Prevention and early treatment of urinary tract infections is important because the neurological symptoms and signs can worsen with intercurrent infection. Checking for a urinary infection is especially important in patients who are about to commence steroids and patients can develop life-threatening sepsis if immunosuppressed while harbouring an infection.

Paroxysmal symptoms

Some patients develop tonic muscle spasms, burning dysaesthetic pains, trigeminal neuralgia, and other brief brainstem symptoms that may be helped by carbamazepine or phenytoin, acting as membrane stabilizers.

Intention tremor

The cerebellar tremor can be quite disabling and can sometimes be reduced with clonazepam.

OTHER CENTRAL DEMYELINATING DISEASES

A number of other rarer diseases can cause demyelination within the CNS but their presentation is very different from MS. These include:

- **Acute disseminated encephalomyelitis – ADEM:** this presents following a viral illness or vaccination. It is fatal in as many as 30% of cases. The areas of white matter change are often confluent and more symmetrical than in MS. Rarely the lesions are haemorrhagic.
- **Progressive multifocal leucoencephalopathy (PML):** caused by JC papovavirus infection, especially in immunocompromised patients, e.g. 4% of patients with HIV.
- **Leucodystrophies:** metachromatic leucodystrophy (disorder of arylsulphatase A enzyme), adrenoleucodystrophy (accumulation of very long chain fatty acids [VLCFAs]).
- **SSPE** (subacute sclerosing panencephalitis): this is a rare and deadly delayed complication of measles virus infection.
- **Vitamin B$_{12}$ deficiency:** can cause central demyelination
- **Central pontine myelinolysis (CPM):** this is associated with too rapid a correction of sodium in patients who are hyponatraemic and often have a history of alcohol abuse.

Systemic disease and the nervous system

Objectives

- Understand the common neurological complications that may arise from rheumatological, endocrine, renal, neoplastic and cardiac disease
- Be aware of the neurological problems that may affect patients in the intensive care unit

NEUROLOGICAL COMPLICATIONS OF ENDOCRINE DISEASE

Diabetes mellitus

Diabetes mellitus is by far the most common endocrinological and metabolic cause of neurological symptoms and signs involving the whole nervous system.

Coma

Coma can result during hypoglycaemia, or during ketotic or non-ketotic hyperglycaemia. Any patient in a coma should immediately have his or her glucose measured.

Cerebrovascular disease

Patients with diabetes have a higher risk of developing cerebrovascular disease than the general population. This includes large-vessel (e.g. middle cerebral artery occlusion) and small-vessel diseases (e.g. pseudobulbar palsy syndrome, gait apraxia and multi-infarct dementia).

Visual loss

Visual loss in diabetes may be due to retinal disease and haemorrhage, cataracts, or vascular disease (e.g. central retinal artery occlusion).

Peripheral nerve lesions

Peripheral neuropathy is a very common finding in diabetes. The most common types of neuropathy are:

- Distal symmetrical polyneuropathy (sensory greater than motor).
- Proximal asymmetrical motor neuropathy ('diabetic amyotrophy'): this syndrome is probably due to a lumbosacral plexopathy.
- Compression mononeuropathies, e.g. carpal tunnel syndrome.
- Multifocal neuropathy ('mononeuritis multiplex'): diabetes is the commonest cause of this syndrome, which may affect peripheral nerves in the limbs or individual cranial nerves, especially the third, sixth, and seventh (see Chapter 19).
- Autonomic neuropathy.

Thyrotoxicosis

Clinical features of Graves' disease often include exophthalmos with ophthalmoplegia. This is due to inflammatory infiltration and oedema of the periorbital fat and connective tissues.

A high-frequency tremor is characteristic and a proximal myopathy may be present. The severe weight loss with muscle atrophy and brisk reflexes that may be present in severe cases can be difficult to differentiate from motor neuron disease. This resolves rapidly with treatment of the hyperthyroidism.

In addition, atrial fibrillation is common and may result in embolic cerebral infarction.

Hypothyroidism

Carpal tunnel syndrome is common in hypothyroidism. Myopathy, neuropathy, and 'myxoedema madness' are extremely rare.

Cushing's disease and syndrome

Whether corticosteroid excess is due to a pituitary tumour, adrenal production, or exogenous steroid therapy, similar neurological features may result. These include proximal myopathy and psychosis.

Addison's disease

Addison's disease causes mental and physical lethargy. A mild proximal myopathy may be present.

Acromegaly

Inititally, there may be an increase in muscle strength but a proximal myopathy follows. Optic chiasmal compression from a macroadenoma causes bitemporal hemianopia. Carpal tunnel syndrome and peroneal nerve entrapment are common. Diabetes mellitus often develops and thus all its neurological sequelae may be seen.

NEUROLOGICAL COMPLICATIONS OF RENAL DISEASE

Encephalopathy

Encephalopathy occurs secondary to uraemia. If the development of uraemia is slow, this results in poor concentration and memory impairment. Misperceptions and visual hallucinations are common. Rapid development of uraemia can cause a severe encephalopathy, with deterioration of conscious level, coma, seizures, and focal signs.

Electroencephalography may show a generalized encephalopathic picture, epileptic activity, or triphasic waves (more common in hepatic encephalopathy).

Movement disorders associated with renal failure

- Myoclonus or limb tremor.
- Asterixis: a non-specific phenomenon in which there is a coarse flapping tremor when the hands are outstretched and the wrists hyperextended. It also occurs with hypercapnia and liver failure.

Other central nervous system signs associated with renal failure

- Transient focal signs: a reversible hemiparesis can occur with dialysis. It can alternate sides and appears to be a metabolic phenomenon rather than ischaemic because it progresses over a few hours.
- Stiffness and rigidity: usually involving axial muscles, with a board-like neck.
- Gait disturbance: usually part of a slowly developing encephalopathy, with marked unsteadiness.
- Seizures: there is a high incidence of seizures associated with renal failure.

Peripheral nervous system involvement in renal failure

Peripheral axonal neuropathy

Peripheral axonal neuropathy begins with burning and tingling pains in the feet, and restless legs. As it progresses, there is the development of a symmetrical sensorimotor neuropathy with absent ankle jerks.

The neuropathy is usually mainly sensory, and profound weakness may be due to another cause (e.g. hyperkalaemia).

There may be reversal or lack of progression of the neuropathy with stabilization of the disease or with transplantation.

Other complications of chronic renal failure

Other complications of chronic renal failure include confusional states and dementia in patients on dialysis, secondary amyloidosis, and side effects of immunosuppression in renal transplant cases. A range of infections may occur, particularly fungal, and lymphoma of the central nervous system develops in 5% of transplant cases. Cyclosporin can cause seizures, encephalopathy, neuropathy, and myopathy.

NEUROLOGICAL COMPLICATIONS OF CONNECTIVE TISSUE DISEASE

A wide variety of conditions cause inflammatory changes in connective tissue, especially of blood vessels. The neurological complications often relate to the vascular changes. All connective tissue diseases can be associated with polymyositis.

Systemic lupus erythematosus

The multisystem disorder systemic lupus erythematosus may be complicated by seizures, psychiatric disorders, cerebrovascular disease (large and small vessel), movement disorders, extraocular muscle palsies, multifocal neuropathy (mononeuritis multiplex), sensorimotor polyneuropathy, and polymyositis.

A central demyelinating variant that mimics multiple sclerosis may also occur.

Rheumatoid arthritis

Rheumatoid arthritis is associated with carpal tunnel syndrome, multifocal neuropathy, muscle atrophy (from disuse), and the serious complication of high cervical spinal cord compression from atlanto-axial subluxation. Cerebral arteritis is very rare.

Treatment with penicillamine causes a myasthenic syndrome in some patients. Prolonged steroid use may cause a proximal myopathy.

Polyarteritis nodosa

Polyarteritis nodosa causes a panarteritis with local thrombosis and occasionally rupture with micro-haemorrhages.

The most common neurological manifestations are due to peripheral nerve infarction, causing multifocal neuropathy. Cranial nerve palsies and cerebrovascular disease are less common.

Polymyositis

This inflammatory muscle disease is discussed in Chapter 25. It is associated with connective tissue disease in up to 25% of cases.

Sjögren's syndrome

A wide variety of neurological manifestations can occur with Sjögren's syndrome, including peripheral neuropathy (mostly sensory affecting joint position sense and vibration), entrapment syndromes, myelopathy, proximal myopathy, and meningoencephalitis. In addition, an isolated trigeminal neuropathy can occur.

NEUROLOGICAL COMPLICATIONS OF NEOPLASTIC DISEASE

Neurological manifestations of neoplasia (apart from primary nervous system tumours) can arise from cerebral metastases, non-metastatic causes (often antibody mediated) otherwise known as 'paraneoplastic' disease, or be due to the side effects of radiotherapy or the drugs used in chemotherapy.

Discussion will be limited to paraneoplastic conditions where there is no evidence of metastases or infiltration of nerves by the tumour.

- **Peripheral neuropathy:** a common finding in a variety of tumours, especially those of the bronchus, breast, and kidney. It is usually sensory involving vibration and joint position sense, but a motor neuropathy can also occur. It is associated with anti-Hu antibodies.
- **Limbic encephalitis:** occurs in small-cell carcinoma of the lung and testicular cancer and is associated with anti-Ma2 antibodies.
- **Cerebellar syndrome:** occurs in ovarian and lung tumours and is associated with anti-Purkinje-cell antibodies (anti-Yo).
- **Dermatomyositis:** is associated with underlying carcinoma (cervix, ovarian, and lung) in up to 15% of cases (see Chapter 25).
- **Lambert–Eaton myasthenic syndrome:** occurs with small-cell carcinoma of the bronchus and is associated with antibodies directed against presynaptic voltage-gated calcium channels (see Chapter 24).

NEUROLOGICAL COMPLICATIONS OF CARDIAC DISEASE

Atrial fibrillation is the most common cardiac risk factor for stroke, especially when there is associated heart failure or left atrial enlargement.

During or following myocardial infarction, cerebral hypoperfusion may occur secondary to left ventricular failure. There may be subsequent embolism from mural thrombus associated with the infarcted heart wall. The routine use of thrombolytic agents reduces the risk of the mural thrombosis but increases the risk of cerebral haemorrhage.

Disease of the mitral and aortic valves increases the risk of cerebral emboli, especially with infective endocarditis.

Congenital heart disease is also associated with neurological disease. There is a high incidence of cerebral aneurysms with coarctation of the aorta. Cyanotic heart diseases can cause chronic cerebral anoxia.

Abrupt changes in cardiac rhythm, usually profound bradycardia, present with presyncope or loss of consciousness (Stokes–Adams attacks). These are typically brief, with more rapid recovery than from seizures. Ventricular tachycardias are a less common cause.

Any patient who undergoes cardiac by-pass (e.g. for valve replacement or coronary artery bypass grafting) is at risk of developing a stroke from thrombus or atheroma that is dislodged during the operation. Patients also develop subtle cognitive changes that may be due to showers of small air and microthrombotic emboli passing into the brain during by-pass.

NEUROLOGICAL COMPLICATIONS ASSOCIATED WITH INTENSIVE CARE

Patients on an intensive care unit (ICU) can have a neurological disease as their primary diagnosis (e.g. respiratory failure in myasthenia gravis or Guillain–Barré syndrome) but any patient can develop one of several neurological complications while in an ICU. Most of these complications are covered elsewhere in the text. Critical illness neuropathy is described in detail below.

Critical illness neuropathy

Epidemiology

Occurs in up to 70% of patients who are in ICU for more than 5 days. The severity is associated with length of stay in ICU.

Clinical features

- Often presents with difficulty in weaning off ventilator.
- Mixed motor and sensory polyneuropathy but motor signs tend to predominate.

Investigations

- Electromyogram (EMG) and nerve conduction: relative preservation of conduction velocities and latencies (primary axonal degeneration). Reduction of amplitude of muscle and sensory compound action potentials. Needle EMG shows fibrillation potentials and positive sharp waves.
- Creatine kinase: normal.
- Cerebrospinal fluid: occasional mildly raised protein.

Prognosis

Most patients who survive their underlying illness will recover nerve function. Clinical recovery may take weeks in mild cases and months in severe cases. Nerve conduction studies may remain abnormal for several years.

Entrapment neuropathies

See Chapter 23, p. 149.

Critical illness myopathy

See Chapter 25, p. 167.

Steroid myopathy

See Chapter 30, p. 167.

Encephalopathy

For example, sepsis, metabolic derangement, hypo-perfusion; see Chapter 2, p. 9.

Seizures

Seizures can develop in ICU due to many factors including sepsis, hypoxia, toxins and drugs.

Myoclonus

This can develop after the patient has had a hypoxic brain injury or after encephalitis.

The effects of vitamin deficiencies and toxins on the nervous system

Objectives

- Understand the common syndromes associated with vitamin deficiencies
- Consider the wide range of drug-induced neurological disorders
- Describe the main neurological syndromes associated with other toxins

VITAMIN DEFICIENCIES

Nutritional deficiencies are particularly common in developing countries but do occur in developed countries due to eating habits, alcoholism, and malabsorption syndromes. The most common conditions will be described below.

Vitamin B$_1$ (thiamine) deficiency

Deficiency of vitamin B$_1$ causes beriberi or Wernicke–Korsakoff syndrome.

Beriberi

Beriberi is caused by a staple diet of polished rice and results in either a polyneuropathy (dry beriberi) or marked generalized oedema with ascites and pleural effusions (wet beriberi).

Wernicke–Korsakoff syndrome

Wernicke–Korsakoff syndrome is more common in the Western world than beriberi and is caused primarily by chronic alcoholism with poor dietary intake of thiamine.

The syndrome is composed of an acute phase (Wernicke's encephalopathy) and a chronic phase (Korsakoff's psychosis).

The typical triad of Wernicke's encephalopathy comprises:

- Ocular signs: with nystagmus and ophthalmoplegia.
- Ataxia: with a broad-based gait, and cerebellar signs in the limbs, especially the legs.
- Confusion: with disorientation, apathy, agitation, amnesia, stupor, and coma.

- In chronic cases, a slower amnestic syndrome develops, with selective impairment of short-term memory, which is made up for by confabulation (Korsakoff's psychosis).

The pathology of Wernicke–Korsakoff syndrome involves symmetrical damage to the mamillary bodies, thalamus, and periaqueductal grey matter.

Treatment for Wernicke's encephalopathy is intravenous thiamine followed by instigation of a normal diet and continued oral thiamine. Korsakoff's psychosis is also treated with oral thiamine and a normal diet, but patients are often left with a severe neurocognitive deficit.

Vitamin B$_6$ (pyridoxine) deficiency

Vitamin B$_6$ deficiency causes a mainly sensory neuropathy and may be precipitated during isoniazid therapy for tuberculosis. Pyridoxine supplements should therefore be given when isoniazid is prescribed.

Vitamin B$_{12}$ deficiency

Deficiency of vitamin B$_{12}$ can, rarely, result from nutritional deficiency (e.g. vegans) but is more often caused by malabsorption. The usual causes are pernicious anaemia, gastrectomy, and diseases of the terminal ileum (e.g. Crohn's disease, coeliac disease blind-loop syndrome). Up to 25% of patients with neurological damage caused by vitamin B$_{12}$ deficiency do not have haematological abnormalities (i.e. macrocytic megaloblastic anaemia).

The condition causes damage to the peripheral nerves, dorsal columns, and corticospinal tracts bilaterally, and is called subacute combined degeneration of the cord (see Chapter 20, p. 136).

Fig. 31.1 Toxins and their neurological effects

Neurological complication	Toxin
Dementia	Alcohol, mercury, lead, manganese, aluminium, solvent abuse, tin
Acute or subacute encephalopathy	Lead, mercury, manganese, thallium, solvent abuse, arsenic, tin
Drug-induced confusional state or psychosis	Antiparkinsonian drugs, steroids, isoniazid, mercury, tricyclics, alcohol withdrawal, lithium, amphetamines, cannabis, lysergic acid diethylamide (LSD), numerous other drugs
Lowered threshold of seizures	Alcohol, amphetamines, neuroleptics, tricyclics, other antidepressants, tin
Parkinsonism	Neuroleptics, flupenthixol, antiemetics, reserpine, amiodarone, manganese, 1-methyl-4-phenyl-1,2,3,6-tetrahydropyridine (MPTP)
Chorea and/or dystonia	L-dopa, dopamine agonists, antiemetics, neuroleptics, phenytoin, benzhexol, manganese
Tremor	β_2-agonists, lithium, sodium valproate, amiodarone, amphetamines, alcohol, levothyroxine, mercury, manganese
Cerebellar syndrome	Alcohol, phenytoin, solvent abuse, mercury, carbamazepine
Ototoxicity	Aminoglycoside antibiotics, quinine, ethacrynic acid, frusemide, overdose of aspirin
Optic neuropathy	Ethambutol, chloroquine, methyl alcohol, chloramphenicol, possibly pipe tobacco
Lens opacities	Steroids, chloroquine, amiodarone
Myelopathy	Nitrous oxide abuse, lathyrism (plant toxins), tin
Peripheral neuropathy	Gold, lead (motor), arsenic, thallium, mercury, alcohol, acrylamide, organophosphates, industrial solvents, drugs including isoniazid, nitrofurantoin, vincristine, metronidazole, disulphiram, clioquinol, dapsone, sulphonamides, emetine, phenytoin, pyridoxine, griseofulvin, cisplatinum, amiodarone, tricyclic antidepressants
Neuromuscular blockade	Botulinum toxin, organophosphate compounds, 'nerve gases', penicillamine, aminoglycosides (and other antibiotics) may exacerbate myasthenia
Myopathy	Steroids, chloroquine, statins, clofibrate, amiodarone, zidovudine (AZT), alcohol

Treatment with intramuscular vitamin B_{12} must be started promptly. If treatment is initiated early, there can be complete recovery; if delayed, the progression may be halted but there is little reversal. The condition can theoretically be made worse by giving folic acid without vitamin B_{12}.

Folic acid deficiency

It has been suggested that deficiency of folic acid (folate) causes neuropathy and dementia. However, the evidence is somewhat conflicting and folate deficiency is often found on a background of either chronic alcohol abuse with poor nutritional intake or malabsorption syndromes, when neurological conditions may be arising from other causes.

Nicotinic acid deficiency

Nicotinic acid deficiency causes pellagra and is found in areas where the staple diet is maize.

The clinical features comprise dermatitis, diarrhoea, and dementia.

Vitamin D deficiency

This is associated with a proximal myopathy with wasting and weakness. It is most commonly seen in the elderly with poor diet and lack of sun exposure. It is also seen in immigrant populations, malabsorption syndrome, treatment with anticonvulsants and in chronic renal failure.

Vitamin E deficiency

Vitamin E is a fat-soluble vitamin that can become deficient in malabsorption syndromes, especially in cystic fibrosis, coeliac disease, and diseases in which there is a reduced bile-salt pool. There is a rare familial fat-malabsorption syndrome with abetalipoproteinaemia associated with vitamin E deficiency.

Vitamin E deficiency causes primarily an ataxic syndrome, with areflexia and loss of vibration sense and proprioception, but sparing of cutaneous sensation. It can resemble Friedreich's ataxia.

Treatment is with oral vitamin E.

TOXINS

There are numerous toxins capable of causing neurological symptoms, many of which are drugs prescribed for other medical conditions. The most common are listed in Fig. 31.1.

In thiamine deficiency, glucose is inadequately metabolized and lactate and pyruvate accumulate. It is therefore essential to give thiamine immediately to any patient with suspected thiamine deficiency, before giving any sugar-containing substance, especially 5% dextrose or dextrose saline.

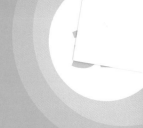

Hereditary conditions affecting the nervous system

Objectives

- Describe the main clinical features of neurofibromatoses, tuberous sclerosis, Sturge–Weber syndrome, the spinocerebellar degenerations, porphyria and Wilson's disease.

Nearly every part of the nervous system can be affected by a genetic disease. As our understanding of the molecular and cell biology of the nervous system progresses, mutations in genes associated with many hereditary diseases are being described. These include mutations in the 'MERLIN' gene in neurofibromatosis type 2, huntingtin or 'IT15' gene in Huntington's disease, frataxin gene in Friedreich's ataxia, PMP 22 gene duplication in Charcot–Marie–Tooth type 1, DYT 1 in early-onset generalized dystonia, CACNA1A in familial hemiplegic migraine and SCN1A in generalized epilepsy with febrile convulsions plus. Many haplotypes that might not necessarily cause the disease but increase the probability of it occurring are being described (e.g. the apo-ε4 allele in Alzheimer's disease). There has also been an expansion in the number of common neurological conditions where a small proportion of the patients have been found to have a family history and the relevant gene has been described (e.g. point mutations in alpha-synuclein causing Parkinson's disease). These discoveries have rapidly advanced our understanding of the cellular processes involved in many neurological diseases and it is hopefully only a matter of time before this translates into pharmacological treatments in the clinical setting.

NON-METABOLIC HEREDITARY CONDITIONS

Neurocutaneous syndromes

A number of inherited conditions involve disorders of organs derived from the ectoderm, causing tumours (benign and malignant), hamartomas (disorganized collections of blood vessels), and lesions in the skin and nervous system. Only the most common are outlined below.

Neurofibromatosis

There are a number of different types of neurofibromatosis, but types 1 (peripheral predominance) and 2 (central predominance) are the most important.

Neurofibromatosis type 1 (von Recklinghausen's disease)

Neurofibromatosis type 1 is an autosomal dominant condition caused by a defect in a gene called neurofibromin on chromosome 17, with an incidence of 1 in 4000.

Clinically, it is characterized (Fig. 32.1) by:

- Neurofibromas: lying along peripheral nerves.
- Café-au-lait spots: multiple pale-brown macules, especially on the trunk. They are found in the normal population, but more than five in an individual is abnormal.
- Cutaneous fibromas (molluscum fibrosum): subcutaneous, soft, often pedunculated, pink tumours, usually multiple.
- Axillary freckling.
- Lisch nodules: small hamartomas of the iris.

Other associated features include:

- Neural tumours: there is a higher incidence of neural tumours than in the general population, e.g. meningioma, vestibular schwannomas on the eighth nerve, gliomas, spinal root neurofibroma.

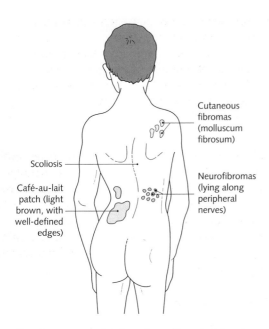

Fig. 32.1 Cutaneous manifestations of neurofibromatosis type 1.

- Skeletal abnormalities: 50% of patients have a scoliosis. There may be bone hypertrophy underlying subperiosteal neurofibromas.
- Endocrine abnormalities: associated phaeochromocytoma, medullary carcinoma of the thyroid.
- Local gigantism of a limb.
- Mental retardation and epilepsy: in 10–15% of patients.
- Renal artery stenosis.
- Obstructive cardiomyopathy.
- Pulmonary fibrosis.

Neurofibromatosis type 2

Neurofibromatosis type 2 is an autosomal dominant condition caused by a defect in the MERLIN gene on chromosome 22, with an incidence of 1 in 50 000. Clinically, it is characterized by few skin and skeletal manifestations and the presence of bilateral eighth nerve vestibular schwannomas ('acoustic neuromas'). Other intracranial and intraspinal tumours are common.

Treatment

Intracranial tumours require excision and, if necessary, radiotherapy. Cosmetic surgery may be required for the cutaneous manifestations. Genetic counselling is important.

Tuberous sclerosis

Tuberous sclerosis is an autosomal dominant condition with an incidence of 1 in 30 000.

It is characterized by skin lesions, especially adenoma sebaceum on the face (Fig. 32.2), epilepsy, and varying degrees of mental retardation.

In addition to the nodular lesions on the cheeks (adenoma sebaceum), skin manifestations include depigmented patches (ash-leaf macule), 'shagreen' patches, and subungual fibromas. Slowly expanding cerebral tumours may occur (hamartomatous 'tubers' and astrocytomas). Systemic tumours may affect the kidney, lung, or muscle.

Treatment

The epilepsy is often quite resistant to treatment. Surgery may be required for large cerebral tumours, especially if hydrocephalus develops. Careful regular evaluation and follow-up of these patients must be made to provide a possibility of early treatment for the neoplastic complications.

Sturge–Weber syndrome

Sturge–Weber syndrome has no clear inheritance pattern. It is characterized by an extensive port-wine naevus or 'stain' on one side of the face (Fig. 32.3), usually within the first and second divisions of the

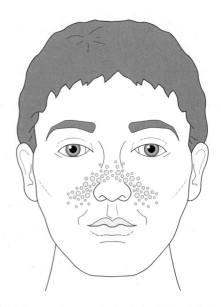

Fig. 32.2 Adenoma sebaceum: classic raised reddish nodules found over the nose and cheeks in tuberous sclerosis.

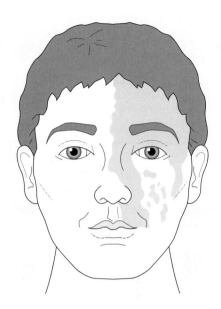

Fig. 32.3 Port-wine naevus in Sturge–Weber syndrome.

trigeminal nerve, and an underlying leptomeningeal angioma. There may be atrophy of the affected hemisphere, epilepsy, and congenital glaucoma.

If epilepsy is sufficiently intractable, lobectomy, or even hemispherectomy may be required. The early removal of the surface lesion remains controversial.

Spinocerebellar degeneration

There are a large number of inherited conditions producing varying clinical pictures of spinocerebellar degeneration. Three of the more common conditions are outlined below but they are all rare.

Friedreich's ataxia

Friedreich's ataxia is an autosomal recessive condition caused by an expanded trinucleotide repeat (GAA) in the intronic sequences of the frataxin gene on chromosome 9. The severity of the disease phenotype depends on the number of trinucleotide repeats. Frataxin is especially found in the spinal cord, heart, and pancreas and not in the cerebellum or cerebrum.

Within the spinal cord there is progressive degeneration of the posterior columns, corticospinal tracts, and dorsal and ventral spinocerebellar tracts.

Clinical features include:

- Ataxia: starting in the legs, spreading to the arms.
- Dysarthria is delayed for at least 5 years.

- Neuropathy: absent ankle jerks, absent joint position and vibration sense.
- Pyramidal signs: upgoing plantar responses (in spite of absent ankle jerks).
- Skeletal abnormalities: pes cavus and scoliosis.
- Cardiomyopathy and arrhythymias.
- Optic atrophy.
- Diabetes

Before the discovery of the frataxin gene, only patients with an earlier onset and severe phenotype were often classified as having the disease but now that gene testing is available, patients in their 60s with a relatively mild phenotype are being diagnosed. Severely affected patients often die from cardiac complications (heart failure and arrhythmias) rather than the neurological complications.

Ataxia telangiectasia

Ataxia telangiectasia is an autosomal recessive disorder causing progressive cerebellar ataxia, ocular and cutaneous telangiectasia, and immunodeficiency. Death is often by the third decade, from infection or lymphoreticular malignancy.

Spinocerebellar ataxias

There is increased recognition of a group of diseases in which the predominant symptom is one of progressive cerebellar ataxia inherited often in an autosomal dominant manner. Many of the genes have now been described and some of them have an expanded CAG triplet repeat similar to Huntington's disease; others are caused by problems in the potassium and calcium channels or 'channelopathies'. The spinocerebellar ataxias may be associated with a wide range of signs including a degenerative retinopathy, spasticity, parkinsonism, and a peripheral neuropathy.

Inherited neuropathies

See Chapter 23

INBORN ERRORS OF METABOLISM

Numerous rare metabolic conditions can cause nervous system abnormalities. Two of these will be discussed briefly and some others are listed in Figs 32.4 and 32.5.

Fig. 32.4 Some examples of rare metabolic encephalopathies

Disorders of phenylalanine
Phenylketonuria
Disorders of sulphur amino acid metabolism
homocystinuria
Disorders of branched-chain amino acids
Maple syrup urine disease
Organic acidaemias
Carnitine deficiency
Methylmalonic acid deficiency
Carnitine palmityl transferase deficiency
Acyl CoA dehydrogenase deficiency
Lactic acidosis
Pyruvate dehydrogenase deficiency
Leigh's disease
Disorders of sugar metabolim
Galactosaemia
Disorders of purine metabolism
Lesch–Nyhan syndrome
Xanthine oxidase deficiency
Disorders of pyrimidine metabolism
Xeroderma pigmentosum
Porphyrias
Lipoprotein deficiencies
Abetalipoproteinaemia
Tangier disease
Disorders of copper metabolism
Wilson's disease
Menke's kinky-hair syndrome
Mitochondrial encephalopathies
MELAS/MERRF/CPEO
Peroxisomal disorders
Infantile Refsum's disease
Adrenoleukodystrophy

Note: CPEO, chronic progressive external ophthalmoplegia; MERRF, myoclonic epilepsy and ragged red fibres; MELAS, mitochondrial encephalopathy, lactic acidosis, and stroke-like episodes

Fig. 32.5 Metabolic storage diseases

Glycogen storage diseases
Pompe's disease
Cholesterol storage diseases
Cerebrotendinous xanthomatosis
Neuronal ceroid lipofuscinois
Late onset (Kufs')
Mucopolysaccharidoses
Hurler's (type I)
Hunter's (type II)
Sphingolipidoses
Gangliosidoses
GM1 gangliosidosis
GM2 gangliosidosis
Niemann–Pick disease
Gaucher's disease
Krabbe's disease
Fabry's disease
Metachromatic leukodystrophy

Porphyria

The porphyrias comprise a heterogeneous group of disorders of haem synthesis, causing overproduction of porphyrins.

Acute intermittent porphyria, an autosomal dominant disorder occurring in adult life, can cause neurological complications. It can be precipitated by certain drugs or alcohol.

Clinical features and their frequency are as follows:

- Abdominal pain: 90%.
- Peripheral neuropathy: 70%; usually an acute motor neuropathy that can present like Guillain–Barré syndrome.
- Hypertension and tachycardia: 70%.
- Psychiatric disturbance: 50%.
- Seizures: 15%.

Diagnosis can be made by screening the urine for porphobilinogen levels. However, testing the blood for reduced erythrocyte porphobilinogen deaminase and raised aminolaevulinic acid synthetase is most sensitive.

Management is largely supportive, with a high carbohydrate intake, narcotics for pain, and haematin infusion. Any drugs that precipitate the condition should be avoided.

Wilson's disease (hepatolenticular degeneration)

Wilson's disease is a rare autosomal recessive disorder of copper metabolism. There is a deficiency of caeruloplasmin, which binds copper, resulting in copper deposition in various organs, especially in the liver and the basal ganglia in the brain.

Clinical features comprise:

- Movement disorder: a wide range of movements can occur, including tremor, early dysarthria, and dysphagia, dystonic movements, and parkinsonism.
- Cirrhosis of the liver.
- Kayser–Fleischer ring (Fig. 32.6): a fine brown deposition of copper in Descemet's membrane of the cornea, which may ultimately form a ring.

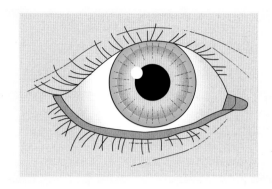

Fig. 32.6 Kayser–Fleischer ring, seen in the cornea of patients with Wilson's disease.

This may be visible to the naked eye but slit-lamp examination is usually necessary.

Diagnosis is by measurement of a low serum caeruloplasmin and total serum copper, with elevated unbound or 'free' copper. There is high urinary copper excretion and liver biopsy may show massive copper deposition.

Treatment involves a lifelong low-copper diet and a chelating agent such as penicillamine. Liver transplantation is sometimes performed.

HISTORY, EXAMINATION AND COMMON INVESTIGATIONS

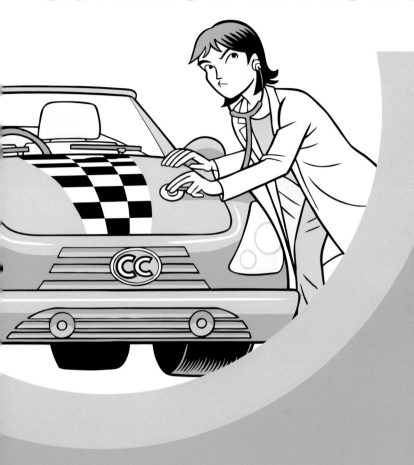

The patient's neurological history often provides more diagnostic information than examination or investigations and it is therefore important to do it well. Many common conditions, such as headache and epilepsy, are diagnosed solely from the clinical history.

General observation of the patient as he or she walks into the examination room, or as you approach the bed, is often important in establishing the diagnosis:

- Does the patient appear unwell?
- Does he or she use any walking aids (sticks, crutches, frame, wheelchair, callipers)?
- Are there any obvious morphological abnormalities (e.g. weakness on one side, drooping of the face, wasting of the muscles, involuntary movements, abnormal gait)?

It is important to gain the patient's trust and to begin to develop a rapport at the initial contact, so that the patient feels comfortable talking about illnesses that might be embarrassing or stigmatizing:

- Introduce yourself.
- Explain who you are.
- Ask if you can talk to and examine the patient.
- Ask the patient's age and occupation.
- Ask whether the patient is right- or left-handed (if you do not ask this at the beginning, you might forget).

Within the first few minutes of the consultation you should be able to make some inferences about the patient's mood and cognitive state:

- Does the patient respond appropriately (indicating probable preservation of important higher mental functioning)?
- Does he or she appear to be depressed (which can either be part of the patient's neurological condition or might indicate a reaction to it) or behaving inappropriately (as in patients who have frontal lobe dysfunction)?
- Is the patient's speech normal?

STRUCTURE OF THE HISTORY

The presenting complaint (PC)

Consider the PC from the patient's point of view. Ask:

- 'What is the main problem?'
- 'What was it that caused you to go to your doctor/come to the hospital?'

When presenting the history to others, use the patient's language (e.g. 'This woman complains of seeing double') not the medical terminology (e.g. 'This woman complains of horizontal diplopia').

History of the presenting complaint (HPC)

Establish the HPC by asking:

- When did the patient first notice it?
- Was the onset sudden (over seconds or minutes), subacute (over hours or days), or insidious and gradual (over weeks, months or years)?
- Is the symptom episodic, constant and progressive, or constant with fluctuations in intensity?
- Has it worsened, improved, or stayed the same since?
- What is the character of the symptom (e.g. headache may be throbbing, stabbing or pressure-like) and its distribution (unilateral, bilateral, frontal, occipital, etc.)?
- Is there anything that makes it better (e.g. medicines, sleep, exercise) or worse (e.g. movement, coughing, posture)?
- Are there any associated symptoms (e.g. vomiting, photophobia, neck stiffness)?
- Have any other symptoms developed since this first complaint was noticed (in particular additional neurological symptoms, e.g. blurred vision, unsteady gait)?
- Has the patient ever had other neurological symptoms in the past? These might be related (e.g. an episode of transient visual loss 5 years

previously in a young woman now complaining of difficulty in walking is indicative of possible multiple sclerosis).
- Have any tests already been performed and if so, where and by whom?

Once the HPC has been elucidated, it is useful to ask general questions pertaining to neurological dysfunction including:

- Problems with double or blurred vision.
- Difficulties in speech, swallowing, chewing.
- Weakness or sensory symptoms in the limbs.
- Sphincter function (bowels, bladder, sexual function).
- A history of falls.
- Difficulties with memory or other cognitive functions.
- Further questions pertaining to the HPC will relate to the differential diagnosis of the main complaint, the most common of which are outlined in Part 1 of the book.

Past medical history (PMH)

Some clinicians prefer to take the PMH before considering the presenting complaint because there might be important background information. The following may be relevant in neurological cases:

- Birth and childhood development, e.g. motor and verbal milestones.
- Infections and seizures during childhood.
- Head injuries.
- Hypertension, ischaemic heart disease, rheumatic fever.
- Diabetes.
- A systemic disorder, e.g. systemic lupus erythematosus.

Drug history (DH)

To determine the DH, find out from the patient:

- Is he or she taking any medicines now, or have any been taken for some time in the past?
- Are there any known drug allergies?

Review of systems (ROS)

Review the following body systems:

- Gastrointestinal: appetite, weight loss or gain, swallowing, change in bowel function.

- Cardiovascular: chest pain, breathlessness, palpitations, claudication.
- Respiratory: cough, breathlessness.
- Genitourinary: bladder function, impotence, sexual function.
- Musculoskeletal: joint pain, stiffness.

Family history (FH)

To determine the FH, find out from the patient:

- Are there any 'family illnesses', especially in relatives under the age of 60 years?
- Are parents, siblings, and children alive and well and, if not, what did they die from and at what age?
- Could the patient's parents possibly be related, i.e. a consanguinous marriage? This is especially important in autosomal recessively inherited conditions when related patients may carry the same defective gene and pass both to their children.

Social history (SH)

To determine the SH, ask the patient about:

- Home circumstances: house or flat, stairs, help from Social Services.
- Smoking history.
- Alcohol intake (units/week): is there a past history of heavy alcohol consumption?
- Diet (vegetarian or vegan).
- Sexual history or orientation: this might be relevant in certain cases.

When presenting the history, always start with the same sequence:
- Name.
- Age.
- Handedness, if relevant.
- Occupation.
- Complaint (in the patient's words).

Then continue with:
- History of presenting complaint.
- Past medical history.
- Review of systems.
- Drug history.
- Family history.
- Social history.
- Summary.

Summary

When presenting the history to colleagues (a very important skill), you need to spend several minutes organizing your thoughts and the structure of the history. It is best to start with a general summary such as: 'Miss Randolph is a 40-year-old, administrator who complains of numbness in the feet.' The HPC, PMH, and ROS should then be described. You do not have to mention all negative points but it is worth pointing out those that are important (e.g. 'She has no history of diabetes' in a patient who has a peripheral neuropathy).

List the patient's medications and any side-effects or benefits they perceive to obtain from them.

Describe the FH, if relevant; if it is not, state: 'There is no relevant family history'.

Describe important social points: 'She drinks only moderate amounts of alcohol and has never smoked'.

You will then move on to your examination findings.

SPEECH

Speech production is organized at three levels:

1. Phonation.
2. Articulation.
3. Language production.

Phonation: dysphonia

Phonation is the production of sounds as the air passes through the vocal cords. A disorder of this process is called dysphonia.

Assessment

Speech will have already been heard during the history taking. Patients who have dysphonia may present with reduced speech volume and the voice may sound hoarse or husky. Aphonia is the inability to produce sound. Coughing may also be impaired in dysphonic patients because this action requires normal vocal cord function. Coughing should be tested in patients in whom there is a possibility of dysphonia.

Articulation: dysarthria

Articulation is the manipulation of sound as it passes through the upper airways by the palate, the tongue, and the lips to produce phonemes. A disorder of this process is called dysarthria.

Assessment

Articulation is assessed from the patient's spontaneous speech during history taking and also, if necessary, by asking a series of additional questions such as the patient's name and address, what he or she had for breakfast and what he or she has been doing recently. Ask the patient to repeat a series of phrases: 'baby hippopotamus', 'West Register Street', 'British Constitution'. The characteristics of the speech can be gained from these phrases and localization of the site of the lesion may be possible based on the type of dysarthria and confirmed by additional signs on formal neurological examination (see Chapter 9).

Although dysarthria can be caused by neurological disorders affecting the muscles of the soft palate, lips, tongue and larynx, a non-neurological cause (such as an inflammatory or infective process affecting the mucosal surfaces) might be responsible and should be sought in the first instance. Ill-fitting or absent dentures can also cause the patient to sound dysarthric.

Dysarthria may result from a lesion of the:

- **Upper motor neuron** (pseudobulbar palsy): slow, high-pitched and forced and often described as 'hot potato' speech' because the patient talks as if they have a hot potato in their mouth.
- **Lower motor neuron** (bulbar palsy): slurred and indistinct with nasal intonation; labial and lingual sounds are affected.
- **Basal ganglia:** rapidly spoken words, low-pitched, and monotonous (akinetic-rigid syndromes); loud, harsh, and with variable intonation (chorea and myoclonus); loud, slow, and indistinct consonants (athetoid).
- **Cerebellum:** slow and slurred, scanning or 'staccato' quality if there is also involvement of the corticobulbar tracts.
- **Muscle and neuromuscular junction:** similar to those of a bulbar palsy. In myasthenia gravis, there might be a deterioration in the quality of speech (fatiguability) during prolonged speech or over the course of the day.

Language production: dysphasia

Language production is the organization of phonemes into words and sentences. It is controlled by the speech centres in the dominant hemisphere (Broca's and Wernicke's areas). A disorder of this process is called dysphasia.

Assessment

To assess language production:

- Establish the patient's handedness: dysphasia is a feature of dominant-hemisphere dysfunction. The left hemisphere is dominant in over 95% of right-handed and about 60% of left-handed individuals.
- Listen to the patient's spontaneous speech, assessing its fluency and content.
- Assess the patient's comprehension by observing his or her response to simple commands, e.g. 'Open your mouth', 'Look up to the ceiling'.
- Assess the patient's ability to name objects: use your wristwatch (face, hands, strap, buckle).
- Assess the patient's ability to repeat sentences, e.g. 'No ifs, ands, or buts'.

An **expressive** dysphasia arises from a lesion of **Broca's** area in the dominant frontal lobe (Fig. 1.1, p. 4). The speech is non-fluent and hesitant, but comprehension mostly intact. The speech may be 'telegraphic' with loss of the conjunctions and articles. Repetition is better than spontaneous speech. The patient has difficulty finding the correct words and often produces an incorrect word. Writing is often also poor. Patients retain insight into their language disturbance.

A **receptive** dysphasia arises from a lesion of **Wernicke's** area in the posterior superior temporal lobe and probably also the adjacent parietal lobe (Fig. 1.1, p. 4). The speech is fluent but the words are partly correct, incorrect but related to the intended word (paraphrasia), or newly created (neologisms). The patient often has poor comprehension of the spoken word and has poor handwriting. The language is therefore mostly unintelligible, but the patient is often unaware of the problem.

Conduction dysphasia occurs when there is damage to the tract called the arcuate fasciculus, that joins Wernicke's and Broca's regions. It causes a syndrome similar to receptive apahasia with fluent speech, abnormal and new words, and loss of repetition but preservation of comprehension.

Nominal dysphasia is the inability to name objects. It can occur following recovery from other types of dysphasia and occasionally as part of a dementia.

Global and mixed dysphasia is often seen in clinical practice where both receptive and expressive defects coexist or only some of the features are seen from each.

The clinical features of the different types of dysphasia are summarized in Fig. 34.1.

MENTAL STATE AND HIGHER CEREBRAL FUNCTIONS

Consciousness

Consciousness is the state of being aware of self and the environment. A number of ill-defined terms are used to describe different levels of consciousness:

- **Alert:** full wakefulness and immediate and appropriate responsiveness. The patient is orientated in person, time, and place.
- **Confusion:** the inability to think with the usual speed and clarity. There may be lack of attention, disorientation in time and place, and impairment of memory. Delirium is a confusional state characterized by hyperactivity. The patient may be agitated, excited, and anxious with visual hallucinations.
- **Obtundation:** the patient is drowsy and indifferent to the environment but responsive to verbal stimuli.
- **Stupor:** the patient is unconscious but rousable when stimulated.
- **Coma:** the patient is unaware of self and the environment and is not rousable.

The terms described above are imprecise and often used differently by different clinicians. The level of consciousness is therefore more objectively assessed using the Glasgow Coma Scale (see Fig. 2.2, p. 13).

Fig. 34.1 Classification of dysphasia

Type	Lesion	Speech fluency	Speech content	Comprehension	Repetition
Expressive	Broca's area	Non-fluent	Impaired	Normal	Variable
Nominal	Angular gyrus	Fluent	Impaired	Normal	Normal
Receptive	Wernicke's area	Fluent	Impaired	Impaired	Impaired
Conductive	Arcuate fasciculus	Fluent	Impaired	Normal	Impaired
Global	Frontal, parietal and temporal lobe	Non-fluent	Impaired	Impaired	Impaired

Appearance and behaviour

Assessment of the patient's mental state begins as soon as you meet the patient. The physical appearance can be helpful. Demented patients may look bewildered but unconcerned, or apathetic and withdrawn. Self-neglect is common but may be masked by caring relatives. The patient's response to your questions during the history taking is important in terms of assessing his or her comprehension and whether he or she retains insight into the problem.

Affect

- Does the patient seem depressed?
- Loss of interest, euphoria or social disinhibition may be signs of frontal lobe dysfunction. Emotional behaviour such as aggression and anger may arise from damage to the limbic system.
- Emotional lability, such as uncontrollable laughing or crying, should prompt further examination to look for upper motor neuron signs associated with a pseudobulbar palsy.

Cognitive function

Mini-mental State Examination

The Mini-mental State Examination is a screening test for several different cognitive functions (Fig. 34.2):

- **Orientation** of person, time, and place establishes full awareness of self and the environment. Further testing requires the patient to be alert.
- **Registration and recall** tests immediate and recent memory respectively. Remote memory may be tested by asking about memories of childhood, work, or marriage. These need corroboration with family or friends to be certain the details are correct. Verbal memory can be tested by asking the patient to remember a sentence or short story and to recall it 15 minutes later. Visual memory can be assessed by asking the patient to memorize three objects on a table and recall them after 15 minutes.

Fig. 34.2 Mini-mental State Examination

Orientation
1. What is the year, season, date, month, day? (one point for each correct answer)
2. Where are we? Country, county, town, hospital, floor? (one point for each answer)

Registration
3. Name three objects, taking 1 second to say each. Then ask the patient to name all three. One point for each correct answer. Repeat the question until the patient learns all three, e.g. 'bus', 'rose', 'door'.

Attention and calculation
4. Serial sevens. One point for each correct answer. Stop after five answers. Alternative: spell 'world' backwards

Recall
5. Ask for names of the three objects asked in question 3. One point for each correct answer

Language
6. Point to a pencil and a watch. Ask the patient to name them for you. One point for each correct answer
7. Ask the patient to repeat 'No ifs, ands, or buts'. One point
8. Ask the patient to follow a three-stage command: 'Take the paper in your right hand; fold the paper in half; put the paper on the floor with your left hand'. Three points
9. Ask the patient to read and obey the following: CLOSE YOUR EYES. (Write this in large letters.) One point
10. Ask the patient to write a sentence of his or her own choice. (The sentence must contain a subject and an object and make some sense). Ignore spelling errors when scoring. One point

Constructional/spatial
11. Ask the patient to copy two intersecting pentagons with equal sides. Give one point if all the sides and angles are preserved and if the intersecting sides form a quadrangle

Maximum score = 30 points

- **Attention** and calculation can be tested by asking the patient to spell a five-letter word backwards and to subtract 7 from 100 and continue to subtract 7 from each answer obtained; if the latter is too complex for the patient's premorbid calculation skills, simple arithmetic can be used.
- **Language** examination tests comprehension of speech and written language and includes tests for dysphasia, dyslexia and dysgraphia.
- **Constructional** ability.

The maximum score is 30. Scores of less than 25 suggest the presence of cognitive impairment. Formal psychometric testing should be performed for all patients suspected of having impaired cognition.

Motor dyspraxia and apraxia

Motor apraxia is the loss and dyspraxia is the impairment of the ability to perform skilled movements in the absence of weakness, sensory loss, incoordination, or impaired comprehension. Motor apraxia and dyspraxia arise from a lesion of the non-dominant parietal cortex and may be confined to the limbs, trunk, or face.

The ability to perform skilled tasks can be tested as follows:

- Upper limbs: the patient's ability to use a pen or comb can be assessed. Dressing can be assessed by asking the patient to put on a shirt.
- Lower limbs: the ability to walk can be tested by examining the gait (see Chapter 14, p. 87).
- Trunk: the patient is asked to sit down and get up from a chair.
- Face: the patient is asked to stick out his or her tongue or to whistle.
- Eyes: the patient is asked to close his or her eyes and to open them on command.

Agnosia

Agnosia is the failure to recognize and interpret a sensory stimulus without the aid of other senses in the presence of intact peripheral sensation (tactile, visual, and auditory). There are several different types:

- **Tactile agnosia (or astereognosis):** the inability to recognize a familiar object placed in the hand with eyes closed, e.g. a patient cannot recognize a key or coin manipulated in the hand with the eyes closed. It arises from a lesion of the contralateral posterior parietal lobe.
- **Visual agnosia:** the inability to recognize a familiar object by looking at it without touching it or hearing any sound from it, e.g. a telephone. It arises from a lesion of the (usually dominant) parieto-occipital lobe.
- **Auditory agnosia:** the inability to recognize a sound such as a bell ringing without seeing or feeling the bell. It arises from a lesion of the dominant temporal lobe.

Clinical syndromes associated with specific focal hemispheric dysfunction

Frontal lobe

Patients who have a lesion of the frontal lobe should be tested for the following:

- A contralateral mono- or hemiparesis and lower facial weakness.
- Broca's expressive dysphasia (see p. 228).
- Behavioural change: alteration in personality or mood and loss of interest and initiative can be observed by watching the patient on the ward and through conversation. This usually occurs more severely with bilateral disease.
- Loss of abstract thought: this can be tested by the patient's interpretation of proverbs, e.g. people in glass houses should not throw stones; and by the patient's ability to identify similarities between pairs of objects, e.g. cow and dog, chair and table.
- Primitive reflexes: the grasp reflex is usually found in infants and consists of flexion of the thumb and fingers on stroking the skin of the palm. The sucking reflex can be elicited by lightly stroking the lips, which produces a sucking response. The palmomental reflex involves a brief muscular twitch on one side of the chin in response to a scratch by the examiner across the patient's palm on the same side.
- Apraxia of gait (see Chapter 14, p. 87).

Parietal lobe

Features of a lesion of the dominant parietal lobe are:

- Contralateral discriminatory sensory impairment: there is impairment of position sense and two-point discrimination, and inability to recognize objects by form and texture (astereognosis) or figures drawn on the hand (agraphasthesia). Pain, temperature, touch, and vibration sensation are intact, but their localization when applied to the body may be impaired.

- Wernicke's receptive dysphasia (see p. 228).
- Visual field deficit: there is a contralateral lower homonymous quadrantanopia.
- Right–left disorientation.
- Finger agnosia: the inability to recognize and identify the fingers of the hand correctly.
- Dyscalculia: calculation is impaired when asked to perform serial sevens or simple arithmetic.
- Dyslexia: there is difficulty with reading.
- Ideomotor and ideational dyspraxia: there is difficulty in carrying out a motor task on request or by imitation.

Features of a lesion of the non-dominant parietal lobe are:

- Constructional dyspraxia: the patient has difficulty drawing a simple object or with constructing an object, e.g. using building blocks.
- Dressing dyspraxia: the patient has difficulty putting on and taking off clothes.
- Geographical dyspraxia: the patient is unable to orientate in his or her environment.
- Contralateral sensory inattention: the patient neglects the opposite side of the body. This may be sensory or visual. Sensory inattention can be tested by asking the patient to close his or her eyes and for the examiner to touch the patient's right or left leg (or arm or face), then to touch both sides together. These patients will identify touch on each side individually but, when touched on both sides, will identify touch only on the side of the lesion, neglecting the contralateral side. Visual inattention may be similarly elicited by testing the visual fields (see p. 233); these patients will have normal visual fields when each side is tested individually but, when both visual fields are tested, the side contralateral to the lesion will be neglected. For similar reasons, a hemiplegic patient may ignore the paralysed side of the body, usually when the right hemisphere is affected.

Temporal lobe

Patients who have a lesion of the temporal lobe should be tested for the following:

- Wernicke's receptive dysphasia (see p. 228).
- Auditory agnosia (see p. 230).
- Visual field deficit: there is a contralateral upper homonymous quadrantanopia.

- Learning difficulties and memory impairment; bilateral lesions result in impaired retention of new information.
- Emotional disturbances: aggression, rage, and hypersexuality can be observed by watching the patient on the ward and through conversation.

Occipital lobe

Patients who have a lesion of the occipital lobe should be tested for the following:

- Visual field deficit: there may be a contralateral homonymous hemianopia (note that a lesion of posterior cerebral artery spares the macula and a lesion of the occipital pole may result in a contralateral macular homonymous hemianopic field defect) (see Fig. 5.2, p. 28); bilateral occipital lesions render the patient blind, but with normal pupillary reflexes (cortical blindness).
- Visual agnosia (see p. 230).

GAIT

Normal gait involves rotating the erect body, supported by one leg at a time, while the other leg swings forward to plant the foot and act as the next support for the body to swing forwards. Only one foot will be on the floor most of the time, although both the heel of the front foot and the toes of the back foot will be on the ground momentarily when the body weight is transferred from one leg to the other. Normal gait requires input from the motor, somatosensory, visual, cerebellar, and vestibular systems.

Assessment

- Ask the patient to walk up and down the examination room, with the arms loose by the side.
- Observe the patient's posture, the pattern of arm and leg movements, and the control of the trunk.
- If gait appears normal, ask the patient to heel–toe walk ('I would like you to walk heel to toe as if you are walking on a tightrope'). Walk alongside to offer support if the patient appears unsteady.
- If gait appears abnormal, classify it into one of the patterns described in Chapter 14, p. 87.

CRANIAL NERVES

The brainstem is a phylogenetically ancient organ that subserves control of basic functions such as breathing, cardiovascular function, consciousness, and thermoregulation. It also acts as a pathway for tracts between the cerebrum and the spinal cord controlling movement and sensation. Finally, it is involved in movement and sensation of the head and neck. Examination of the brainstem provides important prognostic information in the unconscious patient and irreversible damage to the brainstem is the criterion for the legal definition of death.

Olfactory nerve (first, I)

To test the olfactory nerve, first ask the patient about any recent change in the sense of smell or taste. A characteristic-smelling object (e.g. peppermint, clove oil) is held under each nostril in turn while the other is occluded and the patient keeps the eyes closed. An individual who has intact olfaction can not only detect the smell, but also discriminate and name it. The recommended special testing bottles are rarely available when needed and most clinicians perform preliminary assessment with nearby objects such as fruit, a coffee jar, or cigarette packet. Avoid using irritating odours such as ammonia or camphor because these can non-specifically activate fifth nerves receptors in the nasal mucosa.

Unilateral loss of smell is usually asymptomatic. Bilateral loss of smell may be associated with an altered sensation of taste (dysgeusia or ageusia).

When examining patients who have anosmia, it is important to look carefully for frontal lobe signs and evidence of optic nerve or chiasmal damage, as these structures are anatomically close to the pathways that subserve smell.

The most common cause of impaired smell is pathology in the nasal passages or sinuses.

Optic nerve (second, II)

Visual acuity

Visual acuity (VA) is tested using a Snellen chart in a well-lit room. Seat or stand the patient 6 m from the chart. Small, hand-held Snellen charts can be read at a distance of 2 m (Fig. 34.3).

Correct the patient's refractive error with glasses or a pinhole. Ask the patient to cover each eye in turn with his or her palm, and find which line of print the patient can read comfortably. VA is expressed as the distance between the chart and the patient and the number of the smallest visible line on the chart. The numbers associated with each line on the chart correspond to the distance (in metres) at which a normal patient should be able to read that line of letters. So 6/6 is normal and 6/24 means that from 6 metres away the patient can only read letters that a normal individual can read from 24 metres (Fig. 34.3). If the patient is unable to read characters of line 60 (VA less than 6/60), assess his or her ability to count your fingers at 1 m (VA:CF), see your hand movements (VA:HM), or perceive a torch light (VA:PL). If unable to perceive light (VA:NPL), then the patient is blind.

Fig. 34.3 Visual acuity. The patient is able to read line number 24 but not line number 12; visual acuity is therefore 6/24. If the patient could read only three out of the four letters on line number 24 then the visual acuity would be 6/24–1.

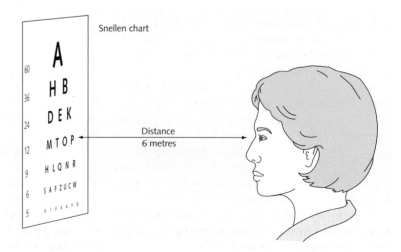

Colour vision

Colour vision is tested using Ishihara plates in a day-lit room. Test each eye separately. If at least 15 out of 17 plates are read correctly, colour vision can be regarded as normal.

This test is designed principally to detect congenital colour vision defects, but is sensitive in detecting mild degrees of optic nerve dysfunction when the red colours are often lost first.

Visual fields

Sit about 1 m from the patient with your eyes at the same horizontal level. Start by testing for visual inattention (see p. 231). Ask the patient to look into your eyes; hold your hands halfway between you and the patient. Stimulate the patient's visual fields by moving each hand separately and then both hands together, and ask the patient to indicate which of your hands has moved each time.

In patients with a non-dominant parietal lobe lesion, a visual stimulus presented in isolation to the contralateral field is perceived, but it may be missed when a comparable stimulus is presented simultaneously to the ipsilateral field.

Visual fields are examined by confrontation, during which you compare your own visual fields with the patient's on the assumption that yours are normal. The patient's visual field will match yours only if your head positions are exactly comparable and if your hand is exactly halfway between you and the patient.

Visual fields in poorly cooperative patients are assessed by the response to visual threat (sudden, unexpected hand movement into the patient's visual field).

Peripheral fields

Examine each eye in turn. To test the patient's right visual field, ask the patient to cover his or her left eye with his or her left palm and to look into your left eye throughout the examination.

Cover your right eye with your right hand, and test the patient's peripheral field by bringing the moving fingers of your left hand into the upper and then the lower quadrants of the patient's temporal fields. Ask the patient to inform you as soon as he or she sees your fingers.

Now cover your right eye with your left hand and examine the patient's nasal fields with your right hand, using the same method.

Lesions of different parts of the visual pathway produce characteristic field defects (see Fig. 5.2, p. 28) and are discussed in Chapter 5.

Blind spot

Routine testing is unnecessary, but enlargement of the blind spot may be an important finding in patients with raised intracranial pressure.

The blind spot is tested using a 10 mm red hatpin. Ask the patient to cover his or her left eye, and move the pin from the central into the temporal field, along the horizontal meridian, having explained to the patient that the pin will disappear briefly and then reappear again, and that he or she should indicate when this happens. Once you have found the patient's blind spot, you can map its shape and compare its size with yours.

Central field

The central field is tested by moving a red hatpin along the central visual field (fixation area) in the horizontal meridian. Ask the patient to indicate if the pin disappears (absolute central scotoma) or if the colour appears diminished (relative scotoma). A central scotoma may extend temporally from the fixation area into the blind spot (centrocaecal scotoma).

Perimetry

Peripheral visual fields are sensitive to a moving target and formally tested with Goldmann perimetery. The patient fixates on a central point and a point of light moves centrally from the periphery. The patient indicates the position of the point of light each time and this is plotted on a chart. Repetitive testing from different directions accurately records the visual fields. Central fields can be tested using this method, but with a less intense light source. Humphrey fields use a static light source. A record of the threshold of the light source with increasing intensity provides information about the central visual field.

Fundoscopy

Ask the patient to fixate on a distant target in dimmed light. Using a direct ophthalmoscope, examine the patient's right eye using your right eye, and the patient's left eye using your left eye.

Adjust the ophthalmoscope lens until the retinal vessels are in focus, and trace them back to the optic disc. Assess the cupping, colour, and contour of the optic disc, and the clarity of its margins. The temporal disc margins are normally slightly paler than the nasal margins. The physiological cup varies in size but does not extend to the disc margins.

The retinal vessels should then be assessed. The arteries are narrower than the veins and more red in colour. The vessels should not be obscured as they cross the disc margins. Look for retinal vein pulsation, which is present in about 80% of normal individuals and is an index of normal intracranial pressure. This is seen best at the disc margins where the veins cross over the arteries. Note the width of the blood vessels and look for arteriovenous nipping at the cross-over points.

Assess the rest of the retina, noting any evidence of discoloration, haemorrhages, or white patches of exudate. Ask the patient to look at the light of the ophthalmoscope, which brings the macula into view.

Classify fundoscopic abnormalities into those affecting the optic disc, the retinal vessels, or the retina (Fig. 34.4).

Oculomotor (third, III), trochlear (fourth, IV), and abducens (sixth, VI) nerves

Eyelids

Ptosis is drooping of the upper eyelid and the drooping is usually partial. A full ptosis (complete closure of the eyelid) is usually due to a third nerve palsy. Examination of pupil responses and eye movements

Fig. 34.4 Common fundoscopic abnormalities

Structure	Abnormality	Pathology
Optic disc	Papilloedema – the optic disc is 'swollen' with blurring of the disc margin and engorgement of the retinal veins; there may be flame-shaped haemorrhages near the disc	Raised intracranial pressure (space-occupying lesions, e.g. tumours, particularly of the posterior fossa, hydrocephalus subsequent to meningitis or subarachnoid haemorrhage), venous obstruction (e.g. cavernous sinus thrombosis), malignant hypertension, idiopathic intracranial hypertension
	Optic atrophy – the disc is paler than usual, particularly on the temporal side, with fewer small vessels crossing its margins	Any cause of chronic optic nerve disease – central retinal artery occlusion, optic neuritis (multiple sclerosis, ischaemia), chronic glaucoma, B_{12} deficiency, toxins (e.g. methyl alcohol, tobacco), hereditary (e.g. Leber's optic atrophy), lesion of the optic chiasm and or tract
Retinal arteries	Silver-wiring, increased tortuosity, arteriovenous nipping	Hypertension
	Gross narrowing with retinal pallor and reddened fovea	Central retinal artery occlusion
	Cholesterol or platelet emboli	Cerebrovascular disease
	New vessel formation (on the surface of the optic disc or retina): new vessels develop subsequent to widespread retinal ischaemia; they do not affect vision, but are fragile and may bleed	Diabetes, central or branch retinal vein occlusion
Retinal veins	Venous engorgement	Papilloedema (see above), central retinal vein occlusion
Retina	Haemorrhages	Superificial flame-shaped and deep dot-shaped (hypertension, diabetes); subhyaloid between the retina and the vitreous (subarachnoid haemorrhage)
	Exudates	'Soft cotton-wool spots' (retinal infarcts) and hard exudates (lipid accumulation within the retina from leaking blood vessels in hypertension and diabetes)
	Pigmentation	Retinitis pigmentosa (e.g. Refsum's disease, Kearns–Sayre syndrome), choroidoretinitis (e.g. toxoplasmosis, sarcoidosis, syphilis), post-laser treatment (diabetes)

provide essential information about the cause of the ptosis (Fig. 34.5).

Pupils

Size and shape

Assess the size and shape of the pupils. They should be circular and symmetrical (see Fig. 6.3, p. 35). A discrepancy between the size if the pupils is called anisocoria. The most common cause of an irregular pupil is secondary to disease or trauma directly to the anterior chamber of the eye (e.g. anterior uveitis or postsurgical). The Argyll Robertson pupil is associated with tertiary syphilis and consists of irregular pupils that have an accommodation reflex but an absent light reflex. This abnormality occurs more often in examinations than in everyday practice.

Light response

Light responses should be assessed using a bright torchlight. Ask the patient to fixate on a distant target, then shine the light into each eye in turn, bringing the torch beam quickly onto the pupil from the lateral side. Observe the direct (ipsilateral) and the consensual (contralateral) responses.

Assess the presence of an afferent pupillary defect by swinging the light from one eye to the other, dwelling 3 seconds on each (see Chapter 6 and Fig. 6.4, p. 37 for further details).

Accommodation

The accommodation reflex consists of two components. The first involves convergence of the eyes, which requires simultaneous adduction of both eyes. The second involves bilateral simultaneous constriction of the pupils. This reflex is required for actions such as reading a book or walking downstairs. To test this reflex, ask the patient to look into the distance and then bring an object to within 10 cm of the patient's eyes and ask him or her to fixate on the object. Both components of the reflex should be observed on near fixation.

Eye movements

Inspect the eyes and note the position of the eyelids and the presence of any strabismus (misalignment of the visual axes). Strabismus is non-paralytic or paralytic (see p. 38). There are two main types of eye movement:

- Pursuit eye movements are used to follow an object smoothly.
- Saccadic ('jump') eye movements are used to look from one object to a distant object without focusing on objects in between.

Conjugate eye movements occur when the visual axes stay correctly aligned during either pursuit or saccadic movements. If the visual axes are misaligned, the patient experiences diplopia. Sometimes, the brain

Fig. 34.5 Assessment of ptosis

Cause	Additional clinical features	Pupil responses	Eye movements
Congenital	Hereditary; unilateral or bilateral	Normal	Normal
Neurogenic 3rd nerve palsy (see p. 37 and Fig. 6.3, p. 35)	Complete ptosis	Dilated pupil, absent response to light and accommodation	Eye looks 'down and out' ophthalmoplegia with diplopia in all positions of gaze
Horner's syndrome	Partial ptosis, apparent enophthalmos; ipsilateral anhidrosis	Constricted pupil, impaired response to light and accommodation	Normal
Myogenic Senile	This is due to degenerative changes in the levator superioris muscle of the upper eyelid	Normal; senile pupil – constricted with impaired dilatation in the dark	Normal
Myasthenia gravis	Fatiguable and therefore variable ptosis	Normal	Variable diplopia and ophthalmoplegia
Myopathy	Associated bulbar/limb weakness	Normal	Abnormal if extraocular muscles involved

tries to correct a partial failure of gaze with a saccadic movement. The cycle of failure to sustain gaze and correction by saccadic movement is called nystagmus.

Pursuit eye movements

To test pursuit eye movements, ask the patient to focus on an object, such as a finger or pen, held approximately 50 cm in front of the patient's nose. Any strabismus, ptosis, or nystagmus in the 'primary position' should be noted. The patient should be asked to follow the object as it describes the shape of an 'H' in front of the patient and to inform the examiner of any double vision. In the presence of diplopia, identify the direction of the maximum separation of images and the two muscles responsible for moving the eyes in this direction (see Fig. 6.5, p. 37). Cover each eye in turn and observe when the outer image disappears. The outer image is always produced by the pathological eye, irrespective of where the double vision occurs. The presence of nystagmus should also be noted, whether it is horizontal or vertical, and in which direction it is maximal. The smoothness and speed of pursuit eye movements should also be noted.

Saccadic eye movements

To test saccadic eye movements, hold a finger approximately 50 cm in front of the patient's nose and a fist approximately 50 cm lateral to the finger. Ask the patient to move his or her gaze rapidly back and forth between the fist and finger. This is repeated in all four directions keeping a finger in front of the patient and moving the fist to the appropriate direction. Assess the velocity and the accuracy of these movements. The presence of slow or absent adduction in the horizontal plane is consistent with an internuclear ophthalmoplegia: (see Fig. 6.10, p. 41). There may also be horizontal gaze-evoked nystagmus in the abducting eye.

If pursuit or saccadic eye movements are absent, the oculocephalic reflex (doll's eye movements) will differentiate between supranuclear and nuclear gaze palsy. The oculocepalic reflex is tested by asking the patient to fixate on your eyes while you rotate his or her head in the horizontal and the vertical planes. The reflex in supranuclear lesions is intact, allowing the patient's eyes to remain fixated on the examiner's eyes. This reflex is intact because the afferent (information from neck muscle and vestibular apparatus) and efferent (nerves and muscles controlling eye movements) loop is intact. If there is a nuclear or more peripheral lesion (i.e. pathology in the brainstem, nerves, or muscles) then the reflex loop is broken and doll's eye movements are absent.

Ocular nerve palsy

Clinical signs and causes of ocular nerve palsy are discussed in Chapter 6.

Nystagmus

Nystagmus is an involuntary, rhythmic oscillation of the eyes caused by lesions affecting the vestibular apparatus, the vestibulocochlear (eighth) nerve, and brainstem centres involved in controlling gaze or the cerebellum. Nystagmus is usually asymptomatic but patients sometimes describe an unpleasant experience of alternating movements of their visual fields, which is called oscillopsia.

In normal individuals a few beats of nystagmus can often be observed at the extremes of gaze. This is not pathological or sustained. It may also occur during voluntary rapid oscillation of the eyes. These physiological movements are called nystagmoid jerks.

Nystagmus should be looked for in the primary position of gaze (i.e. when the patient is looking straight ahead) and also during the testing of eye movements. Nystagmus can be jerky (the oscillation has a fast and a slow phase) or pendular (the oscillation occurs with equal velocity in all directions). The nystagmus may be horizontal, vertical, rotatory, or a mixture of these. The amplitude of the nystagmus and its persistence should be noted. The direction of jerky nystagmus is defined by the direction of the fast phase by convention. Causes of nystagmus are shown in Fig. 34.6.

Trigeminal (fifth, V) nerve

The motor part of the trigeminal nerve is highly robust and is not often affected by the many pathologies that involve the surrounding structures. However, the sensory aspect of the fifth nerve is often affected by local pathologies and loss of the corneal reflex is often one of the first clinical signs of a lesion at the cerebellopontine angle.

Motor

Inspect for wasting of the temporalis muscles, which produces hollowing above the zygoma. Ask the patient to clench his or her teeth and palpate the masseters for contraction and relaxation. Note any loss of bulk. Assess the pterygoid muscles by resisting the patient's attempts to open the mouth. In unilateral trigeminal lesions, the lower jaw deviates to the paralytic side as the mouth is opened.

Fig. 34.6 Causes of nystagmus

Type	Description	Pathology
Pendular	Oscillations of equal velocity	Longstanding impaired macular vision (since early childhood), e.g. albinism, congenital cataracts, congenital nystagmus Lesions in upper brainstem, e.g. MS
Jerky	Fast phase towards the side of the lesion	Unilateral cerebellar lesions
	Fast phase to the opposite side of the lesion	Unilateral vestibular lesions or VIIIn. lesions
	Direction of nystagmus varies with the direction of gaze but fast phase towards side of lesion.	Brainstem pathology
	Upbeat nystagmus	Lesions at or around the superior colliculi (midbrain)
	Downbeat nystagmus	Lesions at or around the foramen magnum
Rotatory	Specific to one head position, and fatigues with repeated testing	Unilateral labyrinthine pathology
Mixed	jerky and rotatory	Brainstem pathology

Jaw jerk

Jaw jerk is a brainstem stretch reflex. Ask the patient to open the mouth slightly. Rest your index finger on the apex of the jaw and tap it lightly with the patella hammer. The normal response is closure of the mouth, which is caused by reflex contraction of the pterygoid muscles. An absent reflex is not significant but the reflex becomes pathologically brisk with upper motor neuron lesions (i.e. bilateral damage to the upper motor neurons (UMNs) to the motor fifth nucleus in the pons).

Sensory

Sensory testing is performed using the techniques described on p. 246. Test light touch, pin-prick, and temperature over the forehead, the medial aspects of the cheeks, and the chin. These correspond to the ophthalmic, maxillary, and mandibular branches of the trigeminal nerve, respectively (see Fig. 7.1, p. 43). It should be noted that the angle of the jaw is not innervated by the trigeminal nerve. A partial loss can be detected by comparing the response to the same stimulus on different areas of the face. The clinical pattern of sensory loss depends on the anatomical site of the lesion (Fig. 34.7).

Corneal reflex is elicited by lightly touching the cornea (not the conjunctiva) with a wisp of cotton wool. Synchronous blinking of both eyes should occur. An afferent defect (fifth cranial nerve lesion) results in depression or absence of the direct and consensual blinking reflex. An efferent defect (seventh cranial nerve lesion) results in an impairment or absence of the reflex on the side of the facial weakness.

Facial (seventh, VII) nerve

Motor

Inspect the patient's face, looking for asymmetry of the nasolabial folds and the position of the two angles of the mouth. Assess the movements of the upper part of the face by asking the patient to:

- Elevate his or her eyebrows.
- Close his or her eyes tightly and resist your attempt to open them. Look for Bell's phenomenon – this is a reflex upward deviation of the eyes in response to attempted but failed forced closure of the eyelids.

Fig. 34.7 Clinical syndromes of the trigeminal nerve

Site of lesion	Pattern of sensory loss
Supranuclear	Contralateral discriminative sensory loss in lesions of the primary somatosensory cortex
Upper pons	Ipsilateral loss of light touch with preserved pain and temperature sensation (spinal tract of trigeminal nerve).
Lower pons, medulla, upper cervial cord (lesion above C2)	Contralateral loss of pain and temperature sensation in an 'onion-skin' distribution; preserved light touch
Cerebellopontine angle	Ipsilateral loss of all modalities
Cavernous sinus	Ipsilateral loss of all modalities in the V_1 and occasionally V_2 distribution
Trigeminal root, ganglion, and peripheral branches of the nerve	Loss of all sensory modalities in the V_{1-3} distributions; there will be a more selective distribution of loss with lesions of the peripheral nerve

Note: JPS, joint position sense; VS, vibration sense.

Movements of the lower part of the face are assessed by asking the patient to:

- Blow out the cheeks with air.
- Purse the lips tightly and resist your attempt to open them.
- Show the teeth.
- Whistle.
- Smile (observe any facial asymmetry).

If you detect any weakness or asymmetry, decide if the weakness is confined to the lower part of the face (upper motor neuron lesion) or both the upper and the lower parts of the face (lower motor neuron lesion) (Fig. 34.8). Do not miss bilateral facial weakness. In this case, the face appears to sag, with lack of facial expression even though it is symmetrical.

Hyperacusis (oversensitivity to noise) is suggestive of a lesion affecting the nerve to the stapedius, which comes off the facial nerve in the facial canal within the petrous bone.

Sensory

Taste (visceral afferent)

Examine taste by applying a solution of salt, sweet (sugar), sour (vinegar), or bitter (lemon) to the anterior two-thirds of the tongue and comparing the response on the two sides. The mouth should be rinsed with water between testing. Lesions of the chorda tympani will cause loss of taste.

A few somatic afferent fibres from the seventh nerve subserve parts of the outer pinna. In Ramsay Hunt syndrome, there may be vesicles in this position with unilateral facial weakness associated with reactivation of herpes zoster in the geniculate ganglion.

Vestibulocochlear nerve (eighth, VIII)

Hearing

Clinical bedside assessment of hearing is not sensitive and can detect only gross hearing loss. Audiometry is usually required for detailed assessment.

Assess each ear separately while masking the hearing in the other ear by occluding the external meatus with your index finger. Test the patient's hearing sensitivity by whispering numbers into their ear and asking them to repeat these.

Determine if the hearing loss is conductive or sensorineural by performing Rinne and Weber's tests (see p. 49).

Vestibular function

There are no satisfactory bedside tests for vestibular function. Examination of the patient's gait and eye movements for nystagmus may be helpful. The findings in a patient who has vestibular dysfunction are summarized in Fig. 8.4, p. 53. The use of caloric testing and the Hallpike manoeuvre for patients

A

B

C

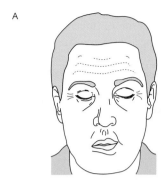

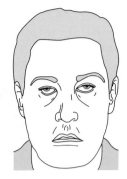

Right UMN weakness

Right LMN weakness

Bilateral LMN weakness

Fig. 34.8 Facial weakness. The patient is asked to close the eyes and purse the lips. Note the defective eye closure and Bell's phenomenon in (B) and (C). LMN, lower motor neuron; UMN, upper motor neuron.

presenting with positional vertigo is discussed on p. 55. A patient suspected of having vestibular dysfunction will sometimes require formal vestibular testing.

Glossopharyngeal (ninth, IX) and vagus (tenth, X) nerves

Motor

Check the patient's speech quality and volume for hoarseness and quietness as well as strength of cough to assess for dysphonia. Nasal intonation of speech arises from palatal weakness and causes a bulbar dysarthria.

Palatal movement can be assessed by:

- Asking the patient to say 'ah' (voluntary activity).
- Touching the posterior pharyngeal wall with the end of an orange stick on both sides (the 'gag' reflex).

Assess the afferent pathway of the 'gag' reflex (ninth cranial nerve) by asking the patient whether sensation is comparable on both sides. Assess the efferent pathway (tenth cranial nerve) by observing the normal response of a symmetrical rise of the soft palate and movement of the pharyngeal muscles; characteristically, a 'gagging' sound is made.

Supranuclear (upper motor neuron) innervation of the palatal and pharyngeal muscles is bilateral. Unilateral lesions will therefore not cause significant and prolonged dysfunction of swallowing and speech. In patients who have bilateral upper motor neuron lesions, the palate cannot be elevated voluntarily, but moves normally when testing the 'gag' reflex. This is part of a syndrome called a 'pseudobulbar palsy' and is associated with a brisk jaw jerk, spastic tongue and speech, and emotional lability.

If the voluntary and reflex movements are bilaterally impaired, then the patient may have a bilateral bulbar palsy (i.e. damage to the lower motor neurons [LMNs] or their nuclei in the brainstem on both sides). If the palate does not elevate on one side, the lesion almost always involves the lower motor neuron because the palate has bilateral UMN innervation. Therefore, in unilateral lower motor neuron lesions, the palate lies slightly lower on the affected side and deviates towards the unaffected side.

Minor and inconsistent deviations of the uvula should be ignored.

Sensory

The posterior pharyngeal wall is innervated by the glossopharyngeal (ninth cranial) nerve and sensation is tested by a wooden probe as described above. The ninth nerve also subserves sensation and taste to the posterior third of the tongue but taste is difficult to test in this location.

Accessory (eleventh, XI) nerve

The spinal part of the accessory nerve is a purely motor nerve that arises from the upper five segments of the cervical cord. It supplies the trapezius and sternocleidomastoid muscles and wasting or weakness of these muscles should be noted on inspection.

The strength of the sternocleidomastoid muscles is assessed by asking the patient to turn his or her head to each side against the resistance of the examiner's hand. Turning of the head to the left involves contraction of the right sternocleidomastoid and vice versa.

Assess the strength of the trapezius muscles by asking the patient to shrug his or her shoulders upwards against resistance and note the bulk of the muscles on palpation.

Hypoglossal (twelfth, XII) nerve

The hypoglossal nerve is a purely motor nerve that supplies the muscles of the tongue. Inspect the tongue as it lies in the floor of the mouth for evidence of wasting (which may be unilateral or bilateral), fasciculations (wriggling movements at the tongue surface) or other involuntary movements. Then ask the patient to protrude the tongue. Abnormalities caused by upper and lower motor neuron lesions are summarized in Fig. 34.9.

The motor system

The examination should start by simply observing the patient. Important information may be obtained through observing the patient during history taking. Is the patient not moving one side of the body? Was the patient unstable when sitting in the chair? The formal examination should be started by assessing the nature of the patient's gait and should then proceed to bedside examination of the motor system.

Gait

The different types of abnormal gait and how to assess gait disorders are discussed in Chapter 14.

Inspection

- **Posture:** look for the characteristic posturing of a patient with a hemiparesis (see Fig. 14.1, p. 88). Ask the patient to hold out both arms in front of the body with eyes closed. If the patient has an UMN lesion, he or she may demonstrate a drift of the arm downwards from the horizontal into a pronated and eventually flexed position. This is called 'pronator drift'. The fingers of the outstretched arm may move spontaneously, as if the patient was playing the piano. This is called 'pseudoathetosis' and is caused by loss of joint-position sense. In cerebellar disease, if the outstretched arms are rapidly displaced, they may oscillate about the horizontal rather than quickly returning to the initial position. This is called 'rebound'.
- **Muscle wasting:** look for the degree and distribution of muscle wasting. This is usually characteristic of LMN disorders, i.e. anterior horn cell, spinal nerve, plexus, or peripheral nerve disorders as well as myopathies.
- **Fasciculations:** these are seen as brief, localized twitches or flickers of movement within the muscle at rest and are also a feature of lower motor neuron disorders. Each muscle should be carefully studied for up to several minutes if there is a strong suspicion of a LMN disorder.
- **Involuntary movements**, e.g. a resting tremor may be evident in patients who have Parkinson's disease (see Chapter 11).
- Atrophic skin changes such as smooth, hairless, purple oedematous skin may be a sign of associated sensory nerve damage in a LMN disorder or from disuse in an UMN disorder.
- Any scars should be noted particularly over the lateral aspect of the foot from a sural nerve biopsy or over the vastus lateralis or triceps from a muscle biopsy. Some patients may have scars from orthopaedic surgery such as arthrodesis at the ankle in foot drop.

Fig. 34.9 Clinical patterns of tongue weakness

Lower motor neuron lesions	Unilateral	Atrophy and fasciculations ipsilateral to the side of the lesion and deviation of the protruded tongue towards the affected side.
	Bilateral	Bilateral atrophy and fasciculations (see bulbar palsy, p. 57 and p. 139)
Upper motor neuron lesions	Unilateral	Slight deviation of the tongue away from the side of the lesion but usually asymptomatic
	Bilateral	Tongue has limited protrusion and appears contracted (see pseudobulbar palsy, p. 57 and p. 139)

Walking sticks, ankle–foot orthoses, and other orthotic devices can often give an early clue as to the patient's main functional difficulty.

Tone

Tone refers to the activity of the stretch reflexes as assessed by the degree of resistance that occurs on stretching a muscle at different velocities.

Some patients have difficulty relaxing during an examination, which can artificially increase stiffness in their limbs. Relaxation can be achieved by asking the patient to loosen up the limbs so that they are limp.

Arm

Pyramidal hypertonia: spasticity

Take the patient's arm and flex and extend the elbow. Spasticity may be especially observed during extension. Then hold the patient's hand, with the elbow flexed, and rapidly pronate and supinate the forearm. If tone is increased, you may feel a 'supinator' or 'spastic catch', which is an interruption of the smooth movement on supination by increased tone of a spastic type. Alternatively, there may be increased tone on extending the elbow, which suddenly gives way to low tone. This is sometimes referred to as the 'clasp-knife' effect. These signs are suggestive of an UMN lesion.

Extrapyramidal rigidity

If there is increased tone throughout movement of a limb this is called 'lead-pipe' rigidity. When the patient has a tremor, which may be subclinical, and lead-pipe rigidity, they may have 'cogwheel' rigidity. These two types of rigidity are typical of idiopathic Parkinson's disease but can occur in many other extrapyramidal syndromes. All extrapyramidal types of increased tone can be enhanced by asking the patient to move the other arm up and down. If this brings out increased tone then the rigidity is said to occur 'with synkinesis'. Extrapyramidal rigidity is best looked for by rotating the wrist in both directions.

Legs

- Rock each leg from side to side on the bed, holding it at the knee. Normally, the foot lags behind the leg. If tone is increased, the foot and leg move stiffly together. If tone is decreased, the foot moves limply from side to side with each movement.
- Passively flex and extend the knee at varying speeds, supporting both the upper leg and the foot.
- With the patient's legs extended on the couch, place your hand under the patient's knee and

quickly lift the knee about 15 cm. The foot will normally stay on the bed as the knee is flexed. If tone is increased, the foot may jump up with the lower leg and if tone is decreased the limb will feel lax and slightly heavier than normal.

'Clonus' describes the rhythmic unidirectional contractions evoked by a sudden passive stretch of a muscle. This is elicited most easily at the ankle. A few beats may be normal but 'sustained clonus' is characteristic of an upper motor neuron lesion.

Power

Power is tested in each of the main muscle groups by the examiner stabilizing the limb proximal to the joint movement that is being tested. Power in each muscle is given a grade as defined by the Medical Research Council (MRC) scale (Fig. 34.10).

The scheme in Fig. 34.11 shows testing of the main muscle groups of the arms. The scheme in Fig. 34.12 shows testing of the main muscle groups of the legs.

Figure 34.13 summarizes the typical pattern of physical signs arising from lesions in different parts of the motor system.

Increased tone may be due to an upper motor neuron or extrapyramidal disorder. Spasticity occurs in patients who have increased tone due to an upper motor neuron lesion – look for a supinator catch, clasp-knife phenomenon and clonus, brisk reflexes, and extensor plantar responses. In patients who have increased tone due to an extrapyramidal disorder, there is characteristic 'lead-pipe' rigidity or 'cog-wheel' rigidity if there is a superimposed tremor. The reflexes are usually normal and plantar responses flexor.

Fig. 34.10 The MRC scale for assessment of muscle power

Grade	Response
0	No movement
1	Filcker of muscle when patient tries to move
2	Moves, but not against gravity
3	Moves against gravity but not against resistance
4	Moves against resistance but not to full strength
5	Full strength (you cannot overcome the movement)

Fig. 34.11 Testing muscle groups of the upper limb. The green arrow indicates the direction of movement of the patient, and the black arrow the direction of resistance by the examiner. Each muscle group should be given a grade as defined by the MRC scale (see Fig. 34.10).

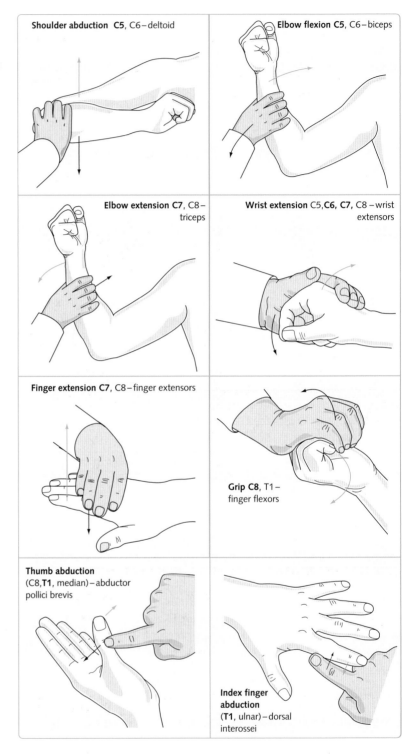

Shoulder abduction **C5**, C6 – deltoid

Elbow flexion C5, C6 – biceps

Elbow extension C7, C8 – triceps

Wrist extension C5, **C6**, **C7**, C8 – wrist extensors

Finger extension **C7**, C8 – finger extensors

Grip C8, T1 – finger flexors

Thumb abduction (C8, **T1**, median) – abductor pollici brevis

Index finger abduction (**T1**, ulnar) – dorsal interossei

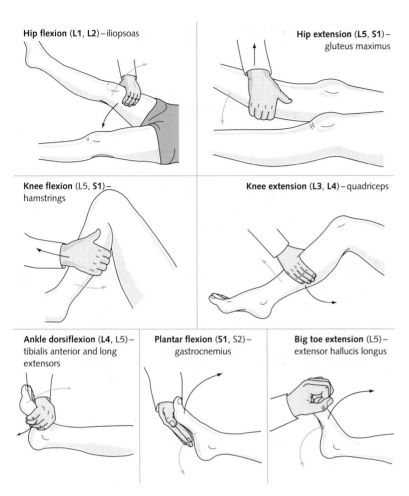

Hip flexion (L1, L2) – iliopsoas

Hip extension (L5, S1) – gluteus maximus

Knee flexion (L5, S1) – hamstrings

Knee extension (L3, L4) – quadriceps

Ankle dorsiflexion (L4, L5) – tibialis anterior and long extensors

Plantar flexion (S1, S2) – gastrocnemius

Big toe extension (L5) – extensor hallucis longus

Fig. 34.12 Testing muscle groups of the lower limb. The green arrow indicates the direction of movement of the patient, and the black arrow the direction of movement of the examiner. Each muscle group should be given a grade as defined by the MRC scale (see Fig. 34.10).

Fig. 34.13 Clinical features of patients presenting with limb weakness

Site of lesion	Wasting	Tone	Pattern of weakness	Reflexes	Plantar response
Upper motor neuron	None	Increased	'Pyramidal' pattern weakness	Increased	Extensor
Lower motor neuron	Present	Decreased	Individual or groups of muscles	Decreased/absent	Flexor or absent
Neuromuscular junction	Uncommon	Usually normal, may be decreased	Bilateral and predominantly of the proximal limb girdle (fatiguable)	Usually normal	Flexor
Muscle	From mild to severe	Decreased in proportion to wasting	Bilateral and predominantly of the proximal limb girdle	Decreased in proportion to wasting	Flexor

Note: Not every patient will have all the features of their syndrome.

Reflexes

Tendon reflexes are most easily determined by briskly stretching the tendon. To perform this, the tendon hammer is held near the end of the shaft and the heavy end is swung onto the tendon directly or onto a finger placed over the tendon (biceps and supinator jerks). The tendon reflexes shown in Fig. 34.14 A and B should be examined. The tendon reflexes may be increased ('brisk'), decreased or absent. If they are absent, this should be confirmed by reinforcement (Fig. 34.14C). Abdominal reflexes can be tested as shown in Fig. 34.14D. The plantar response is elicited by scratching the sole as demonstrated in Fig. 34.14E.

Tendon reflexes are conventionally annotated as shown in Fig. 34.15.

Coordination

The ability of a patient to perform smooth and accurate movements is dependent on power, intact joint-position sense, and coordination. Weakness and loss of joint-position sense may give rise to apparent clumsiness, which may be misinterpreted as incoordination. Cerebellar dysfunction can only be accurately detected if weakness and/or joint position sense loss is mild or there is severe incoordination.

Gait

A wide-based, sometimes lurching gait is seen in cerebellar disease. Unsteadiness is made more obvious if the patient is asked to walk 'heel to toe'.

Arms

Cerebellar dysfunction can be assessed as follows:

- **The finger–nose test:** the examiner places a finger 50 cm in front of the patient's nose and asks the patient to move his or her index finger between the nose and the examiner's finger; both index fingers are tested. In patients who have a cerebellar lesion, on approaching the examiner's finger, the patient's arm may coarsely oscillate. This is called an intention tremor. The inability to perform smooth, accurate, and targeted movements is called dysmetria. If the patient overshoots the intended target, this is called 'past pointing'.
- **Dysdiadochokinesis:** this is the inability to carry out rapid, alternating movements with regularity. It can be tested by asking the patient to alternately pronate and supinate his or her arm and correspondingly tap the palm and then dorsum of his or her hand on the examiner's palm. In cerebellar disease, the movements are irregular in amplitude and speed.
- **The 'rebound phenomenon':** if the wrists are gently tapped when the patient's arms are outstretched, then the arms should rapidly come to the resting horizontal position. In patients with cerebellar disease, the arms oscillate about the horizontal before coming to rest. This is called the rebound phenomenon.

Early stages of an upper motor neuron or extrapyramidal disorder may be picked up by noting impairment of fine finger movements. This can be tested by asking the patient to pretend to play a piano, and to touch each of the fingers in turn with the thumb of the same hand.

Legs

The heel–shin test

Ask the patient to place one heel on the other knee and slowly slide the heel down the shin, then lift the heel off the shin and repeat the test. This test should be performed on each side in turn.

The tapping test

The rapid tapping of the foot is impaired in cerebellar disease. This test should be performed on each side in turn.

The combination of these abnormalities in a patient is called cerebellar ataxia and may be associated with other signs of cerebellar disease such as horizontal jerky nystagmus and slurring dysarthria (see Chapter 10).

THE SENSORY SYSTEM

Patients use various terms to describe sensory disturbance, including numbness, tingling, 'pins and needles', and burning. Medical terms include paraesthesia (tingling), dysaesthesia (unpleasant awareness of touch or pressure), hyperaesthesia (exaggeration of any sensation), and hyperalgesia (exaggerated perception of painful stimuli).

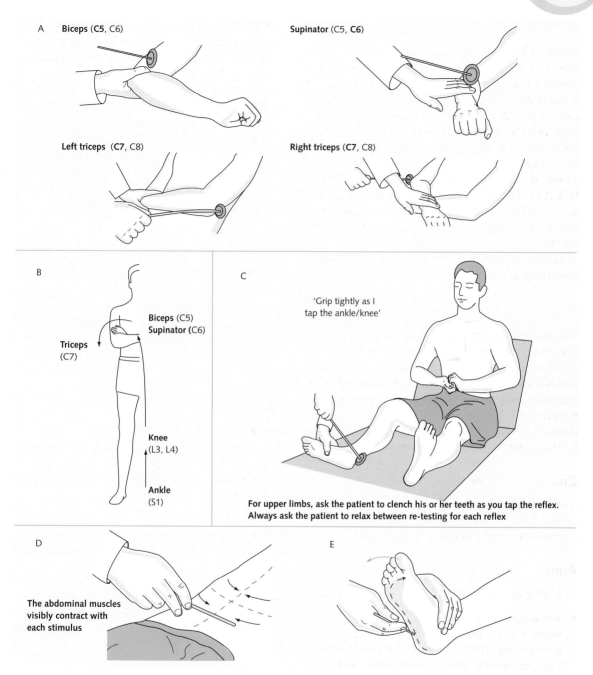

Fig. 34.14 Eliciting reflexes. (A) Upper limb tendon reflexes. (B) A simple way to remember root values of reflexes. (C) Testing ankle jerk reinforcement. (D) Abdominal reflexes: test in the four quadrants shown. (E) Plantar reflex. The normal response is a downgoing hallux. In an upper motor neuron lesion, the hallux dorsiflexes and the other toes fan out (the Babinski response).

Fig. 34.15 Annotation of tendon reflexes

Reduced	+
Normal	++
Very brisk (with associated clonus)	+++
Absent	0
Present with reinforcement only	±

To test the sensory modalities, ask the patient to close his or her eyes and, for all modalities except joint-position sense, apply the test to a reference point such as the skin over the sternum and ask the patient if he or she can feel the sensation normally. Subsequently, test each sensory modality distally to proximally in each limb and ask the patient if it feels the same as the reference point on the chest.

Sensory testing

It is not recommended to spend too much time doing sensory testing because you will exhaust the patient and yourself. It is best to tailor your examination to the patient's complaint.

If the patient complains of loss or impairment of sensation, then start sensory testing in the abnormal area and move out towards the normal area.

Patterns of sensory impairment are discussed in more detail in Chapter 13.

Sensory modalities

Pain
A safety pin or specialized disposable device (e.g. 'neurotip'), and not a hypodermic needle, should be used to test pain sensation. The patient will either feel nothing, a blunt sensation (which is abnormal), or a sharp pain (which is normal). If an abnormal area is found, then its margins should be further defined by moving from the area of reduced sensation to the normal area.

Temperature
A cold object such as the flat surface of a non-vibrating tuning fork can be used to test perception of cold temperature.

Light touch
A wisp of cotton wool is used to test light touch with brief static stimuli. Remember that 'tickle' is carried by spinothalamic fibres.

Joint-position sense

Move the distal interphalangeal (DIP) joint of the index finger/big toe up and down while stabilizing the digit with your other hand. Ask the patient to indicate the direction in which the digit is being moved. If perception of joint position is abnormal then test more proximal joints until the test is normal (e.g. DIP, wrist, elbow, shoulder).

Vibration

A 128-Hz tuning fork should be used to test vibration sense. Start the tuning fork vibrating and place it on the DIP joint of the finger/big toe and ask if the patient can feel it vibrating. If the patient cannot feel these vibrations, move the tuning fork proximally (e.g. lateral malleoli, tibial tuberosity, iliac crest, sternum). The tuning fork should always be touching bony elements under the skin. Vibration sense is often lost early in peripheral polyneuropathies.

Two-point discrimination

Test two-point discrimination with specific compasses. The pulp of the index finger (normal: 2–3 mm) and hallux (normal: 5 mm) are normally tested and ask the patient whether they feel one or two points.

GENERAL EXAMINATION

The conclusion of the neurological examination should include a more general examination of the other body systems.

The blood pressure should be recorded as the patient lies supine and again after standing for a couple of minutes to check for postural hypotension, which can be associated with autonomic dysfunction. The systolic blood pressure usually rises a little on standing and a fall of more than 20 mmHg is abnormal but might not be symptomatic, especially if it has developed progressively over many months or years. The blood pressure of patients who have suspected cerebrovascular insufficiency should be tested in both arms.

There is no single correct way to write a medical clerking, but there are several incorrect ways! Remember that doctors, nurses, physiotherapists and many other health professionals use the medical notes during the course of a patient's medical care. The notes need to last for years and your entries in them may provide valuable information to doctors looking after the patient in several years' time. It is also worth remembering that the medical notes are legal documents that might one day be used as evidence in a court of law.

The basic principles when making entries into the notes are as follows:

- Always write legibly – this sounds obvious but notes are often illegible. Remember, if no one else can read your entry you might as well not write anything.
- A date and time should precede every entry, no matter how brief. At the end of the entry you should sign your name, and, if your signature does not clearly show your name, your surname and initials should be written in capitals below it. There are no exceptions to this rule ever!
- Always be courteous to your patients and colleagues when writing in the notes. Rude or angry entries may give a certain degree of satisfaction when they are made but serve only to make you look unprofessional when read at a later date.
- Write everything down – every time you see a patient an entry should be made in the notes, stating accurately the content and outcome of the consultation. This may sometimes seem pedantic but most qualified doctors will be able to a recall situations when careful documentation resolved a difficult situation.

DOCUMENTATION OF THE HISTORY

The history should always have the following information at the top of the first page:

- Name of patient in full plus at least one other unique identifier (e.g. date of birth or hospital number) – loose sheets often fall out of the notes so all pages of the history should have this information so they are not replaced in the notes of another patient who has the same name.
- Date and time of entry.
- Route of admission – if the patient is being admitted to hospital it is useful to state the route by which the admission came about (i.e. via general practitioner or accident and emergency).

Presenting complaint

This should be a short list of the presenting complaint(s). There is no place in this section for any descriptions.

The purpose of the presenting complaint section is to state clearly the patient's main symptoms so that an initial differential diagnosis can be formulated. It is important that at this stage the list of differential diagnoses is large.

History of the presenting complaint

It is here that information regarding the presenting complaint is expanded. A full description of the presenting compaint(s) in turn should be noted.

Systems review

A full systems review of the other organ systems should be entered here.

It is not necessary to document negatives unless they are particularly relevant.

Once you have memorized the questions they will become second nature and the systems review will be very quick to do. It is worth the initial time-consuming effort to do this properly; after all, you will be taking histories for the rest of your career.

Past medical history

All previous illnesses and operations should be noted, along with details of when they happened and if there were any complications. Patients can be very vague about these details and you may need to speak to the relatives or the general practitioner for more information.

Drug history

All drugs taken should be documented.

Remember, you cannot say you have taken a drug history unless the doses and times of all drugs are written down accurately and legibly.

Allergies

Not only should the drugs that the patient is allergic to be documented, but the type of reaction and when it occurred should be stated.

Many patients say they are allergic to penicillin when they have only experienced some gastric discomfort while taking it. In a situation where a patient is read-mitted with, for example, suspected meningitis, this might influence whether a potentially life-saving dose of benzylpenicillin can be given safely.

Family history

Any diseases that have a potential genetic causation should be documented. The family member who had the disease and whether it was the cause of death should be stated.

Social history

This should include notes on the following:

- Accurate alcohol and drug intake history.
- Smoking – should be carefully documented (i.e. what is smoked, how many, for how long).
- Occupation and possible exposure to industrial dusts or chemicals.

- If HIV infection is a possible differential diagnosis, a thorough history of possible risk factors. This might be embarrassing – both for you and for the patient – but it is important not to miss a diagnosis as serious as this.

DOCUMENTATION OF THE EXAMINATION FINDINGS

There are many ways of documenting the findings on examination and it does not really matter how you do this provided a few rules are obeyed:

- The patient's name and another unique identifier are written on every sheet of paper – this should come as second nature to you.
- Any positive findings are represented in writing – diagrams can be used to aid the description but should never be used alone to document findings because they are likely to be interpreted differently by different people.

AT THE END OF THE CLERKING

The last section is important because it brings together all the information from the clerking. The following should be seen at the end of every clerking:

- A list of differential diagnoses with the most likely diagnosis at the top of the list.
- A list of investigations performed and to be performed – it is good practice to tick those tests that have been done already.
- A plan of action including initial drugs to be given, any intravenous fluids, physiotherapy, specific observations needed (e.g. fluid balance chart or daily weights and any consultant referrals to be made).

This reads like a long list but you do not need to learn it. The only thing you need to remember is that if you do something that concerns a patient then write it down.

SAMPLE MEDICAL CLERKING

Hospital No. X349282

Kopinski, Joanna   29 year old female
29/04/76

20/06/05   14:30
Referred from outpatient clinic following urgent GP referral

PC   Two-week history of difficulty walking

> 1. Presenting complaint should be brief, but it is helpful to mention relevant background information.

HPC   Two-week history of progressive difficulty in walking
          initially: tendency to trip over on left leg — two occasions of catching
          her left foot on kerbstone and falling
          Currently: she is finding it difficult to manoeuvre both legs, and catches
          both feet when climbing kerbstones or stairs
          There is no pain. Her walking has deteriorated gradually.
          No visual symptoms currently (no reduction in visual acuity, central
          field defect, double vision).
          No problems with speech and swallowing.
          No symptoms in her arms.

> 2. Mention only the relevant negatives.

          She has also developed a mild urgency and frequency of micturition over the previous
          week. This is not associated with burning or pain.

          At the age of 20, she had an episode of pain and visual impairment
          in the left eye. This settled after 6 weeks. No treatment was given.
          She was told this was due to 'neuritis'

PMH   1990: appendicectomy
          1996: visual loss - 'neuritis' for 6 weeks

> 3. Always record the dose and frequency of any drugs – remember you'll be writing the drug chart later! Always document that you have asked about drug allergies.

DH   Oral contraceptive pill

Allergies NKDA   smoking — 20 cigarettes per day (since aged 18)
          Occasionally smokes marijuana: no other illicit drugs
          Alcohol — 10 units/week

Fam Hx   No significant FH/no FH of neurological diseases.
          Father, mother and siblings alive and well

Social Hx Works as a secretary
          No pets

Sexual Hx Lives with boyfriend of 8 years; 4 previous sexual partners

Travel Hx Recent travel to Europe only

ROS   General: Marked fatigue recently
CVS: No chest pain/palpitations/orthopnoea/paroxysmal
         nocturnal dyspnoea (PND)
RS: No cough/sputum/wheeze
GIT: Appetite and weight stable
        No change in bowel habit
GUS: Recent urgency and frequency
        No burning/pain
NS: As above
Skin: No rash/pruritis/bruising

> 4. Record your initial observations – they are important. 'Alert and chatty' or 'Distressed and looks unwell' tell you a lot about the patient.

O/E   General; Apyrexial
          Anxious

CVS   'Pulse 80 reg'
         BP 130/70
         Apex beat – 5th ICS midclavicular line
         JVP – not raised
         Heart sounds – normal
         Peripheral pulses – all present
         No bruits

$$\vdash\quad\vdash\vdash\quad\dashv \quad + \text{ NIL}$$
$S_1 \qquad S_2$

RS: Trachea – central
      Expansion – normal
      Breath sounds – vesicular, no added sounds

Chest clear

> 5. You can use diagrams to clarify your examination findings

Abdomen: Soft/non-tender
No liver/spleen/kidneys palpable
Genitalia and rectal examination – not done

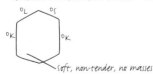
°L   °S
°K   °K
Soft, non-tender, no masses

NS: Alert and oriented
      Higher functions intact

Left relative afferent pupillary defect (L pupil dilates when torch alternated from R to L eye)
Desaturation to red pin centrally in L eye, otherwise normal visual fields.
Fundi: pale disc on L
III/IV/VI Horizontal nystagmus on lateral gaze
No double vision/no internuclear ophthalmoplegia (INO)
V
VII
VIII
IX   Normal
X
XI
XII

Upper limbs: Tone: Normal
Power: 5/5 all muscle groups
Coordination: Intention tremor on finger-nose testing bilaterally (LR)

Lower limbs: Tone: Increased tone bilaterally (LR)
Clonus at both ankles and at the L knee

Power	R	L
Hip flexion	4+/5	4−/5
Hip extension	5/5	5/5
Knee flexion	4/5	3/5
Knee extension	5/5	5/5
Ankle dorsiflexion	4−/5	3/5
Ankle plantar flexion	5/5	5/5

i.e. asymmetrical (LR) pyramidal distribution (flexors weaker than extensors) weakness in the legs
Coordination: Difficult to test heel-shin reliability with the degree of weakness

Reflexes:	R	L
Biceps	+	+
Triceps	+	+
Supinator	+	+
Abdominal	−	−
Knee	+++	+++
Ankle	+++	+++
Plantars	↑	↑

Sensation: Normal light touch (LT), pinprick (PP), joint-position sense (JPS), and vibration (vib) in both upper and lower limbs
Gait: Spastic gait — L worse than R (stiff legs—extended legs circumduct to try and avoid scuffing the toes)

SUMMARY

A 29-year-old lady, with a previous history of temporary visual loss in the left eye, presents with a 2-week history of progressive difficulty in walking. There is unilateral optic atrophy, with nystagmus in both eyes, and mild incoordination in the arms. There is an asymmetrical spastic paraparesis with bladder involvement. The most likely diagnosis is multiple sclerosis.

PROBLEM LIST

1. Confirm diagnosis of multiple sclerosis/ rule out spinal cord compression — magnetic resonance imaging (brain/ spinal cord) lumbar puncture (?positive oligoclonal bands): visual evoked potentials.

2. Treatment — intravenous methylprednisolone (check for urinary tract infection (UTI) and treat if present); physiotherpay

3. Social/psychological factors — discussion about diagnosis, prognosis, and any plans and adaptations that may be required (short or long term)

4. Followup — for further discussion and support, to catch signs of relapse early, to prevent complications of the disease (UTI, pressure sores etc) and to assess suitability for β-interferon.

> 6. Always include a management plan – even when you are still a student. It might not be right but you need to start training yourself to think like a doctor

Turner

TURNER 5092

> 7. Sign your notes, including printed surname and bleep number

ROUTINE INVESTIGATIONS

You should be aware of simple tests of neurological relevance. In this section, five areas of investigation are presented:

- Haematology (Fig. 36.1).
- Biochemistry (Fig. 36.2).
- Immunology (Fig. 36.3).
- Microbiology (Fig. 36.4).
- Cerebrospinal fluid findings.

For each test, normal ranges are given, with neurological differential diagnoses for high and low values.

NEUROPHYSIOLOGICAL INVESTIGATIONS

Electroencephalography (EEG)

EEG measures electrical potentials generated by the neurons lying underneath an electrode on the scalp, and compares these with recordings from either a reference electrode or a neighbouring electrode. The normal trace is symmetrical, and therefore asymmetries, as well as specific abnormalities, may indicate an underlying disorder.

Before accurate brain imaging was possible, EEG was used to detect focal lesions. These are now more commonly picked up with computed tomography (CT) or magnetic resonance imaging (MRI), but EEG remains useful for detecting underlying abnormalities of cerebral function, and especially for:

- Epilepsy (see below).
- Diagnosis of encephalitis (especially herpes simplex infection).
- Coma.
- Aid to diagnosis of Creutzfeldt–Jakob disease.
- Diagnosis of subacute sclerosing panencephalitis.

The main role of EEG is in the assessment of epilepsy. It can help in the following ways:

- Support of the diagnosis: (although this is made primarily on the clinical history and the EEG may be normal in patients who have clearly had seizures) an increased yield of abnormalities may be obtained if recording is made under conditions of sleep deprivation, with hyperventilation, and with photic stimulation.
- Classification of seizure type, which may optimize therapy.
- Assessment for surgical intervention.
- Diagnosis of non-epileptic seizures (especially with simultaneous video recording: 'video telemetry').

'Invasive EEG monitoring' refers to prolonged recording from electrodes inserted directly into the brain, undertaken preoperatively, before surgery to remove an epileptic focus.

Different normal rhythms are characteristically found over different regions of the brain (Fig. 36.5). Other than these rhythmic activities, other abnormal activity may be generated in certain conditions (Figs 36.6 and 36.7).

Electromyography (EMG) and nerve conduction studies (NCS)

EMG and NCS, usually performed together, examine the electrical activity of muscle, neuromuscular junction, and lower motor neurons. They are useful in:

- Determining the cause of weakness, e.g. neuropathy, myopathy, anterior horn cell disease.
- Determining the distribution of the abnormality, e.g. generalized or focal.
- Suggesting the type of myopathy (e.g. dystrophy or myositis) or neuropathy (e.g. axonal or demyelinating), motor, sensory, or sensorimotor.
- Diagnosing myasthenia gravis.
- Assessing baseline deficits before surgery, e.g. carpal tunnel syndrome.
- Objectively assessing the response to medical therapies, especially new treatments currently under trial, e.g. intravenous human immunoglobulin in Guillain–Barré syndrome.

Fig. 36.1 Possible clinical relevance of abnormalities in blood or serum levels of haematological indices. Individual laboratories may have different normal ranges

Test	Normal range	Abnormality	Possible clinical explanation
Full blood count			
Haemoglobin (Hb)	13.5–18.0 g/dL male; 11.5–16.0 g/dL female	Low; anaemia	May cause non-specific neurological symptoms (e.g. dizziness, weakness, faintness); may suggest an underlying chronic illness
		High; polycythaemia	Predisposes to stroke and chorea
Mean cell volume (MCV)	76–96 fL	High; macrocytic	Vitamin B_{12} deficiency (peripheral neuropathy, dementia)
		Low; microcytic	May indicate an underlying chronic illness; associated with idiopathic intracranial hypertension
White cell count (WBC)			
Neutrophils	2–7.5 × 10^9/L	High; neutrophilia	Meningitis or other infection
		Low; neutropenia	Leukaemia or lymphoma (infiltrative disease, space-occupying lesions, peripheral neuropathy) Multiple myeloma (neuropathy, vertebral collapse, hyperviscosity syndrome)
Lymphocytes	1.5–3.5 × 10^9/L	High; lymphocytosis	Viral infection (transverse myelitis, Guillain–Barré syndrome)
		Low; lymphopenia	Leukaemia or lymphoma, as above
Eosinophils	0.04–0.44 × 10^9/L	High; eosinophilia	Hypereosinophilic syndrome (rare)
Platelet count	150–400 × 10^9/L	High; thrombocythaemia	Predisposes to stroke
		Low; thrombocytopenia	Intracranial bleeding
Erythrocyte sedimentation rate (ESR)	20 mm/h	High	Vasculitis (e.g. PAN, SLE, giant-cell arteritis) may cause cerebral, cranial, and peripheral nerve infarcts, confusion and fits)
Coagulation tests			
Activated partial thromboplastin time (APT or PTTK)	35–45 s	High	SLE; antiphospholipid syndrome
Protein C, protein S	Varies with laboratory	Low; deficiency	Inherited predisposition to thrombosis (arterial and venous)
Factor 5 Leiden	Varies with laboratory	Present	Mutation causes a single amino acid substitution in factor 5, which results in activated protein C resistance and predisposition to thrombosis (arterial and venous)
Vitamin B_{12}	>150 ng/L	Low; deficiency	Peripheral neuropathy, myecopathy, confusion/dementia, optic neuropathy, SCDC, ataxia
Folate	4–18 µg/L	Low; deficiency	Peripheral neuropathy, dementia

Note: APT, activated thromboplastin; PAN, polyarteritis nodosa; PTTK, partial thromboplastin time; SCDC, subacute combined degeneration of the cord; SLE, systemic lupus erythematosus.

Fig. 36.2 Possible clinical relevance of abnormalities in blood or serum levels of biochemical indices. Individual laboratories may have different normal ranges

Test	Normal range	Abnormality	Possible clinical explanation
Urea and electrolytes (U and Es)			
Sodium	135–145 mmol/L	High; hypernatraemia low; hyponatraemia	Both may cause weakness, confusion, and fits
Potassium	3.5–5.5 mmol/L	High; hyperkalaemia Low; hypokalaemia	Hyper- or hypokalaemic periodic paralysis
Urea	2.5–6.7 mmol/L	High; renal failure	Confusion, peripheral neuropathy
Creatinine	<120 mmol/L	High; renal failure	Confusion, peripheral neuropathy
Glucose (fasting)	4–6 mmol/L	High; diabetes Low; hypoglycaemia	Neuropathy, coma Confusion, coma, focal signs
Calcium	2.2–2.6 mmol/L	Low; hypocalcaemia	Tetany, seizures
Liver function tests (LFTs) Bilirubin and liver enzymes	Bilirubin range: 3–17 mmol/L; enzyme levels vary between laboratories	High	Liver disease: confusion, tremor, neuropathy
Creatine kinase (CK)	24–195 U/L	High	Muscle disease: myositis, dystrophy
Thyroid function tests Thyroid-stimulating hormone (TSH)	0.5–5.0 mU/L	High T4 Low TSH; thyrotoxicosis	Tremor, confusion, hyperreflexia
Thyroxine (T4)	10–24 pmol/L	Low T4 High TSH; hypothyroidism	Apathy, confusion, hyporeflexia, neuropathy, dementia

Fig. 36.3 Immunology: autoantibodies and their associated syndromes

Test	Associated disorder
Antinuclear factor (ANA)	Systemic lupus erythematosus (SLE): fits, confusion, neuropathy, aseptic meningitis, Sjögren's syndrome: gritty eyes, neuropathies, mixed connective tissue disease (MCTD)
Anti-double-stranded DNA (dsDNA) antibodies	SLE
Rheumatoid factor	Rheumatoid arthritis: cervical spine subluxation, neuropathies, vasculitis
Anti-Ro (SSA), anti-La (SSB) antibodies	Sjögren's syndrome
Antiphospholipid antibodies (e.g. anticardiolipin)	Antiphospholipid syndrome
Anti-ribonucleoprotein (RNP) antibodies	MCTD; myositis, trigeminal nerve palsies
Jo-1 antibodies	Polymyositis and pulmonary fibrosis
Antineutrophil cytoplasmic antibodies (ANCA)	pANCA (peripheral): polyarteritis nodosa cANCA (classical): Wegener's granulomatosis
Anti-acetylcholine receptor (AChR) antibodies	Myasthenia gravis
Anti-GM1 antibodies	Multifocal motor neuropathy, Guillain–Barré syndrome
Anti-GAD antibodies	Stiff-man syndrome
Anti Hu, Yo, Ri antibodies	Paraneoplastic syndromes
Anti voltage-gated potassium channel antibodies	Autoimmune limbic encephalitis

Fig. 36.4 Microbiology: investigations that should be carried out if infections are implicated as the cause of neurological disease

Test	Associated disorder
Bacterial microscopy and culture (including blood, CSF, urine, stool, sputum and wounds)	Bacterial infections can cause a wide range of conditions – septicaemia, meningitis, pneumonia, urinary tract infections, cerebral abscess etc – or are implicated in their pathogenesis, e.g. Guillain–Barré syndrome (Campylobacter pylori)
	Do not forget atypical infections caused by Listeria, Mycoplasma, Legionella etc.; diagnosis of TB requires special stains (Ziehl–Neelsen) and culture media (Lowenstein–Jensen)
Viral serology and culture (blood, CSF)	Viruses can cause a wide range of neurological infections, e.g. meningitis, encephalitis, shingles (herpes zoster)
VDRL (venereal disease reference laboratory) (blood)	Primary syphilis (false positives in pregnancy, systemic lupus erythematosus, malaria)
TPHA (*Treponema pallidum* haemagglutination assay) (blood)	Syphilis, false positives in VDRL and other treponemal infections (yaws, pinta)
Borrelia serology (blood, CSF)	Lyme disease (see Chapter 33)
HIV (blood)	AIDS (see Chapter 33)
HTLV-1 (blood)	Myelopathy

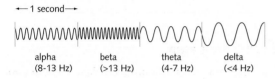

Fig. 36.5 Normal electroencephalographic rhythms.

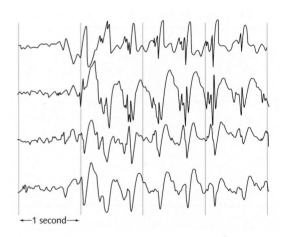

Fig. 36.7 Three-per-second (3/s) spike-and-wave activity, characteristic of typical absence seizure.

Fig. 36.6 Some abnormal electroencephalographic activities

Activity	Interpretation
Generalized slow-wave activity	Metabolic encephalopathy, drug overdose, encephalitis
Focal slow-wave activity	Underlying structural lesion
Focal or generalized spikes, or spike and slow-wave activity	Epilepsy
Three-per-second (3/s), bilateral, symmetrical spike-and-wave activity (Fig 36.7)	Typical absence seizures and other 'primary generalized epilepsy' syndromes
Periodic complexes (generalized sharp waves every 0.5–2.0 seconds)	CJD

EMG

EMG involves the insertion of a needle electrode into muscle.

Normal muscle at rest is electrically silent (apart from actually during needle insertion, 'insertional activity') unless the needle is placed in the region of a motor end-plate (when miniature end-plate potentials are recorded).

In abnormal muscles, either due to primary muscle disease or to denervation of the muscle, spontaneous activity may be seen at rest. The most common types of spontaneous activity include fibrillation potentials, positive sharp waves, and fasciculations.

Fibrillation potentials and positive sharp waves are due to spontaneous contractions of individual muscle fibres, probably due to abnormal rhythmic fluctuations of membrane potential. They cannot be seen clinically through the skin. They are most commonly seen in denervation but may be found in some muscle diseases especially inflammatory muscle disease (e.g. polymyositis).

Fasciculation potentials are much larger than fibrillations and represent the contractions of groups of muscle fibres supplied by a motor unit. They occur following denervation. They may be seen as a clinical fasciculation. They are common in motor neuron disease. Fasciculations may occur as normal phenomenon, especially after excess caffeine or in thyrotoxicosis. However, in these situations the firing rate is far more rapid than in diseases caused by denervation.

During voluntary movement, individual motor unit potentials (MUPs; the activity of a single anterior horn cell) can be seen on the EMG. Common abnormalities of EMG are shown in Fig. 36.8.

Nerve conduction studies

Nerve conduction studies involve stimulating a nerve with an electrical impulse via a surface electrode and recording further along the nerve (sensory studies) or recording the muscle action potential (motor studies).

The amplitude of the response, the latency to the beginning of the response, and the conduction velocity are measured. As a general rule, a reduction in conduction velocity suggests demyelination whereas a reduction in amplitude suggests axonal loss (see Fig. 36.8).

Evoked potentials (EPs)

These use EEG electrodes to record responses centrally to peripheral stimuli:

- Visual EPs (VEPs): these are delayed in patients who have had an episode of optic neuritis (even if this was not clinically symptomatic) and this is therefore a useful test to help confirm a diagnosis of multiple sclerosis.
- Brainstem auditory EPs (BSAEPs).
- Somatosensory EPs (SSEPs).

IMAGING OF THE NERVOUS SYSTEM

Plain radiography

Skull radiography

Skull radiography has a limited role in current neurological practice. The main indication is head injury when more sophisticated imaging is not immediately indicated or available. The standard views are:

Fig. 36.8 Common abnormalities found with electromyography (EMG) and nerve conduction studies (NCS). MUPs, motor unit potentials

Abnormality	Change in electromyographic trace
Denervation	Increased insertional activity; fibrillations, positive sharp waves, and fasciculations; large amplitude, long duration, polyphasic MUPs
Myopathy	Small, short, polyphasic MUPs
Myasthenia gravis	Abnormal decrement of amplitude of response on repetitive stimulation using nerve conduction tests; increased 'jitter' with single-fibre EMG (indicating variable neuromuscular transmission time)

Abnormality	Change in nerve conduction
Axonal neuropathy	Small action potential; normal nerve conduction velocity
Demyelinating neuropathy	Slow nerve conduction velocity; prolonged latency (time to travel from one point to the next); normal or slightly reduced action potential

- Lateral.
- Posteroanterior.
- Towne's view (fronto-occipital).

Spinal radiography

The standard views in spinal radiography are:

- Lateral.
- Posteroanterior.

Computerized tomography scanning

Using an X-ray source and a series of photon detectors housed in a gantry, CT produces a series of consecutive two-dimensional axial brain digital images that show the X-ray density of the brain tissue.

The densities of different brain tissues vary according to their X-ray absorption properties, ranging from low (black: air, cerebrospinal fluid) to high (white: bone, fresh blood).

The diagnostic yield of CT scanning is increased by injecting iodine-containing contrast agents. These enhance the distinction between the different brain tissues and outline areas of breakdown in the blood–brain barrier (around tumours, infarcts, or abscesses).

Magnetic resonance imaging

The term 'nuclear magnetic resonance' describes the interaction between the hydrogen protons in the different body structures and strong external magnetic fields. As the patient lies in the scanner, the naturally spinning hydrogen protons align with the strong magnetic field of the scanner. When a further external magnetic field (radiofrequency pulse) of a specific frequency is applied at a right angle, the protons 'flip' out of the main external magnetic field.

As the protons 'relax' back to their original position, they emit a radiofrequency signal that can be digitally analysed and displayed as an image. This 'relaxation' time has two components, known as T1 and T2, which determine the MRI parameters of the different brain tissues. MRI is especially useful at looking at small detail of intracranial structures, especially in the posterior fossa and spinal column where the surrounding bone distorts the image on CT.

The paramagnetic agent gadolinium-labelled DTPA (diethylene triamine penta-acetic acid, or pentetic acid) is used as contrast agent. Modification of the field conditions can now produce good quality images of the cervical or cerebral blood vessels (either arterial or venous). This is called magnetic resonance angiography.

Despite the better resolution of MRI, CT is faster and cheaper and is often better at examining fresh blood and bony structures.

The advantages of MR imaging are:
- Absence of ionizing radiation.
- The ability to obtain images in coronal and sagittal, as well as axial, planes.
- More sensitive to the pathological changes in the brain tissues.
- Better resolution of structures surrounded by bone, e.g. posterior fossa and spinal cord.

The disadvantages are:
- Cannot be used for patients with pacemakers (the magnetic field interferes with their function).
- Cannot be used for patients with ferromagnetic intracranial aneurysmal clips or implants (they distort the images and could be displaced by the strong magnetic field).
- Patients who suffer from claustrophobia may be unable to tolerate the confined space within the MRI machine, although 'open' MR scanners are now available that are less claustrophobic.

Myelography

This procedure has now been largely supplanted by spinal MRI. A water-soluble iodine-based medium is injected into the subarachnoid space through a lumbar or a cervical approach. This outlines the spinal canal and nerve root sheaths, allowing the assessment of the spinal canal and the nerve roots. Cord compression caused by extramedullary or intramedullary lesions is identified as a compression or interruption of the column of contrast.

Postmyelographic CT scanning provides more detailed images of the nerve roots within the theca.

Imaging of the spinal cord is now performed largely by MR scanning but myelography can be helpful in specific conditions (nerve root lesions, spinal dural arteriovenous malformation) or in patients unable to undergo MRI because of claustrophobia or a cardiac pacemaker.

Catheter arteriography

Serial cranial radiographs are taken after the injection of an iodine-containing contrast agent into a large artery (aorta, carotid, vertebral) to allow the identification of cerebral vessels. Simultaneous digital subtraction of the surrounding soft tissues and bony structures allows the use of more-dilute contrast and a shorter procedure time, although the spatial resolution of the images will be compromised.

Venous digital subtraction angiography is possible but the quality of the images obtained is distinctly inferior to those obtained through the arterial route.

The indications for traditional arteriography are:

- Diagnosis of extracranial atherosclerotic cerebrovascular disease (stenosis, lumen irregularities, or occlusions), when not shown by Doppler study or MR angiography.
- Detailed evaluation of aneurysms and arteriovenous malformations.
- Diagnosis of cerebral vasculitis and other rare angiopathies.
- Assessment of cerebral vessel anatomy and tumour blood supply before neurosurgery.
- Interventional angiography: therapeutic embolization of aneurysms and vascular malformations.

Duplex ultrasonography

Duplex ultrasonography offers a combination of real-time and Doppler-flow ultrasound scanning, allowing a non-invasive assessment of extracranial arteries. It is particularly helpful as a screening test for lesions at the carotid bifurcation, which avoids the need for angiography in many patients. The quality of this technique is dependent on the experience and skill of the operator.

SELF-ASSESSMENT

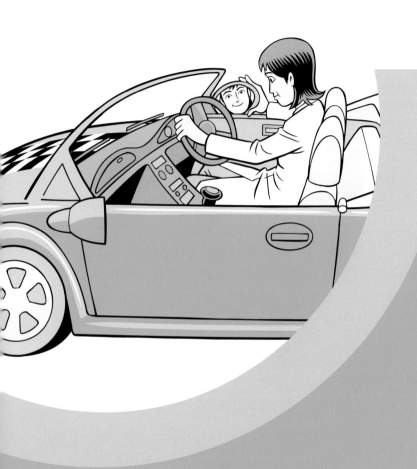

Multiple-choice questions (MCQs)

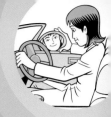

Indicate whether each answer is true or false.

1. **Concerning neuroanatomy:**
   a. The corticospinal tract decussates in the pons.
   b. The oculomotor nerve runs in close proximity to the posterior communicating artery.
   c. The superior colliculus is found in the midbrain.
   d. The trochlear (fouth cranial) nerve supplies the lateral rectus muscle.
   e. The spinal cord ends at the level of the lower border of L3 in the adult.

2. **The following cranial nerves carry parasympathetic fibres:**
   a. Oculomotor.
   b. Trigeminal.
   c. Facial.
   d. Hypoglossal.
   e. Vagus.

3. **Subdural haematomas can cause:**
   a. Dementia
   b. Pupillary change
   c. Bradycardia
   d. Changing level of consciousness
   e. Blood-stained cerebrospinal fluid (CSF)

4. **Myasthenia gravis:**
   a. Is caused by antibodies to the acetylcholine receptor in the majority of cases.
   b. Causes muscle wasting.
   c. May show diurnal variation in symptoms.
   d. Is associated with an improvement in strength after exertion.
   e. May present with ophthalmoplegia.

5. **In a young woman with a spastic paraparesis, the following suggest a diagnosis of multiple sclerosis:**
   a. Delayed visual evoked potentials.
   b. Fasciculations.
   c. Raised CSF protein.
   d. Oligoclonal bands in the CSF.
   e. Periventricular white matter lesions on magnetic resonance imaging (MRI) of the brain.

6. **The causes of a mixed upper and lower motor neuron picture include:**
   a. Guillain–Barré syndrome.
   b. Multiple sclerosis.
   c. Syringomyelia.
   d. Motor neuron disease.
   e. Syphilitic taboparesis.

7. **Unilateral facial weakness is a recognized feature of:**
   a. Herpes zoster infection.
   b. Motor neuron disease.
   c. Acoustic neuroma.
   d. Cholesteatoma.
   e. Syringomyelia.

8. **Bilateral lower motor neuron facial weakness may occur in:**
   a. Sarcoidosis.
   b. Guillain–Barré syndrome.
   c. Lyme disease.
   d. Lymphoma.
   e. Parasagittal meningioma.

9. **The following are true about headaches:**
   a. The headache of raised intracranial pressure is worst at the end of the day.
   b. A normal computed tomography (CT) scan rules out subarachnoid haemorrhage.
   c. Amaurosis fugax may be caused by temporal arteritis.
   d. Neurological signs on examination rules out migraine as a diagnosis.
   e. Cluster headaches are more common in men than in women.

10. **In idiopathic Parkinson's disease:**
    a. There is degeneration primarily of the cells of the globus pallidus.
    b. The classical features include tremor, bradykinesia, and spasticity.
    c. There is an associated vertical gaze palsy.
    d. Anticholinergic drugs are most effective in relieving tremor.
    e. Treatment is aimed at reducing dopamine levels.

11. **The following drugs can produce parkinsonism:**
    a. Chlorpromazine.
    b. Benzhexol (Trihexyphenidyl).
    c. Bromocriptine.
    d. Metoclopramide.
    e. Haloperidol.

12. **The following features suggest that increased tone is due to rigidity:**
    a. Tone is increased equally in flexors and extensors.
    b. Extensor plantar responses.
    c. Associated pill-rolling tremor.
    d. Clasp-knife effect.
    e. Tone increases with synkinesis.

13. Concerning movement disorders:

a. Huntington's chorea presents with progressive dementia and chorea in middle age.
b. Myoclonus is a feature of subacute sclerosing panencephalitis.
c. Infarction of the subthalamic nucleus causes ipsilateral hemiballism.
d. Chorea is commonly found in Cruetzfeldt–Jakob disease.
e. Alcohol reduces benign essential tremor.

14. Causes of a small pupil include:

a. Horner's syndrome.
b. Holmes–Adie syndrome.
c. Tabes dorsalis.
d. Optic neuritis.
e. Pilocarpine eye-drops.

15. Concerning swollen optic discs:

a. There may be a loss of venous pulsation on fundoscopy when caused by papilloedema.
b. There may be enlargement of the blind spot.
c. Intracranial pressure may be normal.
d. Hypocalcaemia is a recognized cause.
e. It is a recognized feature in Guillain–Barré syndrome.

16. Concerning optic neuritis:

a. Visual loss is usually painless.
b. White-matter abnormalities on MRI increase the likelihood of developing multiple sclerosis in the future.
c. After recovery, some impairment of red-green colour vision may remain.
d. Over 90% of patients with a history of optic neuritis go on to develop multiple sclerosis.
e. It causes a delay in visual evoked potentials.

17. Ptosis may be a feature of:

a. Myotonic dystrophy.
b. Horner's syndrome.
c. Abducent nerve (sixth nerve) palsy.
d. Oculomotor nerve (third nerve) palsy.
e. Myasthenia gravis.

18. The following may cause a third nerve palsy:

a. Aneurysm of the posterior communicating artery.
b. Diabetes.
c. Motor neuron disease.
d. Herniation of the uncus of the temporal lobe.
e. Pancoast tumour.

19. Concerning the Brown–Séquard syndrome:

a. There is ipsilateral corticospinal loss below the lesion.
b. There is ipsilateral loss of joint-position and vibration sense below the lesion.
c. A plaque in the spinal cord caused by multiple sclerosis is the commonest cause.
d. There is ipsilateral loss of pain and temperature below the level of the lesion.
e. A central disc lesion at L3 would cause a Brown–Séquard syndrome in the legs.

20. The following typically occur within the first 24 hours of complete cervical cord transection:

a. Upgoing plantar responses.
b. Fall in blood pressure.
c. Loss of bladder control.
d. Brisk reflexes.
e. Gastric dilatation.

21. In motor neuron disease:

a. Fasciculations are required to make the diagnosis.
b. There may be atrophy of the Betz cells in the motor cortex.
c. Electromyography shows chronic partial denervation.
d. There should be no signs of sensory loss.
e. Familial cases account for 50%.

22. Concerning the brachial plexus:

a. In brachial neuritis, severe pain around the shoulder precedes rapid wasting.
b. Klumpke's paralysis causes proximal arm weakness.
c. Erb's palsy is caused by a lesion to C5/C6-derived regions of the brachial plexus.
d. A brachial plexus lesion and an ipsilateral Horner's syndrome may indicate a Pancoast tumour.
e. Vaccination may precipitate brachial neuritis.

23. Causes of a mononeuropathy include:

a. Diabetes.
b. Hereditary motor sensory neuropathy.
c. Polyarteritis nodosa.
d. Guillain–Barré syndrome.
e. Lead poisoning.

24. Causes of a polyneuropathy include:

a. Diabetes.
b. Guillain–Barré syndrome.
c. Renal failure.
d. Amyloid.
e. Multiple sclerosis.

25. Charcot joints:

a. Are often painful.
b. May affect the feet in diabetes.
c. May be caused by neurosyphilis.
d. May affect the shoulders in syringomyelia.
e. Are usually hot and swollen.

26. A lesion to the common peroneal nerve at the fibular head causes:

a. Weakness of eversion of the foot.
b. Decreased sensation over the dorsum of the foot.
c. Weakness of plantar flexion.
d. If long term, wasting of tibialis anterior.
e. Brisk ankle jerk.

27. Hyposmia may arise secondary to:

a. A head injury.
b. Migraine.
c. Seizures.
d. Antibiotic therapy.
e. A frontal meningioma.

28. Criteria for brainstem death include:
    a. Extensor response of the limbs to painful stimuli.
    b. Absent corneal reflexes.
    c. Absent tendon reflexes.
    d. A flat electroencephalogram (EEG).
    e. Absent 'doll's eye' reflexes.

29. The following are causes of acute transient visual impairment:
    a. Retinitis pigmentosa.
    b. Carotid embolism.
    c. Papilloedema.
    d. Migrainous aura.
    e. Glaucoma.

30. A homonymous hemianopia may arise from a lesion of:
    a. The optic tract.
    b. The occipital cortex.
    c. The optic chiasm.
    d. The optic nerve.
    e. The optic radiation.

31. The following may be features of frontal lobe dysfunction:
    a. Altered personality.
    b. Social disinhibition.
    c. Apraxia of gait.
    d. A receptive dysphasia.
    e. A grasp reflex.

32. Dysarthria may result from a lesion of:
    a. The cerebellum.
    b. Broca's area.
    c. The hypoglossal nerve.
    d. The basal ganglia.
    e. The accessory nerve.

33. The following may give rise to a pseudobulbar palsy:
    a. Poliomyelitis.
    b. Motor neuron disease.
    c. Huntington's chorea.
    d. Occlusion of the anterior cerebral artery.
    e. Multiple sclerosis.

34. The following are clinical features of cerebellar dysfunction:
    a. Resting tremor.
    b. Hypotonia.
    c. Dysphasia.
    d. Titubation.
    e. Impaired rapid altering movements.

35. Facial sensory loss may occur with a lesion of:
    a. The cerebellopontine angle.
    b. The facial nerve.
    c. The Gasserian ganglion.
    d. The Geniculate ganglion.
    e. The cavernous sinus.

36. The following clinical features may help differentiate between a syncopal attack and a seizure:
    a. Upright posture at the onset.
    b. Brief convulsive movements of the limbs.
    c. A bitten tongue.
    d. Urinary incontinence.
    e. Prolonged malaise after the attack.

37. Sensorineural deafness may occur secondary to:
    a. Exposure to loud noises.
    b. Gentamicin therapy.
    c. Ménière's disease.
    d. An acoustic neuroma.
    e. Otosclerosis.

38. The following are typical features of a subarachnoid haemorrhage:
    a. Fever.
    b. Thunderclap headache.
    c. Photophobia.
    d. Positive Kernig's sign.
    e. Neck stiffness.

39. Choreic movements are:
    a. Slow and writhing.
    b. Shock-like asymetrical and irregular.
    c. Brief, twitchy and irregular.
    d. A sign of restlessness.
    e. Rhythmical and oscillatory.

40. A physiological tremor is:
    a. Present at rest.
    b. Worsened by anxiety.
    c. Improved by alcohol.
    d. Improved by beta-blockers.
    e. Familial.

41. Features of an upper motor neuron lesion are:
    a. Brisk abdominal and cremasteric reflexes.
    b. Wasted muscles.
    c. Weakness of individual muscles.
    d. Hypotonia.
    e. Fatigable muscle strength.

42. A lesion of the lateral medulla on one side may give rise to:
    a. Ipsilateral facial weakness.
    b. Horner's syndrome.
    c. Ipsilateral weakness of the palate.
    d. Contralateral weakness of the tongue.
    e. Contralateral third nerve palsy.

43. A small pupil may be seen in:
    a. A lesion in the midbrain.
    b. Elderly patients.
    c. Horner's syndrome.
    d. Terminally ill patients taking morphine for analgesia.
    e. A pontine lesion.

265

44. **The following may be seen in a patient with a lesion involving the third nerve or nucleus:**
    a. A fixed dilated pupil.
    b. Ptosis.
    c. Diplopia in all positions of gaze.
    d. A history of diabetes mellitus.
    e. An associated contralateral hemiplegia.

45. **Nystagmus may be seen in:**
    a. A patient with an internuclear ophthalmoplegia.
    b. A lesion of the pons.
    c. A patient who is blind.
    d. A patient with cerebellar dysfunction.
    e. A lesion at the foramen magnum.

46. **In a patient with a sensory ataxia:**
    a. Vibration may be impaired.
    b. The gait is characterized by 'scissoring' posture of the legs.
    c. Romberg's test is usually positive.
    d. A history of alcohol abuse may be implicated in the aetiology.
    e. Clonus may be elicited on examination of the legs.

47. **Clinical features of a unilateral lesion of the cerebellopontine angle may be:**
    a. Conductive deafness on the same side.
    b. An ipsilateral hemiparesis.
    c. Ipsilateral weakness of the lower face.
    d. A pseudobulbar dysarthria.
    e. Vertigo as a prominent early symptom.

48. **A patient with herpes zoster infection of the geniculate ganglion may present with:**
    a. An upper motor neuron facial weakness.
    b. Diplopia.
    c. Hyperacusis.
    d. Altered perception of taste.
    e. Pain from the auditory meatus.

49. **The fibres of the dorsal column pathway:**
    a. Carry information about temperature perception.
    b. Decussate in the midbrain.
    c. Are affected in the deficiency of vitamin B_{12}.
    d. When damaged may result in a positive Romberg's test.
    e. Are spared following occlusion of the anterior spinal artery.

50. **A dissociated sensory loss may be seen in:**
    a. Brown–Séquard syndrome.
    b. Anterior spinal artery occlusion.
    c. A radiculopathy.
    d. Occlusion of a middle cerebral artery.
    e. Compression of the spinal cord by a prolapsed intervertebral disc.

51. **Diabetic polyneuropathy:**
    a. Always produces symptoms.
    b. Usually causes greater sensory than motor loss.

    c. Is unaffected by good blood glucose control.
    d. Is less common in type II diabetes.
    e. May be associated with painless feet ulcers.

52. **Common causes of a painful neuropathy include:**
    a. Diabetes.
    b. Alcohol.
    c. Cryoglobulinaemia.
    d. Charcot–Marie–Tooth disease.
    e. Amyloid.

53. **Causes of a demyelinating neuropathy include**
    a. Guillain–Barré syndrome.
    b. Diphtheria.
    c. Vincristine.
    d. Charcot–Marie–Tooth disease.
    e. Paraproteinaemic neuropathy.

54. **Carpal tunnel syndrome**
    a. Is associated with symptoms only in the hand.
    b. Is associated with hypothyroidism.
    c. Can be treated with night wrist splints.
    d. Often causes severe wasting and weakness of the hand.
    e. Affects the first doral interossei greater than abductor pollicis brevis.

55. **Multiple sclerosis is more likely to have a benign course if the patient:**
    a. Presents with a spastic paraparesis.
    b. Presents with sensory symptoms.
    c. Is young at onset.
    d. Presents with brainstem or cerebellar features.
    e. Presents with optic neuritis.

56. **The following drugs significantly reduce relapse rates in relapsing-remitting multiple sclerosis:**
    a. Beta-interferon.
    b. Glatiramer acetate.
    c. Steroids.
    d. Methotrexate.
    e. Cyclosporine.

57. **In Wilson's disease:**
    a. Total serum copper is raised.
    b. Unrinary 24-hour copper is raised.
    c. Dysphagia and dysarthria are common.
    d. Onset is usually between 10 and 25 years.
    e. Zinc supplementation increases copper excretion in stool and reduces copper absorption in the gut.

58. **Polymyositis:**
    a. Most cases are associated with an underlying malignancy.
    b. Rarely involves muscle of swallowing.
    c. Patients are hyporeflexic.
    d. Distal limb muscles are more involved than proximal muscles.
    e. Some cases are associated with autoimmune disorders.

59. **Myasthenia gravis is associated with:**
    a. Diplopia or ptosis in over 90% of patients at some time in their illness.
    b. Exercise makes symptoms worse.
    c. Older women and younger men.
    d. Type II respiratory failure.
    e. Absent tendon reflexes.

60. **Bilateral extensor plantar responses are associated with:**
    a. Amyotrophic lateral sclerosis.
    b. Cervical myelopathy secondary to cervical spondylosis.
    c. Multiple sclerosis.
    d. Right middle cerebral artery ischaemic stroke.
    e. Subacute combined degeneration of the spinal cord.

61. **Formed visual hallucinations may occur in:**
    a. Ocular blindness.
    b. Temporal lobe epilepsy.
    c. Depressive psychosis.
    d. Migraine aura.
    e. Drug withdrawal.

62. **Fasciculations of muscle may be seen in:**
    a. Motor neuron disease.
    b. Muscular dystrophy.
    c. Thyrotoxicosis.
    d. Parkinson's disease.
    e. Syringomyelia.

63. **Hydrocephalus may result from:**
    a. Tuberculous meningitis.
    b. Cryptococcal meningitis.
    c. Herpes simplex meningitis.
    d. Idiopathic intracranial hypertension.
    e. Subarachnoid haemorrhage.

64. **Petit mal is associated with:**
    a. Normal intelligence.
    b. Prolonged post-ictal confusion.
    c. Drug-resistant seizures.
    d. Post-traumatic epilepsy.
    e. Structural brain lesion on MRI.

65. **Intracranial aneurysms are:**
    a. Multiple in 15% of cases.
    b. Associated with pain and a third nerve palsy when involving the posterior communicating artery.
    c. Associated with intracerebral haemorrhage when on the middle cerebal artery.
    d. More likely to rupture if in the posterior circulation.
    e. Associated with hydrocephalus if they rupture.

66. **Sodium valproate:**
    a. Is the drug of choice in pregnant women.
    b. Can cause severe weight gain.
    c. Is associated with tremor.
    d. Causes hirsuitism.
    e. Is usually the drug of choice in primary generalized epilepsy.

67. **Cerebellar disease is associated with the following features:**
    a. Truncal ataxia with vermal (midline) lesions.
    b. If acute onset should prompt an urgent brain CT.
    c. Often associated with Alzheimer's disease.
    d. Is associated with a potentially irreversible ataxia in association with phenytoin toxicity.
    e. Is a recognized paraneoplastic complication of small cell lung cancer.

68. **Compression of the L4 nerve root:**
    a. Causes pain over the anterior thigh and medial leg.
    b. Causes loss of the knee jerk.
    c. Can be confused with a common peroneal nerve lesion.
    d. Is usually caused by a lateral disc protrusion at L3/L4.
    e. Is associated with wasting of the hamstrings.

69. **In cervical spondylosis:**
    a. May be associated with lower motor neuron signs in the upper limbs.
    b. Pain is particularly severe at night.
    c. In the absence of neurological signs can be treated with a soft collar.
    d. Most patients have neurological signs.
    e. Neck traction may be helpful if the patient has upper motor neuron signs to relieve pressure off the spinal cord.

70. **Temporal arteritis:**
    a. Is more common in men.
    b. Is often associated with systemic symptoms.
    c. Can be associated with scalp tenderness and jaw claudication.
    d. Is ruled out with a normal erythrocyte sedimentation rate.
    e. Steroid treatment should be initiated as soon as the diagnosis is strongly suspected.

71. **The sixth nerve:**
    a. Carries the parasympathetic fibres to the pupil.
    b. May be affected as a 'false localizing' sign.
    c. May be seen in association with papilloedema in idiopathic intracranial hypertension.
    d. Travels through the superior orbital fissure and the cavernous sinus.
    e. Supplies the superior oblique muscle.

72. **The following clinical syndromes typically occur with dominant cerebral cortical lesions:**
    a. Dysphasia.
    b. Dressing apraxia.
    c. Dyscalculia.
    d. Finger agnosia.
    e. Impaired discrimination between left and right.

73. **The radial nerve:**
    a. Is the main continuation of the posterior cord of the brachial plexus.
    b. Supplies the brachioradialis muscle.

c. Runs in the spiral groove on the humerus where it is easily compressed.
d. If damaged usually leaves sensation intact in the hand.
e. Is the main motor nerve to the extensor compartments of the arm and forearm.

74. **Papilloedema:**

a. May produce 'tunnel-vision'.
b. Is a typical feature of idiopathic intracranial hypertension.
c. May resemble papillitis associated with optic neuritis.
d. May be caused by a high CSF protein.
e. Is not a cause of transient loss of vision.

75. **Recognized findings in normal pressure hydrocephalus include:**

a. Urinary incontinence.
b. Papilloedema.
c. Dementia.
d. Difficulty walking.
e. Normal ventricular size on CT.

76. **Multiple sclerosis typically presents with:**

a. Monocular visual loss associated with pain on eye movement.
b. Spastic paraparesis.
c. Homonymous hemianopia.
d. Recurrent sensory symptoms.
e. Seizures.

77. **The headache of raised intracranial pressure typically is associated with:**

a. Worsening with coughing, sneezing or bending over.
b. Fortification spectra.
c. Stabbing or shooting pains.
d. Worse on waking and better on standing.
e. Progressive nausea and vomiting.

78. **The following statements are correct:**

a. The ulnar nerve supplies most of the muscle in the flexor compartment of the forearm.
b. The ulnar nerve supplies most of the intrinsic muscles of the hand.
c. The median nerve supplies most of the muscles in the hypothenar eminence.
d. The radial nerve supplies the dorsal interossei.
e. Most of the intrinsic hand muscles are supplied by nerves from the T1 spinal root.

79. **A CSF protein greater than 1g/L is often seen in:**

a. Stroke.
b. Guillain–Barré syndrome.
c. Neoplastic meningitis.
d. Tuberculous meningitis.
e. Viral meningitis.

80. **Temporal lobe epilepsy is associated with:**

a. Visual and olfactory hallucinations.
b. 'Trance-like' states.

c. Jerking of the upper limbs.
d. Repetitive conjugate eye movements.
e. Lip smacking.

81. **Involuntary movements of the face or tongue are characteristic of:**

a. Huntington's disease.
b. Levodopa-treated Parkinson's disease.
c. Neuroleptic treatment.
d. Motor neuron disease.
e. Blepharospasm.

82. **Seizures are recognized complications of:**

a. SIADH.
b. Cerebral venous thrombosis.
c. Withdrawal of long-term barbiturate therapy.
d. Subdural haematoma.
e. Antidepressant therapy.

83. **In subarachnoid haemorrhage:**

a. Lumbar puncture is contraindicated because of the risk of coning.
b. Severe hypertension should be treated immediately with antihypertensive agents.
c. A Berry aneurysm is more often found in the posterior rather anterior circulation.
d. CT head scan detect 70% of haemorrhages.
e. There is a 20% chance of rebleed within the first two weeks.

84. **Alzheimer's disease:**

a. Commonly presents with disorientation in time and place.
b. Relatives are more aware of the degree of memory loss than the patient.
c. Typically presents with disinhibition and apathy.
d. Geographical apraxia and language deficits are often early features.
e. Anticholinesterase inhibitors can delay symptom progression by 6 months.

85. **Idiopathic trigeminal neuralgia:**

a. Is associated with an absence of neurological signs.
b. Is usually bilateral.
c. Often responds to carbamazepine.
d. Is a constant pain.
e. Is associated with depression.

86. **Autonomic dysfunction is associated with:**

a. Diabetes.
b. Early idiopathic Parkinson's disease.
c. Small-cell lung cancer.
d. Guillain–Barré syndrome.
e. Myasthenia gravis.

87. **Post-lumbar puncture headache:**

a. Is related to the gauge of the needle used.
b. Often resolves spontaneously within one week.
c. Can be accompanied by neck stiffness and nausea.
d. Improves dramatically on lying flat.
e. Is related to draining greater than 10 mL of CSF.

88. **A diagnosis of tension-type headache is favoured by:**

    a. Continuous daily headache.
    b. Mild to moderate severity.
    c. Ability to continue working through the headache.
    d. Difficulty sleeping.
    e. Tight, band-like pain around the whole of the head.

89. **The following are associated with anterior circulation (carotid territory) transient ischaemic attacks (TIAs):**

    a. Diplopia.
    b. Weakness in all four limbs.
    c. Loss of vision in one eye (amaurosis fugax).
    d. Dysphasia.
    e. Vertigo.

90. **Myasthenia gravis:**

    a. Is associated with antibodies to the terminal axon.
    b. May worsen transiently during treatment with steroids.
    c. Often improves after removal of a thymoma.
    d. Edrophonium is used to help make the diagnosis.
    e. Weakness is usually in the distal upper limbs.

91. **A low CSF glucose is seen in:**

    a. Alzheimer's disease.
    b. Ischaemic stroke.
    c. Multiple sclerosis.
    d. Guillain–Barré syndrome.
    e. Sarcoidosis.

92. **Stroke is associated with:**

    a. Hemiparesis due to a lacunar infarct in the anterior limb of the internal capsule.
    b. Silent infarcts in the frontal lobes.
    c. A right incongruous hemianopia caused by a left occipital infarct.
    d. Seizures more common in the acute phase if they are haemorrhagic and not ischaemic.
    e. Gerstmann's syndrome is associated with constructional and geographical apraxia.

93. **Cerebrospinal fluid:**

    a. Is only produced in the lateral ventricles.
    b. Is absorbed by the arachnoid granulations.
    c. Is produced at a rate of 500 mL per day.
    d. Is normally at a pressure of less than 15 cmH$_2$O.
    e. May normally contain up to 4 lymphocytes/mm^3.

94. **In myotonic dstrophy:**

    a. Myotonia may be worse in cold weather.
    b. Exhibits genetic anticipation.
    c. Conduction defects may require a pacemaker.
    d. Males are often sterile and demonstrate early frontal balding.
    e. Anaesthetic complications occur.

95. **In Duchenne muscular dystrophy:**

    a. Is fatal in most patients before the age of 30.
    b. Is associated with a high CK.
    c. Gower's sign is positive.
    d. Is X-linked.
    e. Spares ocular, facial, bulbar and hand muscles.

96. **Benign essential tremor:**

    a. Often improves with alcohol.
    b. Worse at rest than on action.
    c. May be treated with propranolol.
    d. May be familial.
    e. Is sometimes functionally disabling.

97. **Primary intracerebral haemorrhage:**

    a. Is associated with polycystic kidney disease.
    b. Usually causes meningism.
    c. Is often less clinically dangerous if in the posterior fossa.
    d. Is usually within the cerebral cortex in hypertensive patients.
    e. Is best treated with emergency surgical evacuation.

98. **Herpes meningoencephalitis:**

    a. Is never associated with a low CSF glucose.
    b. The CSF is often normal.
    c. Imaging may show haemorrhage in the temporal lobes.
    d. EEG shows slowing over one or both temporal lobes.
    e. Is associated with severe behavioural disturbance.

99. **Prion diseases:**

    a. Are caused by slow viruses.
    b. The infectious particles are easily destroyed by conventional sterilization techniques.
    c. Can be genetically inherited.
    d. Have a quicker clinical progression in the new variant than the sporadic form.
    e. May have characteristic findings on MRI.

100. **Migraine with aura:**

    a. There is often a family history.
    b. Is usually straightforward to differentiate from TIA.
    c. Sumatriptan is an excellent agent for migraine prophylaxis.
    d. Is typically associated with EEG abnormalities.
    e. Patients are often agitated and cannot get to sleep.

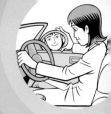

1. Name the site of the lesion causing the following visual field defects:

    a. Right central scotoma.
    b. Bitemporal hemianopia.
    c. Left homonymous hemianopia.
    d. Right upper homonymous quadrantanopia.
    e. Left lower homonymous quadrantanopia.
    f. Right homonymous hemianopia with macula sparing.

2. Describe the fundoscopic appearances of optic atrophy and name four causes.

3. List the features of a third cranial nerve (oculomotor nerve) palsy and name three causes.

4. List four causes of a ptosis and important associated features of each.

5. What features in the examination would help you to differentiate Bell's palsy, upper motor neuron facial weakness, and a cerebellopontine angle tumour?

6. Differentiate the features of an upper motor neuron lesion from those of a lower motor neuron lesion and indicate where in the nervous system each type of lesion might be found.

7. What is the Brown–Séquard syndrome? What is the most common cause and what signs are found?

8. Which pathways convey the various modalities of sensation within the spinal cord and where do they decussate?

9. List five causes of absent ankle jerks with extensor plantars.

10. Name the different types of neuropathy that can occur as a complicating feature of diabetes mellitus.

11. Describe the clinical features of a cerebellar syndrome and give four causes.

12. What are the clinical features of a Horner's syndrome? Discuss the possible sites of the lesion and give a cause at each site.

13. What are the features of a lesion of the cerebellopontine angle? What causes should be considered?

14. A patient presents with a resting tremor of the right arm. What additional signs would support the diagnosis of Parkinson's disease?

15. What clinical signs would you expect in a patient who has a 'pseudobulbar palsy'? In which conditions can this occur?

16. What is Lhermitte's phenomenon? What diagnoses should be considered?

17. What are the signs of a common peroneal nerve palsy? What are the most common causes?

18. What are the clinical features of lateral medullary syndrome?

19. What are characteristics that differentiate the increased tone of an upper motor neuron lesion and that of an extrapyramidal syndrome?

20. What are the clinical features of Wernicke's encephalopathy? How is the condition treated?

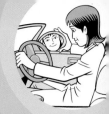

1. Options:

a. Tension-type headache
b. Migraine with aura
c. Migraine without aura
d. Stroke
e. Subarachnoid haemorrhage
f. Bacterial meningitis
g. Tuberculous meningitis
h. Viral meningitis
i. Low-pressure headache
j. Raised intracranial pressure headache

For each of the following patients with headache, select the most likely answer from the list of options.

1. A 22-year-old man presents to casualty with a severe headache that came on 12 hours ago and is increasingly severe. He has vomited twice. On examination, he is confused, photophobic, and has a stiff neck. Kernig's sign is positive but the rest of the neurological examination is normal. His lumbar puncture shows an opening pressure of 23 cmH$_2$O, 160 polymorphs, 10 red cells, a protein of 1.2 g/L and a CSF glucose of 2 mmol/L (serum 5.4 mmol/L).

2. A 68-year-old smoker presents to clinic with a 3-week history of a progressive headache, which is increasing in severity. It is worse in the morning and after his afternoon nap. Over the past few days, he has been feeling increasingly nauseated and his right hand is becoming slow and clumsy. His wife feels that he is 'not himself' and that 'he cannot get his words out'. On examination, he has pyramidal weakness in the right arm and an expressive dysphasia. His optic disc margins are slightly indistinct.

3. A 24-year-old woman has recently started the contraceptive pill, and has noticed that three or four times per month she gets a numbness in her face which resolves in 20 minutes and is followed by numbness in her arm, which also resolves in 20 minutes. She then develops a bilateral retro-orbital and throbbing headache that makes her feel sick, although she does not usually vomit. She has to come home from work and rest in her bedroom with her curtains drawn but it is usually better by the next day. Her mother says that she had a few similar attacks in her teens but 'never as severe as her daughter's'.

4. A 40-year-old man comes to casualty with a 3-hour history of severe headache, which is now improving slightly. He normally gets headaches when he is stressed but he has never had anything as bad as this headache. On examination, he has slight neck stiffness, a right-sided ptosis, double vision on looking to the left and up as well as a slightly bigger pupil on the right compared to the left, but he is otherwise well now. His CT head is normal and his lumbar puncture shows an opening pressure of 25 cmH$_2$O, with 500 red cells and 3 lymphocytes. The protein is 0.8 g/L and the glucose is normal. He is kept in for observation overnight and during the night he alerts the nurses because his severe headache has returned. He subsequently becomes drowsy and has a tonic clonic seizure.

5. A 72-year-old man with diabetes presents to casualty with a 12-hour history of dull right-sided headache associated with acute onset of left-sided weakness. On examination, he is moderately drowsy but has a GCS of 15. He also has a left hemiparesis and a left homonomous hemianopia. His headache seems to be dull and nagging but he has no neck stiffness or photophobia. He is pyrexial to 37.4 °C. His wife tells you that 2 weeks ago the left side of his body went numb but it went away within a few hours.

2. Options:

a. Vasovagal syncope
b. Cardiogenic syncope
c. Complex partial seizure
d. Tonic-clonic seizure
e. Non-epileptic seizure
f. Narcolepsy
g. Hypoglycaemia
h. Absence seizure
i. Postural hypotension
j. Subarachnoid haemorrhage

For each of the following patients with impairment of consciousness, select the most likely answer from the list of options.

1. A 13-year-old girl is noticed by her teacher at school to be 'not concentrating on her work'. The teacher describes episodes where she stares into space for approximately a minute and returns to normal

rapidly. The girl is otherwise very well and has a normal neurological examination. She had one febrile convulsion as a child.

2. An 18-year-old man complains of episodes where he suddenly collapses to the ground and starts to shake both upper limbs. He feels slightly 'distant' while the shaking occurs but remembers people around him being concerned. The attacks last 30 seconds to 5 minutes and have occurred up to 10 times in a day. When the shaking stops, he complains of feeling slightly tired but can resume his activities. He is due to sit his A-levels in 4 months. There is a family history of epilepsy in his younger sister after she had meningitis as a baby.

3. A 24-year-old woman presents with episodes of loss of consciousness for a few minutes and recently one of the attacks was followed by some mild stiffening in all her limbs and urinary incontinence. The episodes tend to happen at the end of the day when she is standing on the train coming home. She is aware that she feels slightly nauseated before the attacks and feels as if a curtain is coming over her vision before she loses consciousness. Normally, she recovers fully in a few minutes after being given a seat by another passenger.

4. A 25-year-old woman has lapses of consciousness that occur anytime of the day. There are no associated movements or incontinence. She has also found that she has been feeling extremely tired throughout the day, despite having a good night's sleep. The attacks last from seconds to minutes and she does not get any warning they are going to occur. She also describes vivid 'dream-like' images on going to sleep and feels she cannot move her body on waking up for several minutes.

5. A 35-year-old man complains of episodes of confusion. His wife tells you that he will suddenly 'go blank and stare into space' for several minutes. He often wanders around the room and picks up and puts down objects repeatedly. His wife tells you he does not respond appropriately to her concerns during the attack, and he often feels extremely tired once they have finished. He sometimes gets a 'strange, horrible taste' in his mouth prior to the attacks.

3. Options:

a. Alzheimer's disease
b. Frontotemporal dementia
c. Normal pressure hydrocephalus
d. Acute confusional state
e. Non-convulsive status epilepticus
f. Multi-infarct dementia
g. Subcortical ischaemic leucoencephalopathy
h. New variant Creuztfeldt–Jakob disease

i. Vitamin B$_{12}$ deficiency
j. Pseudodementia

For each of the following patients with impairment of memory, select the most likely answer from the list of options.

1. A 60-year-old man lives in a nursing home after suffering a severe subarachnoid haemorrhage 5 years ago. Recently, his carers have noticed that his walking is becoming much slower and he is becoming slightly confused and forgetful. They have also noticed that, despite regular toileting, he has become incontinent of urine. On examination, he has old left-sided pyramidal signs, but coordination in his right side and sensory examination are normal. When he tries to stand up he slips backwards into his chair. His mini-mental test score is 21 out of 30, whereas 2 years ago it was noted to be 28. He informs you that he is simply unaware of needing to pass urine.

2. A young woman aged 20 dropped out of university recently because of a depressive illness. She has noticed that in retrospect she has also had strange sensations in her arms and legs over the past 2 months. In spite of treatment for her depression, her parents have noticed that she is becoming forgetful, disorientated, and clumsy.

3. A 75-year-old hypertensive patient had a small stroke 1 year ago, from which he made a good recovery although he was left with mild weakness on the left side and mild confusion. Since then, he has had two further acute episodes of slurred speech and then dysphasia, which have partially resolved but have left him functionally disabled. He is now very forgetful and shuffles when he walks. His wife suggests to you in confidence that he is 'not the man I used to know'. On examination, he has a pseudobulbar palsy, brisk but symmetrical reflexes, and extensor plantar responses with mild left-sided pyramidal weakness.

4. A 70-year-old woman comes to clinic with her daughter. The patient admits to having problems with her memory, which is frustrating for her, but she is mostly unaware of her difficulties. Her daughter then suggests that actually her mother has been becoming increasingly 'muddled and forgetful'. Two weeks previously, her mother was found wandering lost in her local shops. Two months before that the patient decided to stop attending her social meetings because she found it difficult to keep up with the conversation. She had also forgotten recent family events. Neurological examination was normal apart from a mini-mental test score of 22 out of 30.

5. A 82-year-old man presents to clinic with a 5-month history of 'apathy, loss of interest, and forgetfulness'. He has withdrawn from all his social engagements following the death of his

wife 6 months previously. He recently had a small house fire because he left a chip pan on, but he was able to call the fire brigade. He has lost a significant amount of weight recently because he claims he is never hungry. He is often seen wandering around his local shops alone but his daughter claims his cupboards are empty and his house is in a bad condition. Neurological examination is normal and his mini-mental test score is 28 out of 30, but he was very slow in giving his answers.

4. Options:

a. Idiopathic Parkinson's disease
b. Multisystem atrophy
c. Huntington's disease
d. Wilson's disease
e. Benign essential tremor
f. Spasmodic torticollis
g. Physiological tremor
h. Levodopa-induced dyskinesias
i. Hemiballismus
j. Pseudoathetosis

For each of the following patients with abnormal movements, select the most likely answer from the list of options.

1. A 30-year-old woman presents to clinic with difficulty drinking a cup of tea because of a tremor. It is absent at rest but she also notices it as she is writing. She has noticed that it rarely affects her when she goes out at the weekend for a few drinks. On examination, she has a postural tremor of the upper limbs.

2. A 21-year-old man presents with a 1-year history of slurring of his speech and difficulty swallowing. More recently, he has noticed that his legs and arms can go into 'spasms' and have become tremulous.

3. A patient with Parkinson's disease has been managed successfully by his GP for the past 6 years but recently he has been experiencing writhing movements of his tongue, face, neck, trunk, and limbs that is worst 2 hours after he takes his dose of levodopa but resolves by the time he goes 'off'. It is now difficult for him to do anything during these episodes.

4. A 70-year-old hypertensive woman has a sudden onset of wild flailing movements of her right arm and leg. She is otherwise well.

5. A 42-year-old man, who has recently lost contact with his family because of 'differences', has noticed that his arms will suddenly jerk. He functionally copes with the jerking but finds it frustrating and he has noticed that he loses his temper more frequently. He did not know his father very well because he had an unknown neurological illness that led to his father's early death.

5. Options:

a. Multiple sclerosis
b. Parkinson's disease
c. Spinal cord compression
d. Peripheral neuropathy
e. Normal pressure hydrocephalus
f. Subcortical ischaemic leucoencephalopathy
g. Progressive supranuclear palsy
h. Polymyositis
i. Acute confusional state
j. Motor neuron disease

For each of the following patients with imbalance, select the most likely answer from the list of options.

1. A 74-year-old man presents with a 1-year history of feeling as if he is 'walking on stones'. He now has numbness and weakness, which involve both legs and recently he has had some numbness in the tips of his fingers. He recently fell over when he tried to get up during the night. On examination, he has weakness and sensory loss to the knees and he has lost all his tendon reflexes in his lower limbs. Plantars are flexor. His random glucose is 7 and his serum electrophoresis demonstrates an IgM paraprotein.

2. A 65-year-old woman has noticed that over the last 3 months she has had increasing difficulty climbing stairs and standing from her chair. Over the past 2 weeks, her swallowing has also deteriorated. On examination, she has weakness around the shoulder and hip girdle and her swallow is slow. Her reflexes are slightly brisk but symmetrical. She has no sensory loss. Her creatine kinase is 3000.

3. A 24-year-old woman presents acutely with slurred speech, double vision, vertigo, and imbalance on walking. On examination, her right optic disc is pale and she has a right relative afferent pupillary defect. She also has horizontal gaze-evoked nystagmus, which is worse on looking to the left, with a left internuclear ophthalmoplegia. On examination of her limbs, she has left-sided dysmetria, brisk but symmetrical reflexes and extensor plantar responses. Her gait is slightly broad and unstable. Five years previously she had an episode of blurred vision in her right eye and pain behind the eye for a few days but it has since returned to normal.

4. A 75-year-old hypertensive woman presents to casualty with a 1-week history of difficulty walking. She has not passed urine or opened her bowels for the past 48 hours and she puts this down to the fact that she has not been eating

much lately. On examination, she has reduced tone in her legs with only slight movement with gravity at the hip. Her reflexes are brisk in the legs and her abdominal reflexes are absent. She has lost pin-prick and vibration sensation to her upper chest. Her anal tone is reduced and her bladder is palpable. Her cranial nerves and arms are normal. She also informs you that she had a mastectomy over 10 years ago for breast cancer, but a recent check-up was 'all clear'.

5. A 52-year-old man is referred to you from the ENT doctors because of imbalance, which was initially thought to be due to inner ear disease. He gives a 1-year history of falling over. His wife suggests that he is also becoming slower in everything he does and that he often cries or laughs at things he never used to feel emotional about. On examination, he has reduced down gaze, a brisk gag reflex, a starring face, prominent grasp reflexes, and symmetrical mild bradykinesia. As soon as you try and stand him up, he falls back into his chair.

6. Options:

a. Multiple sclerosis
b. Posterior interosseous nerve palsy
c. Motor neuron disease
d. Carpal tunnel syndrome
e. Brachial neuritis (neuralgic amyotrophy)
f. Ulnar nerve palsy at the elbow
g. Radial nerve palsy in the spiral groove.
h. Lower brachial plexus lesion
i. Ulnar nerve palsy at the wrist
j. Cervical radiculopathy

For each of the following patients with symptoms in their arms, select the most likely answer from the list of options.

1. A 74-year-old male smoker has developed severe pain and weakness in his right hand; he also describes some numbness over his right arm. On examination, he has wasting and power loss in his hand involving both thenar and hypothenar eminences as well as sensory loss over the C8 and T1 dermatomes. Closer inspection suggests that his right eyelid is drooping and he has a small right pupil. He has also lost a stone in weight over the past month.

2. A 25-year-old woman has noticed that, over the last 3 months, she has had increasing pain in her left arm and occasionally in her right. The pain wakes her up at night-time and she shakes her hands to relieve her symptoms. She has not noticed any weakness in her hands although she has recently been commenced on thyroxine replacement for hypothyroidism. Neurological examination is normal apart from a positive Phalen's test on the left.

3. A 46-year-old man had an acute onset of severe right shoulder pain which prevented him from working 6 weeks ago. Since then, he has noticed that his right shoulder has become weak. On examination, he has severe wasting and weakness of his deltoid, supraspinatus, rhomboids, and biceps. His reflexes in the right arm are all diminished. He has some slight numbness over his shoulder but it is relatively minor.

4. A 59-year-old secretary has noticed that her typing was not as good as it used to be 5 months ago and took early retirement. Recently, she has noticed that she has difficulty with getting dressed because her hands feel weak. Her swallowing has also become a problem, especially when drinking tea. She suffers from cramps at night-time in her legs and sometimes her arms. On examination, her tongue is small and possibly has some fasciculations in it. She has a brisk gag reflex and jaw jerk. She has fasciculations in her hands, biceps, quadriceps, and calves associated with wasting in her hands and forearms. Her reflexes are all brisk and her plantars are extensor.

5. A 62-year-old woman has recently been developing severe pain, especially at night, in her neck. She has also noticed that she gets shooting pains down her right arm, especially when she flexes her neck. On examination, she has weakness of her right elbow flexion and some numbness over the lateral surface of the arm. Her right biceps jerk is absent. You incidentally notice that her walking is slow and that her triceps, knee, and ankle jerks are brisk and her plantars are extensor.

7. Options:

a. Lacunar infarction of the internal capsule
b. Total right middle cerebral infarction
c. Total left middle cerebral infarction
d. Basilar artery thrombosis
e. Lateral medullary syndrome
f. Cerebellar haemorrhage
g. Partial left middle cerebral artery infarction
h. Transient ischaemic attack
i. Posterior cerebral artery infarction
j. Internal carotid artery occlusion

For each of the following patients with stroke, select the most likely answer from the list of options.

1. A 74-year-old hypertensive man developed an acute onset of severe weakness in his right side involving his lower face, arm and leg. On examination, he has a right hemiplegia with no sensory loss.

2. A 25-year-old woman was involved in a car accident and suffered a severe 'whiplash injury and shock' but was otherwise well. The following day she presents to casualty with weakness on her

right side, confusion, and incomprehensible speech. On examination, she has a left-sided Horner's syndrome, a dense right hemiplegia, dysphasia, and probably a right homonomous hemianopia. Unfortunately she becomes very drowsy and obtunded over the next 24 hours and dies on ITU. ☐

3. A 66-year-old man had an acute onset of right lower facial weakness and his wife tells you that he had severe difficulties 'in stringing his words capsule together'. It has slowly improved over the past 4 days and, when you see him, he is only complaining of slight difficulties in expressing himself fully but he knows what he wants to say. On examination, he has a left carotid bruit and a mild expressive dysphasia. ☐

4. A 59-year-old type 2 diabetic presents to casualty with acute onset of vertigo and imbalance. He also has problems swallowing and his right side of his face 'feels strange'. On examination, he has a right-sided Horner's syndrome, right-sided loss of pain and temperature sensation, his uvula moves to the left and he has pooling of his secretions in his pharynx. He has mild left-sided weakness and right-sided dysmetria. Over the next 2 weeks he almost makes a full recovery. ☐

5. A 62-year-old hypertensive woman presents to casualty with a 4-hour history of rapidly progressive drowsiness. Her husband informs you that, prior to her becoming drowsy, she complained of a severe pain in the back of her head and she vomited twice. She tried to walk but was too unsteady. On examination, she has a Glasgow Coma Scale of 6 out of 15 and has a grossly dilated left pupil. There are no other obvious cranial nerve signs. She is too confused and drowsy to properly examine her but she appears to be moving all her limbs. Her reflexes are brisk but symmetrical and her plantars are extensor. ☐

8. Options:

a. An isolated third nerve palsy
b. An isolated fourth nerve palsy
c. An isolated sixth nerve palsy
d. Myasthenia gravis
e. Ocular myopathy
f. Third and fourth nerve palsy
g. A lesion in the cavernous sinus
h. Pontine lesion
i. A frontal lesion
j. An occipital lesion

For each of the following patients with difficulties in moving their eyes, select the most likely answer from the list of options.

1. A 64-year-old diabetic man developed an acute onset of double vision. On examination, his right eye is looking down and out and he has a ptosis of the right eyelid. The outer image is lost when he covers his right eye. The pupils are normal. The rest of the examination is normal. ☐

2. A 26-year-old woman has slowly developed worsening double vision over the past 4 weeks associated with a headache and nausea. On examination, she has gross papilloedema and failure of abduction of the right eye. ☐

3. A 30-year-old woman presents with worsening intermittent double vision over the past 2 weeks. She has noticed that it usually comes on when she is tired at the end of the day. On examination, she has limitation of movements in most directions except on looking down with the right eye and abducting the left eye. Her pupils are normal but she has bilateral ptosis, which gets worse on sustained upgaze. She is otherwise well and is a well-controlled type 1 diabetic for 16 years. ☐

4. A 59-year-old man presents with a 1-month history of progressive double vision and a 2-week history of deteriorating vision in the right eye and numbness over his right upper face. On examination, he has visual acuities of 6/6 on the left and 6/36 on the right. He has a partial right ptosis, slight movement of upgaze in his right eye but otherwise complete restriction of movement and loss of sensation in the ophthalmic and maxillary branches of the fifth nerve. ☐

5. A 62-year-old diabetic, hypertensive woman presents to casualty with sudden onset of left-sided weakness. On examination, she has a dense left hemiplegia and both her eyes deviate laterally to the right. She is drowsy and moderately confused. ☐

9. Options:

a. Optic neuritis
b. Giant cell arteritis
c. Parietal lobe lesion
d. Occipital lobe lesion
e. Pituitary macroadenoma
f. Temporal lobe lesion
g. Orbital tumour
h. Craniopharyngioma
i. Leber's optic neuropathy
j. Idiopathic intracranial hypertension

For each of the following patients with loss of vision, select the most likely answer from the list of options.

1. A 64-year-old man presents acutely with left-sided weakness and sensory loss. On examination, he has a left hemiplegia and hemisensory loss but also a left inferior homonymous quadrantinopia. ☐

2. A 24-year-old man develops worsening vision in his right eye over several days associated with pain on

moving the eye. On examination of the affected eye, his visual acuity is 6/18 and he has lost perception of colour in the centre of his vision. His pupil is sluggish to react to a direct but not a consensual light stimulus and his fundi are normal. Over the next 4 weeks, his vision returns to normal.

3. A 30-year-old woman presents with tiredness and lethargy and is found to have diabetes. You notice that her facial features are coarse and enlarged. The size of her hands and feet has increased over the past 5 years and colleagues at work have commented that she has a deep voice. She has also recently been developing tingling of her hands at night. On neurological examination, she has a bitemporal upper quadrantinopia and carpal tunnel syndrome.

4. A 79-year-old woman has been feeling lethargic for 6 months and recently has developed severe right-sided headaches, which last most of the day and night. She finds it difficult to touch the right side of her face because of pain. Last night, she noticed that the vision in her right eye suddenly deteriorated and she has been left with a 'black area' at the bottom of her vision in the right eye. On examination, she has an altitudinal defect affecting the inferior portion of her right visual field.

5. A 25-year-old man presents with episodes of brief loss of vision in both eyes. He is markedly overweight. On examination, he has peripheral restriction in his visual fields and swollen optic discs with a few peripapillary haemorrhages.

10. Options:

a. Idiopathic Parkinson's disease
b. Huntington's chorea
c. Peripheral neuropathy
d. Cerebellar syndrome
e. Spastic paraparesis
f. Spastic hemiparesis
g. Subcortical ischaemic leucoencephalopathy
h. Functional disorder
i. Common peroneal nerve lesion
j. Myopathy

For each of the following patients with abnormal gaits, select the most likely answer from the list of options.

1. A 35-year-old man has had progressive weakness in his shoulder and pelvic girdle for 10 years. When he walks he has a 'waddling' gait.

2. A 25-year-old man has had difficulties walking all his life. When he walks, his legs 'scissor' across one another. On examination, he has very stiff legs and clonus at the ankles. His reflexes are brisk and his plantars are extensor.

3. A 30-year-old alcoholic presents with difficulty walking. On examination, he has a broad-based gait and is severely imbalanced.

4. A 79-year-old hypertensive woman has recently had difficulty walking. Her gait is slow and shuffling and she takes very little steps. Even when she starts walking, she cannot speed up and easily comes to rest. On examination, she has a pseudobulbar palsy, brisk tendon reflexes and extensor plantars.

5. A 27-year-old man presents with episodes of sudden inability to walk. The attacks occur up to 10 times per day and are associated with twitching of his shoulder. He has fallen many times but not hurt himself. When you ask him to walk, he collapses to the floor, even though his bedside examination was normal. When he starts to walk, his gait is slow, intermittently clumsy and he has an asymmetrical posture with hunching of his right shoulder. He describes his feet as being 'stuck to the floor'.

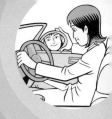

Patient-management problems (PMPs)

1. A 65-year-old woman is seen in the Accident & Emergency Department having woken with no vision in her left eye. She had had two episodes of short-lived visual loss in the same eye, lasting a couple of minutes, within the previous 2 weeks, but had not sought medical advice.

   Three months previously, she had become aware of aching and stiffness of her shoulders and hips, which was most pronounced in the mornings. She had found it increasingly difficult to get up out of a low chair, to climb stairs, and to brush and wash her hair. This had been diagnosed as arthritis and she had gained a little relief from non-steroidal anti-inflammatory drugs.

   One month before admission, she had begun to develop headaches. These were initially mild and localized to the left temple, but subsequently the severity and distribution increased and she had marked scalp tenderness.

   Examination reveals no perception of light in the left eye. The left pupil is dilated with no direct light reflex but there is a normal consensual response to light in the right eye. Fundoscopy shows general pallor of the retina and swelling of the optic nerve head. Proximal muscles are tender, but otherwise the neurological examination is normal. Palpation of the temples causes pain.

   a. What does the history of aching muscles suggest?
   b. What is the probable cause of the headaches?
   c. What is the mechanism of the visual loss?
   d. What investigations are indicated?
   e. What is the treatment for this condition?
   f. What is the prognosis for her vision?

2. A 55-year-old male accountant presents with a 2-year history of increasing difficulty in walking. Initially, when he walked over half a mile, he would develop pain in his buttocks, which spread down the posterior aspect of his legs to his feet. If he rested for a few minutes, the pain would settle. Subsequently, he could only manage to walk about 400 yards before the pain would spread. He began to notice that the pain was associated with numbness and tingling. Resting would partly relieve the symptoms, as would bending forwards. He could, however, ride his bicycle for indefinite distances without the symptoms developing. On several occasions, when trying to walk through the symptoms, he became incontinent of urine. He had no significant past medical history or family history. He was a smoker.

   Examination at rest is normal. All peripheral pulses were palpable.

   a. What is the differential diagnosis of exertional pain in the legs?
   b. What points in the history indicate a neurological cause?
   c. What additional test might be helpful to carry out during the examination in a patient with a history such as this, especially with a normal examination at rest?
   d. What investigation would confirm the diagnosis?

3. A 21-year-old woman presents to her GP in a distressed state as she had woken that morning with difficulty speaking and thought she had had a stroke. The previous day she had developed pain around the right ear, which had kept her awake part of the night. In the morning, she found that she had dribbled on her pillow and her speech had become slurred. Her boyfriend had told her that her mouth had become twisted and that her right eye was not closing when she blinked. She had no other symptoms.

   Examination reveals severe weakness of all right-sided muscles of facial expression.

   a. What is the most likely diagnosis and what is the differential diagnosis?
   b. What other functions should be examined?
   c. What investigations are indicated?
   d. What is the treatment?
   e. What is the prognosis?

4. A 46-year-old man presents complaining of nocturnal incontinence. Five times in the previous 6 months he had awoken in the morning with a wet bed, having been incontinent of urine. Each time he had gone to bed feeling well and had not taken any drugs or excessive quantities of alcohol. Bladder function during the day is normal. He lives alone. Two years previously he had been in a road traffic accident, when he lost consciousness briefly. Examination is normal apart from a slight spastic catch in his left arm, with slightly brisker jerks on the left side and an upgoing left plantar.

   a. What is the probable cause of the nocturnal incontinence?
   b. What might be the underlying cause?
   c. What investigations are indicated?

5. A 64-year-old executive chauffeur had been noted to be confused when he arrived at the central office to clock in and had been sent home. His wife was concerned and had brought him to Casualty. In the department, he had recovered. As far as he was concerned, he had got up, washed and dressed, and then remembered nothing until being in Casualty. He had actually had breakfast, driven to work, clocked on, and then had driven home after being noted to be acting oddly by his boss.

When assessed, he scored fully on a mini-mental test, with normal orientation and memory apart from loss of memory of events between 8 a.m. and 11 a.m. His blood pressure was 160/100 mmHg. There were no bruits and the remaining examination was normal.

a. What is the differential diagnosis?
b. What investigations are indicated?
c. Is treatment required?
d. What is the prognosis?

6. A 58-year-old man presents with a history over several months of tingling in both feet. He is noted to have an abnormal gait. There is no weakness in his limbs, but his ankle and knee jerks are diminished.

a. What is the most likely diagnosis?
b. Describe further the signs that may be found on clinical examination.
c. Discuss the pertinent features in the history and examination that would help elucidate the aetiology and guide further management.

7. A 63-year-old woman presents with unilateral transient visual loss. Discuss what features in the history and examination would help in differentiation of the diagnosis.

8. A 34-year-old woman presents with a 1-week history of pain in the legs, pins and needles in the feet and to a lesser degree the hands, then progressive weakness of the legs. She had previously been well apart from a mild episode of diarrhoea a couple of weeks before this current presentation.

a. What is the most likely diagnosis?
b. What clinical signs would you expect to find on examination?
c. Discuss the investigations and further management of the patient.

9. A 45-year-old man presents to casualty with a 3-day history of fever, headaches, and vomiting. He had been been treated by the haematologists for acute lymphatic leukaemia 6 months ago with a bone marrow transplant. He has been told that he is in remission but has developed moderate graft-versus-host disease and continues to take a small dose of prednisolone. On examination, he is drowsy and confused with a GCS of 13 out of 15. He has neck stiffness and a pyrexia. There is no obvious rash. He has no other obvious neurological signs. As you are examining him he has a generalized tonic-clonic seizure.

a. What is the most probable diagnosis?
b. What would your immediate management be?
c. Which specialties would you discuss his case with and why?

10. A 65-year-old man presents to casualty with a 2-day history of difficulty breathing and is referred to your medical team. He is noted to be using his accessory muscles and on auscultation of his chest, his breath sounds can be just heard. He has been a smoker in the past. His chest X-ray and ECG are normal. An arterial blood gas demonstrates a high carbon dioxide, a borderline low oxygen, a normal pH and base excess and slightly raised bicarbonate. When you review him, he informs you that he has been having some difficulty swallowing recently and having episodes of double vision, especially towards the end of the day. On examination, he has mild bilateral ptosis, full range of eye movements, a very poor swallow and slurred speech. His upper limbs are also mildly weak, especially proximally. His reflexes are present and symmetrical and his plantars are flexor. There are no fasciculations.

a. What is the most probable diagnosis/diagnoses?
b. What other aspects of the examination would you perform that may help in confirming this?
c. What investigations would you perform?
d. What would be your management plan?

1. a. F–The corticospinal or 'pyramidal' tract decussates below the pyramids on the inferoventral surface of the medulla.
   b. T–Expansion of a Berry aneurysm of the posterior communicating artery can cause compression of the oculomotor nerve and therefore a 'painful third nerve palsy'.
   c. T–The superior colliculus lies on the dorsal surface of the midbrain and it and other more ventral nuclei (pretectal) receive fibres from the optic nerve to coordinate light reflexes and eye movements.
   d. F–The lateral rectus muscle 'abducts' the eye and is supplied by the sixth or 'abducens' nerve. The fourth nerve or 'trochlear nerve' innervates the superior oblique muscle which hooks around the trochlear protruberence below the upper margin of the eye socket.
   e. F–The spinal cord ends at L1/2 in adults.

2. a. T–Cranial nerves III, VII and X and S3–5 spinal nerves carry parasympathetic fibres.
   b. F–The trigeminal nerve carries somatic motor and sensory fibres.
   c. T–see 2(a).
   d. F–The hypoglossal nerve only carries somatic motor fibres.
   e. T–see 2(a).

3. a. T–Chronic subdural haematomas can present with dementia.
   b. T–Acute subdural haematomas can present with signs of raised intracranial pressure including a dilated pupil due to third cranial nerve compression.
   c. T–Cushing's reflex (bradycardia and hypertension) is uncommonly associated with raised intracranial pressure.
   d. T–Acute rises in intracranial pressure can cause drowsiness.
   e. F–Blood is contained between the dura and arachnoid mater and does not leak into the subarachnoid space.

4. a. T–Up to 80% of patients have antibodies to the acetylcholine receptor.
   b. F–The axons to the muscles affected are not damaged and so wasting is not a prominent feature.
   c. T–As acetylcholine is released during the day, there is a gradual reduction at the motor end-plate leading to fatigability that is worst towards the end of the day.
   d. F–Lambert–Eaton myasthenic syndrome is associated with a transient improvement after exercise but patients with MG get worse after exercise because of reducing levels of acetylcholine at the end-plate.

   e. T–Ocular involvement occurs in 90% of patients at some time in their illness and diplopia is a common symptom at presentation. 15% of patients present only with ocular involvement – 'ocular myasthenia'.

5. a. T–VEPs can be delayed when a demyelinating process affects the optic nerve suggesting a previous episode of optic neuritis which the patient may or may not have been aware of.
   b. F–Fasciculations are a lower and not an upper motor neuron sign and MS nearly always affects only the upper motor neurons in the CNS.
   c. F–During acute attacks, the CSF protein and lymphocyte count can be slightly elevated but an isolated rise in CSF protein has no diagnostic specificity.
   d. T–Intrathecal production of a few clones of IgG is suggestive of MS but it is also seen in other inflammatory processes involving the CNS.
   e. T–The periventricular area, corpus callosum, brainstem, cerebellum and cervical cord are regions often affected by MS plaques which can be visualized on MRI.

6. a. F–Guillain–Barré is a polyneuropathy and therefore a purely lower motor neuron syndrome.
   b. F–MS is a disease of the CNS and therefore is only associated with upper motor neuron signs.
   c. T–The anterior horn cells and the corticospinal tracts at the level of the syrinx may be involved.
   d. T–MND is associated with degeneration of the anterior horn and upper motor neuron cell bodies.
   e. T–Syphilitic taboparesis, B_{12} deficiency and a conus medullaris lesion may also affect both LMN and UMNs. The commonest cause however is a mixture of cervical myelopathy secondary to cervical spondylosis or a stroke and a peripheral neuropathy which are common in the elderly.

7. a. T–Herpes zoster causes facial weakness as part of Ramsey–Hunt syndrome.
   b. F–Motor neuron disease does not tend to cause unilateral lower motor neuron weakness, but can cause wasting in the facial muscles (lower motor neuron) as well as slow movements of the face and brisk facial reflexes (upper motor neuron).
   c. T–Acoustic neuromas occur on the vestibular portion of the VIII nerve which is adjacent to the seventh nerve as it exits the brainstem at the cerebellopontine angle. The facial nerve is often only mildly involved initially but may have to be sacrificed during surgery to remove the tumour.

d. T–A cholesteatoma can infiltrate towards the brainstem and affect the facial nerve.

e. F–It is 'syringobulbia' not 'syringomyelia' that is associated with cranial nerve palsies although syringobulbia is very rare.

8. a. T–Bilateral seventh nerve lesions is one of the commoner neurological presentations of sarcoidosis.

b. T–Facial weakness usually occurs with limb weakness in Guillain–Barré syndrome.

c. T–Chronic stage 3 Lyme disease can be associated with many neurological complications.

d. T–Lymphoma can cause a basal meningitis and affect the cranial nerves.

e. F–A parasagittal meningioma causes damage to the leg area of both primary motor cortices and therefore causes upper motor neuron weakness of the legs.

9. a. F–Headaches of raised intracranial pressure are worse in the morning when the patient has been lying down all night.

b. F–90% of CT scans demonstrate free blood in subarachnoid haemorrhage. Sometimes blood is not seen because the bleed is too small or the scan is performed too late.

c. T–Any disease process which blocks off the ophthalmic artery or its branches, e.g. embolism or in situ thrombosis, can lead to transient loss of vision in one eye or 'amaurosis fugax'.

d. F–The aura associated with migraine may be associated with neurological signs usually for up to 48 hours after the headache including sensory disturbance, dysarthria, visual field loss and occasionally weakness.

e. T–Cluster headaches are about 7 times more common in men than women whereas migraine is more common in women.

10. a. F–Parkinson's disease (PD) is caused by a loss of dopaminergic neurons in the substantia nigra which is in the ventral midbrain.

b. F–Spasticity is a feature of hypertonia associated with upper motor neuron lesions and is not a feature of PD. Rigidity, either lead-pipe or cogwheel, is the form of hypertonia associated with PD.

c. F–Supranuclear vertical gaze palsies in the context of parkinsonism tend to occur with progressive supranuclear palsy.

d. T–Anticholinergic drugs such as trihexyphenydyl (benzhexol) are often better at treating tremor than L-dopa.

e. F–The prime aim of treatment is to replace the loss of dopamine with its precursor L-dopa or stimulate dopamine receptors with dopamine agonists.

11. a. T–Chlorpromazine is a neuroleptic used in the treatment of psychosis and is a dopamine antagonist.

b. F–Trihexyphenydyl (Benzhexol) is used to treat tremor.

c. F–Bromocriptine is a dopamine agonist and was used to treat PD until other agonists were developed.

d. T–Metoclopramide is a dopamine antagonist used as an anti-emetic and can cause several extrapyramidal side-effects including parkinsonism.

e. T–Haloperidol is another dopamine antagonist neuroleptic which can cause parkinsonism.

12. a. T–Rigidity is increased tone caused by extrapyramidal disease such as PD. Tone is increased throughout all movement whereas in spasticity, tone tends to be higher in the flexors in the upper limbs and extensors in the lower limbs.

b. F–Extensor plantar responses are an upper motor neuron and not extra-pyramidal sign.

c. T–A pill rolling tremor is typical of PD which is an extra-pyramidal disease.

d. F–The clasp-knife effect is an upper motor neuron and not extra-pyramidal sign.

e. T–Increased tone with synkinesis, i.e. during movement of the contralateral limb, is typical of extra-pyramidal diseases.

13. a. T–Huntington's disease often starts with subtle cognitive changes which do not present to doctors. This is followed by chorea and dementia in middle age.

b. T–Myoclonus is seen in many diseases including SSPE and sporadic CJD.

c. F–The subthalamic nucleus is involved in controlling contralateral movements.

d. F–Sporadic CJD typically presents with a rapidly progressive dementia and myoclonus, not chorea.

e. T–Alcohol reduces benign essential tremor and is a good predictor of response to a β-blocker.

14. a. T–Horner's syndrome consists of meiosis, ptosis and anhidrosis and is seen in lesions of the sympathetic supply to the eye.

b. F–A Holmes–Adie pupil is usually larger than normal in standard light.

c. T–Tabes dorsalis is associated with an Argyll–Robertson pupil which is small and irregular.

d. F–Optic neuritis can lead to a relative afferent pupillary defect with a sluggish reacting pupil, not small pupils.

e. T–Pilocarpine is a directly acting parasympathomimetic and therefore constricts the pupil.

15. a. T–Papilloedema is caused by raised intracranial pressure which can prevent the retinal veins near the disc from pulsating. The presence of venous pulsation makes raised intracranial pressure highly unlikely.

b. T–Papilloedema is associated with an enlarged blind spot due to swelling of the optic disc.

c. T–The optic disc may be swollen due to causes other than raised CSF pressure, e.g. inflammation of the anterior part of the optic nerve or 'papillitis'.

d. T–Hypocalcaemia can cause a swollen optic disc.

e. T–Guillain–Barré syndrome is associated with a raised CSF protein which may also cause swelling at the optic disc.

16. a. F–Optic neuritis is often painful especially on eye movement.

b. T–The probability of developing MS in the future is lower if there are no white matter lesions on MRI brain and higher if there are typical lesions.

c. T–Vision usually recovers with some residual loss of red–green colour perception and sometimes a reduction in visual acuity.

d. F–The probability of going on to develop MS is approximately 70% not 90%.

e. T–The demyelinating process often leaves a delay in the visual evoked potentials.

17. a. T–Ptosis is common in myotonic dystrophy secondary to the associated myopathy.

b. T–Horner's syndrome is associated with anhydrosis, meiosis and ptosis due to damage of the sympathetic supply to levator palpebrae superioris.

c. F–The abducent nerve has no role in controlling the eyelid.

d. T–The oculomotor nerve carries fibres which innervate levator palpebrae superioris and control voluntary eye closure.

e. T–Neuromuscular junction transmission is affected in myasthenia gravis. Some patients present only with ptosis which is often bilateral. The ptosis often becomes worse with use and throughout the day, i.e. it fatigues.

18. a. T–Berry aneurysms of the posterior communicating artery often cause of painful third nerve palsy.

b. T–Diabetes causes a cranial mononeuropathy usually by microvascular damage to the nerve.

c. F–Motor neuron disease does not cause any ophthalmoplegia.

d. T–Herniation of the uncus through the tentorial hiatus commonly causes third nerve compression due to raised supratentorial pressure.

e. F–A Pancoast tumour often infiltrates the lower part of the brachial plexus and cause weakness and wasting of the hand in association with a Horner's syndrome.

19. a. T–Brown–Séquard syndrome is associated with damage to half the spinal cord. The corticospinal tracts carry fibres from the same side of the body and cross in the inferior part of the brainstem.

b. T–The dorsal columns carry information regarding joint position and vibration and cross in the brainstem.

c. T–MS is the commonest cause. The clinical signs are often only partial as the inflammatory plaque does not exactly involve half of the spinal cord.

d. F–Pain and temperature fibres cross a few levels above the entry into the spinal cord and ascend in the contralateral spinothalamic tract.

e. F–The spinal cord ends at L1/2 and so a central L3 disc will cause a cauda equina syndrome.

20. a. F–In the acute phase of severe damage to the spinal cord, the typical upper motor neuron signs are often not seen for up to several weeks. Usually within 48 hours the reflexes become brisk, the plantar responses become extensor and spasticity slowly develops.

b. T–The loss of reflexes to vessels in the lower limbs often leads to venous pooling and reduced peripheral resistance which can cause hypotension.

c. T–Patients often become constipated and develop urinary retention which manifest as abdominal pain and/or overflow incontinence due to a loss of higher order control.

d. F–The reflexes often absent in acute lesions to the upper motor neuron.

e. T–Reflexes to the GI tract are also affected and gastric dilatation is common.

21. a. F–Motor neuron disease can present with purely upper motor neuron signs and lower motor neuron signs may be present even in the absence of fasciculations, e.g. severe wasting.

b. T–The Betz cells are one of the main types of upper motor neurons in the primary motor cortex.

c. T–EMG often shows denervation within wasted and non–wasted muscles.

d. T–Patients often complain of sensory symptoms and cramps but do not have objective sensory loss.

e. F–Between 5 and 10% of cases are familial.

22. a. T–Severe pain preceding wasting is typical of brachial neuritis.

b. F–Klumpke's paralysis affects mainly the distal upper limb, especially the hand and is caused by lesions to the lower brachial plexus.

c. T–Erb's paralysis affects the upper part of the plexus (C5, 6) and causes the classical 'waiter's tip' posture of the arm with sparing of the hand and forearm.

d. T–The brachial plexus lies in close proximity to the apex of the lung and the first rib and therefore tumours can spread to involve the lower roots including T1 which contains sympathetic fibres to the pupil.

e. T–Brachial neuritis may occur after a viral infection or vaccination.

23. a. T–Diabetes causes microvascular infarcts in individual nerves, e.g. abducent nerve.

b. F–HMSN is a polyneuropathy affecting the longest nerves in the body initially.

c. T–PAN is a vasculitis and can cause infarction of individual nerves.

d. F–Guillain–Barré syndrome is a polyneuropathy.

e. T–Lead poisoning can cause multiple mononeuropathies especially of the radial nerves.

24. a. T–Diabetes can cause polyneuropathies and mononeuropathies.

b. T–Guillain–Barré syndrome is a polyneuropathy but often affects the motor greater than the sensory system and proximal rather than distal muscles.

c. T–Chronic renal failure can cause a polyneuropathy.

d. T–Amyloid often causes a painful polyneuropathy.

e. F–MS is a disease of the central and not the peripheral nervous system.

25. a. T–Diabetes can be associated with a small fibre neuropathy which causes painless ulcers and joint damage.

b. F–Charcot joints are caused by repeated painless trauma to a denervated joint often resulting in bony ankylosis (fusion) of the joint. Denervation makes the joint painless.

c. T–Charcot joints typically used to occur in patients who had tertiary syphilis.

d. T–Syringomyelia initially affects the decussating spinothalamic fibres especially around the upper limbs.

e. F–Charcot joints do not show signs of acute inflammation and are painless but functionally often disabling.

26. a. T–The common peroneal nerve innervates the anterior tibialis which dorsiflexes the ankle and the peronei which evert the foot.

b. T–The common peroneal nerve supplies sensation to the lateral aspect of the leg and dorsum of the foot excluding the lateral border of the foot.

c. F–Plantar flexion is mediated by soleus and gatrocnemius which are innervated by the tibial nerve.

d. T–A common peroneal nerve lesion is a lower motor neuron disorder and therefore wasting of the muscles supplied by the nerve occurs, including the tibialis anterior.

e. F–The ankle reflex involves the tendon of soleus and gatrocnemius and is therefore not involved in common peroneal lesions. Tibial nerve lesions would cause a reduced, not brisk, ankle reflex.

27. a. T–Hyposmia often follows head injuries as the delicate nerve fibres in the first nerve are sheared as they pass through the cribriform plate.

b. F–Migrainous aura may be associated with olfactory hallucinations but not hyposmia.

c. F–Temporal lobe epilepsy may be associated with olfactory hallucinations but not hyposmia.

d. T–Antibiotic therapy can cause a reversible loss of smell.

e. T–Any expanding frontal lesion can affect the first nerve.

28. a. F–Extensor plantar responses reflect upper motor neuron damage and are not involved in the brainstem reflexes. They are often extensor, however, because lesions that cause brainstem death often involve the upper motor neurons as they pass through the brainstem.

b. T–The brainstem reflexes involve all the cranial nerves except I, XI and XII. The corneal reflex involves the fifth (sensory) and seventh (motor).

c. F–Absent tendon reflexes represent a lower motor neuron disorder and are not involved in the brainstem reflexes.

d. F–A flat EEG has many causes including diffuse cerebral cortical damage and deep anaesthesia but this is not a criterion for brainstem death. A patient's brainstem reflexes can be fully intact but the patient may be unconscious and unresponsive because of diffuse cortical damage.

e. T–Doll's eye movements involve proprioceptive information from the neck muscles, visual input (second cranial nerve) and vestibular input (eighth) as well as output to the extraocular muscles (third, fourth and sixth).

29. a. F–Retinitis pigmentosa causes progressive visual loss which usually starts in the peripheral visual field and spreads to involve central vision.

b. T–Amaurosis fugax is transient visual loss caused by a blockage, from whatever cause, of the ophthalmic artery or its branches to the retina. This includes carotid embolism.

c. T–Papilloedema due to raised intracranial pressure can also cause progressive visual loss starting at the periphery but can also cause transient visual loss called 'visual obscurations' which is a warning of rising intracranial pressure.

d. T–Migrainous aura is associated with both positive and negative visual phenomena which usually travels across the vision for up to 1 hour prior to the onset of the headache.

e. T–Closed angle glaucoma can be associated with transient visual loss preceding chronic visual failure.

30. a. T–Homonymous hemianopia arises from lesions in the optic pathway posterior to the optic chiasm.

b. T–as answer 30 (a).

c. F–Lesions in the optic chiasm cause bitemporal hemianopia.

d. F–Lesions in the optic nerve cause visual defects ranging from complete monocular blindness to a central scotoma to impairment of red–green perception only, but not homonymous defects.

e. T–as answer 30 (a).

31. a. T–The frontal lobes represent 50% of the cerebral cortex but patients with frontal lobe disease often have few obvious clinical signs because the bulk of the frontal lobes deal with functions that are difficult to quantify such as personality.

b. T–Patients often find it difficult to inhibit or be aware of socially inappropriate behaviour.

c. T–A region anterior to the primary motor cortex is concerned with coordinating the movements that enable walking.

d. F—The most posterior part of the dominant frontal lobe is the primary motor cortex and anterior to this is Broca's area which is involved in producing speech. If this is damaged, the patient may have an expressive dysphasia. Receptive dysphasia occurs with damage to the posterosuperior part of the dominant temporal lobe or Wernicke's area.

e. T—The grasp reflex is one of the 'primitive reflexes' and is probably one of the most accurate primitive reflexes in localizing pathology to the frontal lobes.

32. a. T—Dysarthria may result from damage to the cerebellum due to its involvement in the control of movements as they occur.

b. F—Broca's area is concerned with language production and causes a dysphasia if damaged.

c. T—The hypoglossal nerve controls tongue movements. The tongue is manipulated to produce different sounds. The facial and vagus nerves are also involved in controlling the muscles involved in articulation.

d. T—The basal ganglia are involved in movement control including the articulating movements of speech.

e. F—The accessory nerve innervates the sternocleidomastoid and trapezius muscles in the neck and is not involved in articulation.

33. a. F—Pseudobulbar palsy refers to a syndrome where both sets of upper motor neurons to cranial nerve nuclei are damaged, i.e. bilateral upper motor neuron lesions. Poliomyelitis only damages the lower motor neurons.

b. T—Motor neuron disease is the commonest cause of a pseudobulbar palsy due to bilateral involvement of the upper motor neurons.

c. F—Huntington's disease is mostly associated with disease of the basal ganglia.

d. F—Occlusion of the anterior cerebral artery causes weakness in the contralateral leg.

e. T—MS is associated with widespread damage to the white matter tracts bilaterally and can therefore damage both sets of corticobulbar fibres leading to pseudobulbar palsy.

34. a. F—Cerebellar disease causes action and not resting tremor.

b. T—Muscle tone is reported as being reduced in cerebellar disease but this is often not a prominent feature.

c. F—Dysphasia is a disorder of the production or understanding of speech and not failure of articulation or dysarthria which is seen with cerebellar disease.

d. T—Titubation (a head tremor) often occurs in cerebellar disorders which have been inherited.

e. T—Patients with cerebellar disease often find it difficult to perform rapid alternating movements.

35. a. T—The cerebellopontine angle lies in close proximity to the fifth, seventh and eighth cranial nerves.

b. F—The facial nerve does supply a very small region of somatic sensation to the outer ear but not the face.

c. T—The cells bodies of the sensory nerves lie in the Gasserian ganglion for the fifth nerve.

d. F—The cells bodies of the sensory nerves lie in the geniculate ganglion for the seventh nerve.

e. T—The first and second divisions of the fifth nerve run in the cavernous sinus.

36. a. T—Syncope is often associated with patients standing whereas seizures can occur in any position.

b. F—Convulsive movements can be seen after a syncopal episode but they are usually not prolonged or rhythmical.

c. T—A bitten tongue or inside cheek usually indicates a seizure.

d. F—Urinary incontinence is often not helpful diagnostically as it occurs in both syncope and seizures.

e. F—Malaise is often more prolonged after a seizure but can also occur after a syncopal attack.

37. a. T—Excess prolonged noise damages the cochlear hair cells.

b. T—Gentamicin can damage both the auditory and vestibular components of the inner ear.

c. T—Ménière's disease is associated with recurrent attacks of vertigo, tinnitus and nausea which eventually results in deafness due to damage within the cochlea.

d. T—An acoustic neuroma develops on the vestibular portion of the eighth nerve and causes progressive unilateral deafness.

e. F—Otosclerosis is associated with reduced compliance in the bony ossicles and is therefore a form of conductive deafness.

38. a. F—Fever can occur but not typically.

b. T—The headache is often described as the worst the patient has ever experienced.

c. T—Meningeal irritation by blood products is one cause of photophobia.

d. T—Kernig's sign is caused by irritation of the meninges due to stretch.

e. T—Neck stiffness is also a feature of meningism.

39. a. F—Slow and writhing movements are called athetosis or dystonic movements.

b. F—Shock-like jerks are myoclonic.

c. T—Chorea is rapid, brief, twitchy movements.

d. F—Restlessness occurs with chronic neuroleptic usage and is called akathisia.

e. F—Rhythmical oscillatory movements are usually associated with tremors.

40. a. F—Tremors at rest are often pathological. A physiological tremor is present on holding a posture or on action.

b. T—Many tremors are worse with anxiety.

c. T—Both physiological and essential tremor can respond to alcohol.

d. T–Both physiological and essential tremor can respond to β-blockers.

e. F–Some tremors, e.g. benign familial tremor, are familial. Physiological tremor occurs in everyone to varying degrees.

41. a. F–The cutaneous reflexes, such as the abdominal reflexes, are reduced in an upper motor neuron syndrome.

b. F–Wasting of muscles, especially individual muscles innervated by one nerve, is a lower motor neuron sign.

c. F–Upper motor neuron weakness causes a pattern of weakness called 'pyramidal', which affects the extensors more than the flexors in the upper limbs and the flexors more than the extensors in the lower limbs. Focal weakness is typical of lower motor neuron syndromes.

d. F–Hypotonia is a lower motor neuron sign although in the initial stages of an upper motor neuron lesion, the tone may be reduced.

e. F–Fatigability is a sign of a problem at the neuromuscular junction, especially myasthenia gravis.

42. a. F–Ipsilateral facial spinothalamic sensory loss not weakness. The facial nucleus and nerve are in the pons.

b. T–Involvement of the sympathetic tract can give rise to a Horner's syndrome.

c. T–The nucleus ambiguus, which is often involved in disorders of the lateral medulla, innervates the soft palate via the vagus nerve.

d. F–The hypoglossal nucleus is a paramedian structure in the medulla and is therefore not affected in a lateral lesion.

e. F–The third nerve nucleus is mostly in the midbrain and is therefore not affected.

43. a. F–A lesion in the pons, not midbrain, can give small 'pin–point' pupils.

b. T–The commonest cause of a small, poorly reactive pupil is old age.

c. T–Horner's syndrome results from damage to the sympathetic fibres to the pupil and includes meiosis.

d. T–Opiates cause meiosis.

e. T–as 43 (a).

44. a. T–The third nerve carries parasympathetic fibres to the constrictor pupillae which constrict the pupil.

b. T–The third nerve innervates levator palpebrae superioris which enable voluntary opening of the eye.

c. T–The third nerve innervates all the extraocular muscles except the lateral rectus and superior oblique and is often associated with diplopia in all positions of gaze.

d. T–Diabetes cause damage to the small blood vessels which supply the third nerve. These vessels can block and cause infarction of the nerve.

e. T–In the context of a midbrain infarct a third nerve palsy can cause contralateral hemiparesis or 'Weber's syndrome'.

45. a. T–INO can be associated with horizontal jerky nystagmus in the 'normal' abducting eye.

b. T–The vestibular nuclei are in the pons and if disrupted can result in nystagmus.

c. T–Patients who are blind can often develop pendular nystagmus as opposed to jerky nystagmus.

d. T–Cerebellar dysfunction can lead to jerky nystagmus.

e. T–Lesions at the foramen magnum classically cause downbeat vertical jerky nystagmus.

46. a. T–The dorsal columns of the spinal cord carry sensory information regarding discriminating sensory experiences such as vibration and joint position sense. These fibres continue into peripheral nerves as 'large fibre' axons and if they or the dorsal columns are damaged then the patient may develop a 'sensory ataxia', i.e. incoordination of movement due to lack of proprioceptive information.

b. F–A scissoring gait is typical of a spastic paraparesis.

c. T–Romberg's test examines the function of the dorsal columns and large sensory fibres.

d. F–Alcohol usually causes a cerebellar and not a sensory ataxia.

e. F–Clonus is seen in lesions of the upper motor neuron.

47. a. F–The deafness is sensorineural and not conductive.

b. F–The ipsilateral corticospinal tracts can be involved which causes contralateral weakness because the lesion is superior to the pyramidal decussation.

c. F–Lower facial weakness is an upper motor neuron deficit. Lesions at the CP angle affect the facial nerve and therefore cause lower motor neuron weakness, i.e. whole of the face.

d. F–Pseudobulbar dysarthria occurs in bilateral upper motor neuron deficits. A lower motor neuron bulbar dysarthria may occur due to involvement of the tenth cranial nerve.

e. F–Vertigo tends to occur with acute rather than slowly progressive lesions of the vestibular system.

48. a. F–Ramsey–Hunt syndrome is caused by reactivation of herpes zoster within the geniculate ganglion of the seventh nerve. The upper motor neurons are not involved. A lower motor neuron seventh nerve lesion occurs.

b. F–Diplopia does not tend to occur as the third, fourth and sixth nerves are spared.

c. T–The nerve to stapedius, which if damaged causes hyperacusis, can be affected.

d. T–The chorda tympani, which provides taste sensation to the anterior two-thirds of the tongue, can be affected.

e. T–A small sensory branch from the seventh nerve supplies a portion of the auditory meatus and painful vesicles can occur.

49.
a. F–The dorsal columns carry information regarding joint position and vibration sense.
b. F–The dorsal columns decussate in the lower, not the upper brainstem.
c. T–B_{12} deficiency can cause subacute combined degeneration of the spinal cord involving the dorsal columns and the corticospinal pathways.
d. T–Romberg's test looks for a sensory ataxia associated with dorsal column damage.
e. T–The spinal cord is mostly supplied by one anterior spinal artery which has poor anastomoses and is vulnerable to occlusion. The posterior cord, including the dorsal columns, is richly supplied by a posterior network of vessels and is therefore rarely involved following anterior spinal artery occlusion.

50.
a. T–In a unilateral spinal cord lesion (Brown–Séquard syndrome) the two modalities of sensation are truly dissociated, with each being affected on opposite sides of the body.
b. T–The dorsal columns are usually spared.
c. F–A radiculopathy results in a dermatomal loss of sensation to all modalities.
d. F–Middle cerebral artery infarcts usually cause cortical sensory loss and often involve all modalities although if only the cortex and not the thalamus is involved, there is often relative sparing of pain and temperature sensation.
e. F–A prolapsed intervertebral disc compressing the spinal cord will cause a myelopathy and affect all modalities.

51.
a. F–Many patients are asymptomatic and only recognize something is wrong when they are examined.
b. T–The most common finding is absent ankle jerks and some distal sensory loss, especially to vibration sense without gross wasting or weakness.
c. F–There is evidence from trials that good blood glucose control slows or even slightly improves diabetic polyneuropathy.
d. F–Diabetic polyneuropathy is common in both type I and II diabetics.
e. T–Small pain-carrying fibres are often affected and therefore trophic ulcers can easily occur especially because microvascular and macrovascular arterial disease leads to ischemia in the feet.

52.
a. T–Painful neuropathies are caused by damage to the small unmyelinated 'slow' fibres in peripheral nerves that carry pain and temperature sensation. Conventional electrophysiology is often normal when patients have an isolated small fibre neuropathy. Patients often can not tolerate even bed sheets touching their legs and may have spontaneous 'dysaesthetic' pain or pain only on touching the affected region. Diabetes is a common cause of small fibre neuropathy.
b. T–Alcohol is also a common cause.
c. T–Cryoglobulinaemia (antibodies that precipitate in the cold), often in association with chronic hepatitis C infection, can cause a very painful neuropathy.
d. F–Charcot–Marie–Tooth disease is usually insidious and painless in onset.
e. T–Amyloid is a rare cause of painful neuropathy.

53.
a. T–It is important to recognize demyelinating neuropathies as some of them are potentially treatable. Guillain–Barré is the most common cause of an acute demyelinating neuropathy. Prolonged and/or severe demyelination may eventually cause axonal loss and therefore the patterns are often mixed.
b. T–Diphtheric polyneuropathy is much more likely than Guillain–Barré to have a bulbar onset and progress to respiratory failure. It often evolves more slowly and can have a biphasic course. Death and long term disability are also more common.
c. F–Vincrinstine and other cytotoxic agents typically cause an axonal neuropathy with a poor prognosis.
d. T–CMT type 1 is the most common demyelinating form of CMT and can be associated with enlarged nerves.
e. T–Paraproteinaemic neuropathies are often associated with IgM paraprotein and may resemble chronic inflammatory demyelinating polyneuropathy.

54.
a. F–Patients with carpal tunnel have parasthaesia confined to the hand but pain often extends right up the arm.
b. T–Any condition associated with an increase in soft tissues or reduction in the size of the carpal tunnel can cause this syndrome. This includes hypothyroidism and acromegaly.
c. T–Many patients may feel some symptomatic relief by maintaining their wrists in a slightly extended and fixed position with splints.
d. F–Elderly patients often do not complain of any sensory symptoms and may present with profound weakness of one or both hands. Most patients have only sensory symptoms.
e. F–The median nerve is affected which primarily supplies the thenar eminence including abductor pollicis brevis. The first dorsal interossei is supplied by the ulnar nerve.

55.
a. F–Patients presenting with a spastic paraparesis have a poorer prognosis.
b. T–Patients who present with sensory symptoms are more likely to have a relatively benign course.
c. T–Patients who present before the age of 45 are more likely to have a relatively benign course.
d. F–Patients presenting with sphincter disturbance, brainstem or cerebellar signs have a poorer prognosis.
e. T–Patients who present with optic neuritis are more likely to have a relatively benign course.

56. a. T Beta-interferon reduces relapses by approximately 30%.
     b. T—Glatiramer acetate also reduces relapses by approximately 30%.
     c. F—Steroids may speed up the recovery of a single episode but do not change the overall prognosis.
     d. F—There is no convincing evidence that methotrexate helps in MS.
     e. F—There is also no convincing evidence that cyclosporine helps in MS.

57. a. F—Total serum copper is reduced in Wilson's disease because of a deficiency in the serum copper binding protein, caeruloplasmin.
     b. T—The reduction in caeruloplasmin leads to an increase in free, unbound copper, which is filtered at the glomerulus and therefore urinary copper levels are raised.
     c. T—Patients often present with bulbar dysfunction and dystonia.
     d. T—Onset is usually between the ages of 10 and 25.
     e. T—Zinc competes for copper absorption in the gut and therefore raises stool levels to help reduce dietary copper intake.

58. a. F—Polymyositis can be associated with an underlying malignancy especially in the elderly but it is relatively uncommon and trends to occur with dermatomyositis.
     b. F—Impairment of swallowing is not uncommon and patients often need parenteral feeding.
     c. F—Patients are often hyperreflexic and not hyporeflexic possibly due to the inflammatory changes in the muscle leading to hyperexcitability.
     d. F—Proximal muscles are more severely impaired in the upper and lower limbs.
     e. T—Polymyositis probably has an autoimmune aetiology and is associated with the development of other organ specific autoimmune diseases.

59. a. T—Ocular involvement in myasthenia gravis occurs in the majority of patients at some time in their disease.
     b. T—Symptoms are often worse towards the end of the day and after exercise and are associated with fatigable weakness of the proximal muscles of the upper limbs and cranial nerves.
     c. F—There are two incidence peaks in myasthenia: old men and young women but any patient of any age or sex can be affected.
     d. T—Patients can develop type II respiratory failure due to neuromuscular weakness surprisingly quickly and measurement of the vital capacity is an absolute requirement in any new patient presenting with bulbar myasthenia.
     e. F—Tendon reflexes should be present unlike Lambert–Eaton myasthenic syndrome where they are often absent at rest.

60. a. T—Patients must have lesions involving both corticospinal ('pyramidal') tracts, between the primary motor cortex down to the spinal cord in order to develop bilateral extensor plantars. Amyotrophic lateral sclerosis is associated with bilateral degeneration of both upper and lower motor neurons.
     b. T—Any cause of myelopathy can cause extensor plantar responses.
     c. T—Multiple sclerosis is associated with diffuse white matter involvement which often involves both corticospinal tracts at some point in their long pathway.
     d. F—Bilateral stokes can cause bilateral extensor responses but not usually a unilateral stroke.
     e. T—B$_{12}$ deficiency can cause demyelination in both corticospinal tracts as well as the dorsal columns.

61. a. F—Visual hallucinations can occur in ocular blindness but they tend not to be well-formed.
     b. T—Visual hallucinations can occur with lesions anywhere within the visual system but formed visual hallucinations of people, animals and objects often occur with diseases affecting the temporal lobes.
     c. T—Psychosis especially depressive psychosis can be associated with morbid formed visual hallucinations.
     d. F—Migrainous aura is associated with fortification spectra and lights that move across the visual field.
     e. T—Drugs/alcohol are often associated with formed visual hallucinations which are typically insects. Acute confusional state from any cause can also cause formed hallucinations.

62. a. T—Fasciculations are spontaneous contractions of a group of muscle fibres innervated by one axon or a 'motor unit'. Fasciculations tend to occur when the axons are damaged or the muscle becomes hyperexcitable, e.g. thyrotoxicosis.
     b. F—Processes that affect the central nervous system (unless it involves the anterior horn cell) or muscle do not tend to cause fasciculations.
     c. T—see 62 (a).
     d. F—Parkinson's disease affects the basal ganglia in the central nervous system.
     e. T—Syringomyelia can affect the anterior horn cells and therefore cause fasciculations.

63. a. T—Any process that causes a blockage in the passage of CSF between the choroid plexus and arachnoid granulations can cause hydrocephalus.
     b. T—Basal meningitis caused by *Mycobacterium tuberculosis* and some fungi and bacteria can block the passage of CSF around the fourth ventricle and basal cisterns.
     c. F—Viral meningitis does not tend to block the passage of CSF.
     d. F—Idiopathic or 'benign' intracranial hypertension causes an increase in total brain water which increases intracranial pressure but does not cause hydrocephalus.
     e. T—Subarachnoid haemorrhage can cause blockage of the arachnoid granulations or basal cisterns to cause hydrocephalus.

64. a. T–Petit mal is a form of generalized epilepsy that occurs in children and often resolves spontaneously with age. Children of normal intelligence can underperform at school when the absence episodes become frequent.
    b. F–The seizures tend to be short (seconds) and are not associated with prolonged post-ictal confusion.
    c. F–The seizures tend to be relatively easily treatable.
    d. F–There is no association with previous head injury unlike grand mal seizures.
    e. F–There is no association with an underlying structural lesion.

65. a. T–Berry aneurysms are often multiple in 15% of cases.
    b. T–Aneurysms of the posterior communicating artery can cause pain in the eye and an associated third nerve palsy.
    c. T–Intracerebral and intraventricular haemorrhage are relatively common with MCA aneurysms.
    d. T–aneurysms are less common in the posterior circulation than the anterior circulation but are more likely to rupture.
    e. T–Blood can block the passage of CSF through the arachnoid granulations and basal cisterns causing hydrocephalus.

66. a. F–Sodium valproate has a high incidence of teratogenicity and should be avoided in women of child-bearing age.
    b. T–Weight gain is a common problem.
    c. T–A coarse tremor can develop with valproate.
    d. F–Phenytoin and carbamazepine can cause hirsuitism but valproate causes hair loss.
    e. T–It is usually the drug of choice in primary generalized epilepsy.

67. a. T–Patients with midline cerebellar disease may initially appear to have a paucity of cerebellar signs but on careful examination they often have difficulty in walking due to truncal imbalance.
    b. T–An acute cerebellar syndrome is of concern as it may be due to a space occupying lesion in the posterior fossa which can cause brainstem compression and death. A CT scan should therefore be performed as an emergency in patients with an acute cerebellar syndrome.
    c. F–Alzheimer's disease does not tend to affect the cerebellum but other neurodegenerative diseases such as multiple system atrophy can cause a severe cerebellar syndrome.
    d. T–Anticonvulsants, especially toxic levels of phenytoin can cause irreversible damage to the cerebellum.
    e. T–Small cell lung cancer as well as gynaecological malignancies can cause a severe cerebellar syndrome often in association with anti Yo antibodies.

68. a. T–Compression of the L4 nerve root causes pain into the thigh and medial leg rather than L5 and S1 lesions where the pain can extend into the foot.
    b. T–The knee jerk is supplied by L3 and L4 and can therefore be reduced.
    c. F–Foot drop is associated with lesions of the common peroneal nerve which is innervated by L4 and partly L5 and therefore L4 root lesions can mimic the motor signs of a common peroneal nerve palsy but the sensory deficit is very different.
    d. T–Degenerative disc disease is a common cause of lumbar radiculopathies.
    e. F–The hamstrings are supplied by the sciatic nerve from L5/S1 roots. Tibialis anterior may be wasted with L4 root lesions.

69. a. T–Cervical spondylosis can cause compression either of the cervical spinal cord causing a cervical myelopathy or the cervical roots causing lower motor neuron signs in the arms.
    b. T–Pain is often worse at night.
    c. T–In the absence of neurological signs and compressive disc lesion a soft collar can be used in combination with analgesia.
    d. F–Most patients do not have neurological signs but have neck pain.
    e. F–Neck traction is contraindicated as it can lead to destabilization of the neck and subsequent cord compression.

70. a. F–Temporal arteritis is five times more common in women and rarely affects patients below 50.
    b. T–It can be associated with a systemic inflammatory disease called polymyalgia rheumatica in up to 20% of cases.
    c. T–Ischaemia of the scalp and muscles of mastication can cause jaw claudication and scalp tenderness.
    d. F–Up to 30% of biopsy-proven temporal arteritis have a normal ESR.
    e. T–If the history is highly compatible with the diagnosis, steroids should be commenced and an ESR and temporal artery biopsy then commenced.

71. a. F–The third nerve carries parasympathetic fibres to the pupil.
    b. T–Raised intracranial pressure may cause downward displacement of the brain and pressure on the fragile sixth nerve leading to a sixth nerve palsy. This is said to be a 'false localizing sign' because the anatomical site of the sign is distant to the site of the initial lesion.
    c. T–A sixth nerve palsy may be seen in idiopathic intracranial hypertension as a false localizing sign.
    d. T–The sixth or abducent nerve travels from the brainstem through the cavernous sinus and superior orbital fissure into the orbit.
    e. F–The sixth nerve supplies the lateral rectus muscle which abducts the eye.

72. a. T–The dominant cerebral cortex is on the left in the majority of right-handed people and is specifically involved in reading, maths, writing and language.

b. F–Apraxias involving visuospatial tasks, e.g. dressing and drawing shapes, is a symptom of dysfunction in the non–dominant right hemisphere.

c. T–as 72 (a).

d. T–More subtle functions of the dominant parietal lobe include naming fingers and left–right discrimination.

e. T–as 72 (d).

73. a. T–The radial nerve is the main branch of the posterior cord of the brachial plexus.

b. T–It supplies most of the muscles on the extensor surface of the arm and forearm including brachioradialis.

c. T–It can be easily damaged as it runs in the bony spiral groove of the humerus especially by pressure from misplaced crutches and by leaning an arm over a chair.

d. F–Most of the sensation to the hand is supplied by the ulnar and median nerves but the 'anatomical snuff box' on the dorsum of the hand is usually numb if the radial nerve is damaged.

e. T–as 73 (b).

74. a. T–Chronic papilloedema can cause damage to the optic nerve which usually involves the fibres that supply peripheral vision initially but can extend to involve all fibres.

b. T–It is often seen in idiopathic intracranial hypertension.

c. T–Papillitis caused by optic nerve inflammation can resemble the swollen disc seen in raised intracranial pressure. Papillitis is often associated with pain on eye movement, a reduction in visual acuity and impaired red–green colour vision.

d. T–A high CSF protein, as seen in Guillain–Barré, can cause papilloedema probably through a local effect on the flow of CSF.

e. F–It can also be associated with transient blurring or loss of vision or 'visual obscurations'.

75. a. T–Normal pressure hydrocephalus is seen in elderly patients who have hydrocephalus but with normal CSF pressures. It is associated with urinary incontinence, gait apraxia and dementia.

b. F–The ventricles are enlarged but patients do not have papilloedema.

c. T–as 75 (a).

d. T–as 75 (a).

e. F–The ventricles are enlarged out of proportion to any coincidental atrophy. Therapeutic trial of draining at least 30 mL of CSF can often improve function and help diagnosis, but a ventriculoperitoneal shunt may need to be inserted if the history and examination are consistent with the diagnosis in spite of an absence of effect following LP drainage.

76. a. T–Loss of vision in one eye associated with pain on moving the eye is typical of optic neuritis and is a common initial presentation.

b. T–A spastic paraparesis is common in MS.

c. F–Hemianopias are surprisingly uncommon in MS.

d. T–Recurrent sensory symptoms are very common in MS and often cause a lot of pain and distress to patients. The symptoms may be highly complex such as water dripping down the leg and a tight band.

e. F–Seizures are relatively uncommon in MS but do occur.

77. a. T–Coughing, sneezing and bending over all increase intracranial pressure and worsen the headache.

b. F–Fortification spectra are typical of aura associated with migraine headache.

c. F–Patients with raised pressure often have a dull progressive, headache.

d. T–The headache is worse on waking in the morning and on prolonged lying flat and better with standing in contrast to low-pressure headaches seen after LP.

e. T–Nausea and subsequently vomiting are common symptoms of increasing intracranial pressure.

78. a. F–The median nerve supplies most of the muscles in the forearm.

b. T–The ulnar nerve supplies all the intrinsic hand muscles, including all the interossei, except the lateral two lumbricals, abductor pollicis brevis, opponens pollicis and flexor pollicis brevis which are supplied by the median nerve.

c. F–The hypothenar eminence is supplied by the ulnar nerve – the median nerve supplies most of the thenar eminence.

d. F–The radial does not supply any of the intrinsic hand muscles.

e. T–The intrinsic hand muscles are mostly supplied by T1 but C8 has a smaller contribution.

79. a. F–Stroke does not typically cause a very high CSF protein but it is often slightly raised.

b. T–Guillain–Barré and CIDP cause inflammatory neuropathies with proximal root involvement within the dura. This can cause an associated high CSF protein without many inflammatory cells.

c. T–Neoplastic involvement of the CSF is typically associated with extremely high CSF protein values, low glucose ratios and an inflammatory cellular reaction. A large-volume fresh cytology sample should be examined on at least two occasions.

d. T–Tuberculous and fungal meningitis may also cause a raised CSF protein, with a low glucose ratio and inflammatory cells.

e. F–Viral meningitis rarely causes a highly elevated CSF protein.

80. a. T–Temporal lobe epilepsy can be associated with formed visual, olfactory and gustatory hallucinations.

b. T–Patients do not fall to the ground but can wander or stare into space.

c. F–Patients who shake only the upper limbs and have repetitive conjugate eye movements often have pseudoseizures but these can reflect seizures in the frontal lobes and be difficult to diagnose.

d. F–as 80 (c).

e. T–Movements of the tongue and mouth including 'lip-smacking' is often associated with temporal lobe seizures.

81. a. T–Patients often have dyskinesias including chorea of the face, tongue and neck.

b. T–Dyskinesias are seen as a late complication of levodopa-treated Parkinson's disease.

c. T–Neuroleptic treatment characteristically causes dyskinesias and dystonia around the mouth and tongue.

d. F–Motor neuron disease causes a small, wasted, fibrillating, slow-moving tongue and a staring, expressionless face.

e. T–Blepharospasm is a focal dystonia of the muscles around the eyes causing repetitive opening/closing. Any disorder of the basal ganglia can cause abnormal movements in the face or tongue.

82. a. T–SIADH can cause hyponatraemia which can cause seizures and other neurological complications especially when rapid.

b. T–Cerebral venous thrombosis causes venous ischaemia and infarction of the brain which can lead to seizures.

c. T–The rapid withdrawal of barbiturates such as phenobarbitone, is especially likely to cause seizures.

d. T–Most space occupying lesions in the cranium, including subdural haematomas, can cause seizures.

e. T–The tricylic antidepressants are especially associated with causing seizures in predisposed individuals. Lithium toxicity can also cause seizures.

83. a. F–The raised pressure in subarachnoid haemorrhage (SAH) is usually communicating and it is therefore safe and sometimes necessary to perform a LP to aid diagnosis.

b. F–Patients often become hypertensive and only when it becomes malignant with signs of end-organ damage or greater than 240 mmHg systolic should hypertension be treated.

c. F–Berry aneurysms are more common in the anterior circulation but are at a greater risk of rupturing in the posterior circulation.

d. F–Approximately 90% of SAH can be detected on CT.

e. T–The highest incidence of rebleeding is within the first two weeks and therefore many surgeons and radiologists advocate early treatment of aneurysms.

84. a. F–Patients who are acutely confused present with disorientation, but patients are often initially quite well-orientated in Alzheimer's disease. Later in the disease, patients become disorientated.

b. T–Patients are often unaware of the degree of memory loss but can retain some insight into their illness in the initial stages of the disease.

c. F–Alzheimer's disease typically involves the parietal (including apraxias and aphasias) and temporal lobes initially and therefore spares the frontal lobes at presentation.

d. T–Alzheimer's disease typically involves the parietal lobes causing dyspraxia and dysphasia as well as the temporal lobes in the initial stages. The disease becomes more global as it progresses.

e. T–Patients can be treated symptomatically by increasing brain acetylcholine levels but this does not treat the underlying neurodegenerative process.

85. a. T–By definition, idiopathic trigeminal neuralgia should not be associated with neurological signs.

b. F–It is usually unilateral – if bilateral then other conditions which affect the trigeminal nuclei and exit zone of the nerve need to be considered, e.g. MS.

c. T–It usually responds better to carbamazepine and lamotrigine but less well to other anticonvulsants such as phenytoin, gabapentin and sodium valproate.

d. F–The pain is often paroxysmal and is triggered by touching particular parts of the face and mouth, e.g. during chewing and shaving.

e. T–The pain is severely debilitating and can make patients very depressed and lose weight.

86. a. T–Autonomic dysfunction causes with postural hypotension, cardiac arrhythmias, gastric stasis, paralytic ileus, anhydrosis and pupillary abnormalities. It usually presents as postural hypotension or erectile dysfunction in diabetes.

b. F–If patients present with parkinsonism and severe autonomic failure then the diagnosis of idiopathic Parkinson's disease is highly unlikely and multi system atrophy is more probable.

c. T–Small cell lung cancer can be associated with a variety of paraneoplastic syndromes including an autonomic neuropathy.

d. T–It can be life-threatening and is a major cause of mortality in Guillain–Barré syndrome.

e. F–Lambert–Eaton myasthenic syndrome not myasthenia gravis is associated with an autonomic neuropathy.

87. a. T–The post-LP low-pressure headache is probably related to ongoing CSF leakage after the needle has been removed and therefore larger gauge needles which make a bigger hole in the dura and repeated unsuccessful attempts are the primary cause.

b. T–The headache usually resolves within 48 hours although it may continue for several weeks.

c. T–Patients may develop slight neck stiffness, dizziness and nausea, especially on standing, and some patients vomit.

d. T–A low pressure headache is worse on standing and is mostly relieved on lying flat.

e. F–Up to 500 mL of CSF are produced by the choroid plexus daily and therefore draining 10 mL of CSF will not cause the headache.

88. a. T–The chronic form of tension-type headache occurs most days in the month unlike migraine which tends to occur periodically.

b. T–Tension-type headache is mild to moderate severity. It is rarely severe enough to warrant admission to casualty unlike migraine or other more malignant headaches, e.g. subarachnoid haemorrhage.

c. T–Patients are often able to continue working through the headache unlike migraine.

d. T–Difficulty sleeping is a common problem with tension-type headache and tricyclic agents such as amitryptiline often have beneficial sedative effects.

e. T–A tight band-like pain around the head is the typical character of the headache.

89. a. F–Diplopia can be caused by TIAs involving the pons and midbrain supplied by the posterior circulation.

b. F–Weakness of all four limbs or 'tetraparesis' is usually caused by TIAs involving the basilar artery which supplies both corticospinal tracts in the brainstem.

c. T–Amaurosis fugax is due to blockage in the ophthalmic artery or its branches. It is especially common in the elderly and may be associated with temporal arteritis.

d. T–Dysphasia results from lesions to the dominant frontal, parietal or temporal lobes which are supplied by the middle cerebral artery.

e. F–Vertigo can be caused by lesions to the pons or cerebellum supplied by the posterior circulation.

90. a. F–Myasthenia gravis (MG) is associated with antibodies to the acetylcholine receptor.

b. T–Steroids may temporarily worsen the symptoms but are often necessary to control the disease.

c. F–The removal of thymomas is to remove the potential risk of malignant transformation and not to improve the underlying disease.

d. T–Edrophonium or 'tensilon' can be used as a short-acting acetylcholinesterase inhibitor which increases the amount of acetylcholine at the post-synaptic membrane and improves symptoms temporarily in MG.

e. F–Weakness usually is fatigable and affects the proximal upper limbs as well as the extraocular muscles, neck flexion, swallowing and speech.

91. a. F–A low CSF glucose occurs in conditions where there are cells or organisms in CSF that consume large quantities of glucose as part of their metabolism such as bacteria, fungi, TB, and neoplastic cells but not viruses or inflammation although very high white cell counts and viral loads in the CSF can reduce the CSF glucose.

Alzheimer's disease is a neurodegenerative disorder and does not cause a low CSF glucose.

b. F–Ischaemic stroke can be associated with a mildly raised CSF protein but not a low glucose.

c. F–During acute attacks of multiple sclerosis the lymphocyte count and protein can be raised but this is not associated with a low glucose.

d. F–Guillain–Barré is typically associated with a high CSF protein in isolation due to inflammation of the proximal nerve roots.

e. T–Neurosarcoidosis can cause a raised CSF protein, cell count and ACE, and in 20% a low glucose.

92. a. F–Hemiparesis is the commonest syndrome resulting from a lacunar infarct of the posterior limb of the internal capsule.

b. T–The frontal lobes can often be affected by strokes that are clinically silent.

c. F–Incongruous, i.e. not the same amount of visual field affected, hemianopias typically occur following damage to the optic tract.

d. T–Seizures are relatively common in the acute phase of haemorrhagic stroke whereas they are not common in the acute phase of ischaemic stroke.

e. F–Gerstmann's syndrome is often caused by a stroke involving the dominant parietal lobe and results in finger agnosia, left/right discrimination difficulties, dysgraphia and dyscalculia.

93. a. F–CSF is produced from the choroid plexus which is mostly in the lateral, third and fourth ventricles.

b. T–CSF circulates through the ventricular system and then through foramina in the roof of the fourth ventricle to the subarachnoid space. The CSF is then absorbed via the arachnoid granulations into the sagittal sinus.

c. T–CSF is produced at a rate of up to 500 mL/day from the choroid plexus.

d. T–Following a lumbar puncture in the lateral decubitus position, the opening CSF pressure is usually less than 15 cmH$_2$O but in anxious patients can be higher and still be normal. Pressures above 30 represent significant intracranial hypertension.

e. T–The CSF may contain up to 4 lymphocytes but should not contain any neutrophils or 'polymorphs'.

94. a. T–Myotonia typically is worse in the cold.

b. T–Myotonic dystrophy (MD) is one a several neurodegenerative conditions that has been found to be associated with an expanded trinucleotide repeat sequence which demonstrate 'anticipation'. This is where the disease is more severely inherited from the father than the mother due to greater trinucleotide expansion in sperm than eggs. The disease therefore occurs earlier in life and/or more severely in the next generation. In MD, the trinucleotides are the bases 'CTG' and the disease is worse when inherited from the mother.

c. T–Myotonia is a failure or slowing of relaxation following contraction of a muscle and patients not only have a myopathy with myotonia but also dysfunction of other organ systems, e.g. cardiac conduction defects and diabetes.

d. T–Frontal balding and sterility are common especially in male patients.

e. T–Patients with myotonia are often difficult to anaesthetize due to affects on the respiratory muscles.

95. a. T–It usually causes a severe and progressive myopathy resulting in death by the third decade.

b. T–The creatine kinase (CK) is often in the 1000s due to death of muscle fibres.

c. T–It causes a severe proximal symmetrical myopathy resulting in the patient having to use their arms to push on their thighs in order to stand from sitting on the ground. This is called 'Gower's sign'.

d. T–Duchenne muscular dystrophy is an X-linked disorder that affects a protein called dystrophin.

e. T–It tends to spare the muscles in the head and neck as well as the hands.

96. a. T–Benign essential tremor is often seen in patients in their middle age and usually affects the upper limbs, sometimes the head and neck and spares the lower limbs. It often improves with alcohol.

b. F–It is a course 6–8 Hz tremor which is worse on holding a posture or performing specific actions, typically on trying to drink from a cup. It often improves at rest.

c. T–The tremor may respond to propranolol, primidone, clonazepam or anticholinergic drugs.

d. T–It may be familial and several genes have been associated with the condition.

e. T–It may be only socially embarrassing but in some patients it may cause severe functional disability.

97. a. F–A number of conditions including polycystic kidney disease and coarctation of the aorta are associated with subarachnoid not primary intracerebral haemorrhage.

b. F–Meningism only occurs if the haemorrhage extends into the subarachnoid space.

c. F–A cerebellar haemorrhage in the posterior fossa is a neurological emergency and if suspected clinically a CT head should be performed as the patient can rapidly deteriorate because of the proximity of the brainstem.

d. F–Patients who are hypertensive tend to have subcortical haemorrhages in the basal ganglia, internal capsule or thalamus.

e. F–Surgical evacuation is only really indicated if the haemorrhage is in the posterior fossa or is on the convexity of the brain and is having a pressure effect.

98. a. F–Herpes meningitis is associated with a low CSF glucose in only 20% of patients.

b. F–The CSF is very rarely normal.

c. T–The virus has a predilection for the temporal lobes and may be associated with haemorrhagic changes within the temporal lobes.

d. T–There may be slow waves or epileptiform discharges over the temporal regions on the EEG.

e. T–Some patients present with severe memory disturbance or personality change and have little clinical evidence of meningitis.

99. a. F–Prion diseases are caused by a novel infectious agent called a 'prion'; prions are abnormally conformed proteins that do not contain RNA or DNA.

b. F–The infectious particle is highly resistant to all usual methods of sterilization and requires special techniques to inactivate it. Surgical instruments used on an infected patient should therefore not be used again.

c. T–There are several rare forms of inherited prion disease but most are sporadic with no known cause.

d. F–Recently, there has been a link between a prion disease that affects cows or 'bovine spongiform encephalopathy' and a new variant of a human form of prion disease called 'new variant Creutzfeldt–Jakob disease' or 'nvCJD'. This form is slower in onset than the sporadic form and often presents with psychiatric features.

e. T–MRI may show characteristic changes in both new variant and sporadic CJD.

100. a. T–Migraine with aura is often associated with a positive family history and recently several genes have been described.

b. T–The aura of migraine may be similar to a TIA but TIAs usually come on within seconds where as aura symptoms progress and spread over 20–60 minutes.

c. F–The 'triptan' group of drugs including sumatriptan are used for the acute phase of migraine treatment and not prophylaxis.

d. F–EEGs performed during an attack may be non–specifically abnormal.

e. F–Patients who are agitated and cannot sleep often have tension-type headache, whereas migraines often are relieved by sleeping.

1. a. Right optic nerve.
   b. Optic chiasm.
   c. Right optic tract, radiation or occipital cortex.
   d. Left temporal lobe (optic radiations).
   e. Right parietal lobe (optic radiations).
   f. Left calcarine cortex (occipital lobe).

2. The disc is pale and clearly delineated. Causes include:

   - Multiple sclerosis – following an episode of optic neuritis.
   - Compression of the optic nerve or following papilloedema, e.g. by a tumour or aneurysm.
   - Anterior ischaemic optic neuropathy.
   - Vitamin B_{12} deficiency.
   - Tobacco–alcohol amblyopia.
   - Friedreich's ataxia.
   - Leber's optic neuropathy.

3. Features include unilateral ptosis, dilated pupil, and deviation of the eye inferolaterally. However, in diabetes and other non-compressive causes, there may be sparing of the pupil (i.e. pupil not dilated). Causes comprise:

   - Aneurysm of the posterior communicating artery.
   - Herniation of the uncus of the temporal lobe.
   - Mononeuritis multiplex – especially that due to diabetes.

4. Causes and associated features are as follows:

   - Third nerve palsy – dilated pupil, deviation of the eye inferolaterally.
   - Horner's syndrome – small pupil (miosis), ± decreased sweating ipsilaterally.
   - Myasthenia gravis – fatiguable weakness worse at the end of the day, ± ophthalmoplegia with diplopia (may be variable or fixed), ± swallowing difficulties, ± respiratory difficulties.
   - Myotonic dystrophy (dystrophia myotonica) – ptosis (usually bilateral and symmetrical), frontal balding, myopathic facies, myotonia (e.g. difficulty releasing grip), ± cataracts, ± distal limb wasting and weakness (worse in cold), ± diabetes.

5. In Bell's palsy, there is a lower motor neuron distribution of facial weakness, with ipsilateral weakness of the upper and lower parts of the face. Weakness of eye closure and lifting eyebrows, in this context, as well as weakness of the mouth, indicates a lower motor neuron lesion. There may be pain behind the ear just prior to the onset of the facial weakness.

   In upper motor neuron weakness, the facial weakness is confined to the lower part of the face because of bilateral cortical innervation of the upper face. There may also be an accompanying hemiparesis and hemisensory loss. All the signs are contralateral to the lesion.

   In a cerebellopontine angle tumour, as well as a lower motor neuron distribution of facial weakness, one would expect damage to the eighth (vestibulocochlear) and fifth (trigeminal) cranial nerves ± the cerebellar connections (i.e. ipsilateral reduction in hearing, tinnitus, reduced facial sensation (including the corneal response) ± poor coordination in the limbs on the same side.

6. Features of an upper motor neuron lesion include:

   - Increased tone (spasticity).
   - No significant wasting.
   - No fasciculations.
   - Weakness in a pyramidal distribution (extensors weaker in the arms, and flexors weaker in the legs).
   - Brisk reflexes.
   - Extensor plantars.

   Features of a lower motor neuron lesion include:

   - Reduced tone (flaccidity).
   - Wasting of muscles.
   - ± Fasciculations.
   - Weakness not pyramidal in distribution.
   - Reduced or absent reflexes.
   - Flexor plantar response.

   The lesion in an upper motor neuron defect can be anywhere from the pyramidal cells in the motor cortex, through the corticospinal tracts in the brainstem and spinal cord, down to, but not including, the anterior horn cells. The lesion in a lower motor neuron defect can be anywhere from the anterior horn cell, through the spinal roots (radiculopathy), to the peripheral nerve.

7. The Brown–Séquard syndrome results from a strictly unilateral lesion of the spinal cord. The most common cause is a focal plaque of multiple sclerosis. The clinical picture consists of the following features:

   - Ipsilateral spastic weak leg with brisk reflexes and extensor plantar response (corticospinal tract).
   - Ipsilateral loss of joint-position sense and vibration (dorsal columns).
   - Contralateral loss of pain and temperature sensation (spinothalamic tract).

8. Touch can divided into accurate localization of light touch, two-point discrimination, and poorly localized touch. Accurate touch and two-point discrimination are carried in the dorsal columns, which decussate in the medulla. Poorly localized touch is conveyed in the ventral spinothalamic tract and crosses close

to the point of entry. (Because touch is conveyed in two pathways, it is unusual for gross touch to be completely abolished in cord disease, apart from complete transection.)

Pain and temperature are conveyed in the lateral spinothalmic tract. The afferents enter the spinal cord, then ascend two or three segments before they cross the cord anterior to the central canal.

Joint-position sense and vibration are carried in the dorsal columns and decussate in the medulla.

9. Absent ankle jerks with extensor plantars can be caused by:
   - Spondylotic cervical myelopathy and mild polyneuropathy in elderly people.
   - Subacute combined degeneration of the cord (vitamin B$_{12}$ deficiency).
   - Motor neuron disease.
   - Friedreich's ataxia.
   - Tabes dorsalis (syphilis).
   - Conus medullaris lesion.

10. Types of neuropathy that can occur as a complicating feature of diabetes mellitus include:
   - Distal symmetrical polyneuropathy.
   - Proximal asymmetrical motor neuropathy (diabetic amyotrophy).
   - Mononeuritis multiplex.
   - Entrapment neuropathies.
   - Autonomic neuropathy.

11. The following features may be present in a patient with a cerebellar syndrome:
   - Hypotonia.
   - A wide-based gait with difficulty walking heel-to-toe.
   - Ataxia of the limbs manifested by an intention tremor, finger–nose incoordination, dysdiadokokinesis, and heel–shin incoordination.
   - Pendular knee jerks.
   - Disordered eye movements with horizontal nystagmus, jerky pusuits, and overshooting of eye movements on attempted fixation.
   - Dysarthria.
   - Titubation.

Causes include:
   - Multiple sclerosis.
   - Lesions of the posterior fossa – abscess, tumours, trauma, infarction.
   - Toxins – alcohol, anticonvulsants.
   - Inherited ataxias – Friedreich's ataxia.
   - Viral encephalitis.
   - Developmental deformities – Arnold–Chiari malformation.
   - Metabolic – myxoedema.

12. The clinical features of a Horner's syndrome are:
   - Pupil constriction.
   - Ptosis (usually partial).

   - Ipsilateral anhidrosis of the face (lesion proximal to the carotid bifurcation) or medial side of the forehead only (distal to the bifurcation).
   - Apparent enophthalmos.

Interruption of the sympathetic pathway gives rise to a Horner's syndrome. The sympathetic fibres arise in the hypothalamus and descend uncrossed to the midbrain, pons, medulla, and lower cervical/upper thoracic spinal cord where they synapse with the lateral horn cells. From the latter arise preganglionic fibres, which exit the cord in the anterior roots of C8 and T1 and pass through the stellate ganglion to synapse in the superior cervical ganglion.

Postganglionic fibres course along the internal carotid artery through the cavernous sinus to the long ciliary nerve, which innervates the dilator pupillae. Some fibres follow the external carotid artery and innervate Müller's muscle of the eyelid, the blood vessels, and sweat glands of the face (apart from fibres responsible for sweating of the medial aspect of the forehead, which follow the internal carotid artery).

A Horner's syndrome therefore occurs from a lesion at the following levels:
   - Brainstem – multiple sclerosis, infarction, tumour.
   - Cervical cord – syringomyelia, tumour, e.g. ependymoma.
   - T1 root – Pancoast tumour, cervical rib.
   - Sympathetic chain – neoplastic infiltration or surgical damage in the neck involving the larynx, pharynx, thyroid; carotid artery lesions such as a dissection or trauma.

13. The clinical signs associated with a lesion of the cerebellopontine angle are:
   - Damage of the ipsilateral fifth, seventh, and eighth cranial nerves; late involvement of the sixth, ninth, and tenth nerves.
   - Ipsilateral cerebellar signs in the limbs.
   - Contralateral 'pyramidal' weakness, if the brainstem is compressed.

The following causes should be considered:
   - Acoustic neuroma.
   - Meningioma.
   - Metastatic deposits.
   - Granulomatous disease – tuberculosis, sarcoidosis.

14. The clinical features of Parkinson's disease include:
   - A resting, coarse, 'pill-rolling' tremor – this may be present in the upper and lower limb. In idiopathic Parkinson's disease, the tremor is usually asymmetrical.
   - Rigidity in the limbs and axially – there is increased tone equally in the extensor and flexor muscles of the limbs throughout the range of movement.
   - Bradykinesia – of the limbs, immobile facies, swallowing difficulties may develop.
   - Hypophonic (quiet) speech, which may later become dysarthric.

- Characteristic stooped posture.
- Shuffling, 'festinant gait', loss of arm swing.
- Difficulty initiating and alternating movements.
- Dementia may occur at a later stage of the disease.

15. The speech of a 'pseudobulbar palsy' is slow, indistinct, and strained. On examination, the tongue may appear contracted with limited protrusion. Look for upper motor neuron signs – spasticity in the limbs, brisk reflexes, in particular a brisk jaw jerk, and extensor plantar responses. Additionally, there may be emotional lability. A bilateral lesion is required to produce the dysarthria.

    Conditions in which this may occur include:
    - Multiple sclerosis.
    - Motor neuron disease.
    - Bilateral subcortical ischaemic lesions.

16. Lhermitte's phenomenon – an 'electric' or tingling feeling passing down the spine (less commonly into the lower extremities) on neck flexion. It is a sign of pathology of the cervical spinal cord.

    Causes include:
    - Multiple sclerosis – the most common cause.
    - Cervical spondylosis.
    - Tumour of the cervical spinal cord.
    - Subacute combined degeneration of the cord.

17. There is wasting of the anterior and peroneal group of muscles and weakness of dorsiflexion and eversion of the foot. As a result, there is 'foot drop' and a steppage gait. Sensation is diminished on the anterolateral border of the shin and dorsum of the foot.

    Damage to the nerve usually occurs at the head of the fibula (e.g. due to minor trauma, fracture, compression by a tight plaster cast or bandage, prolonged squatting, or leg crossing).

18. Lateral medullary syndrome results from infarction of a small region of the lateral medulla, classically due to occlusion of the posterior inferior cerebellar artery. The clinical features are:
    - Sudden-onset vertigo, nausea, vomiting (vestibular nuclei).
    - Ipsilateral diminished facial pain and temperature (descending tract and nucleus of the fifth nerve), diplopia (sixth nerve), palatal paralysis and diminished gag reflex (there may also be dysphagia and hoarseness from involvement of the ninth and tenth nerves), cerebellar signs (cerebellum and its connections), Horner's syndrome (descending sympathetic tract).
    - Contralateral diminished pain and temperature sensation of the trunk and limbs (spinothalamic tract).

19. The increased tone of an upper motor neuron lesion is more marked in the flexors of the arms and extensors of the legs. This is more obvious early during the movement, the so-called 'clasp-knife' phenomenon. Clonus may be elicited at the ankles or patellae; the reflexes are brisk and the plantar responses extensor. One of the most common signs is of a 'spastic catch'. This can occur at most joints, but is typically seen on supination at the elbow.

    The increased tone of an extrapyramidal syndrome is equal in the flexors and extensors with the increased tone apparent throughout the range of movement. There is no clonus, the reflexes are normal, and the plantar responses flexor.

20. Features of Wernicke's encephalopathy include ocular abnormalities as follows:
    - Nystagmus – vertical and horizontal.
    - Abnormal eye movements – most commonly bilateral lateral rectus muscle weakness. Abnormalities of horizontal gaze are more common than of vertical gaze. Complete loss of ocular movement in a direction can occur.
    - Pupillary abnormalities – the pupils are usually spared. However, in advanced stages, the pupils may become miotic and non-reacting.

    Other features are:
    - Ataxia – the gait is broad based and there is ataxia of the limbs, particularly of the lower limbs on heel–shin testing. In milder cases the ataxia may only be manifest on tandem walking, which is carried out with difficulty.
    - Disturbance of consciousness and mental state – the patient may present with a confusional state. There is apathy, disorientation, and agitation. Memory and learning are impaired. The patient may progress from this condition to a state of stupor, coma, and death within 1–2 weeks if untreated or they may survive with the persistent severe amnesia of Korsakoff's syndrome.

    Wernicke's disease is due to a deficiency of thiamine. It is seen most commonly in developed countries in individuals with alcohol dependence, usually in association with a poor nutritional intake. It is a medical emergency and requires prompt recognition and treatment.

    Treatment is with intravenous thiamine followed by intramuscular supplements until a normal diet is resumed. Oral thiamine supplements may be given thereafter. Thiamine is required for the glycolytic pathway; alcoholics may exhaust their body stores of thiamine within 2 months. In this situation, glucose administration without previous replenishment of thiamine can precipitate Wernicke's disease or cause rapid progression of the condition if it is present in a milder form.

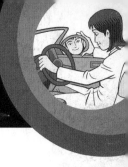

1. 1. F The CSF confirms that the patient has a bacterial meningitis, although he should have been given broad-spectrum antibiotics based on the history alone without waiting for the CSF results.

2. J The features of raised intracranial pressure combined with a progressive course suggest a space-occupying lesion such as a neoplasm and, since he is a smoker, it is likely to be lung metastases.

3. B The recent onset of the contraceptive pill can precipitate migraine in a susceptible individual.

4. E The patient has had a partial third nerve palsy with a sentinel bleed from a Berry aneurysm of the posterior communicating artery.

5. D Patients who have had a stroke often complain of a headache even when it is ischaemic and not haemorrhagic.

2. 1. H Absence attacks are rare in adulthood and often patient's attacks will disappear as they get older. Poor performance at school is one possible presentation, although relatives and patients often recognize that there is a problem before this occurs.

2. E Non-epileptic seizures are common even in patients with epilepsy. The awareness during the event and the shaking of only the upper limbs with rapid return to normality are suggestive but occasionally strange episodes can occur as part of frontal lobe seizures.

3. A Vasovagal syncope often has a prodrome of impending loss of consciousness and patients can even have some myoclonic jerking of the limbs and urinary incontinence especially if they are kept upright which delays the return of normal cerebral blood flow.

4. F Narcolepsy often presents with excessive daytime sleepiness and hallucinations on going to sleep (hypnagogic hallucinations).

5. C This is a typical complex partial seizure of temporal lobe origin.

3. 1. C The triad of dementia, gait apraxia, and urinary incontinence, especially when there is a previous history of subarachnoid haemorrhage, suggests normal pressure hydrocephalus.

2. H New variant CJD has a slower onset than sporadic CJD and often starts non-specifically with psychiatric features and non-specific sensory symptoms.

3. F A stepwise progressive deterioration in neurological function in an elderly patient with vascular risk factors suggests multi-infarct dementia, although there is considerable cross-over with ischaemic leucoencephalopathy.

4. A This is a typical presentation of Alzheimer's disease.

5. J The patient has an excellent MMSE score and is actually able to walk to the shops and call the fire brigade but is too depressed to take an active part in life.

4. 1. E Essential tremor may be responsive to alcohol.

2. D Any progressive abnormal movements in young patients especially with bulbar dysfunction suggests Wilson's disease.

3. H Most patients with idiopathic Parkinson's disease who are treated with levodopa develop peak-dose dyskinesias within 5–10 years of commencing treatment.

4. I This is usually caused by a lacunar infarct in the contralateral subthalamic nucleus.

5. C Huntington's disease typically starts with cognitive and psychiatric features and progresses to a movement disorder. Patients often have no family history even though it is autosomal dominant because their affected parent was becoming symptomatic when they were conceived.

5. 1. D A 'glove and sock' loss of sensation and power in a patient with a paraprotein suggests a peripheral neuropathy.

2. H The proximal weakness with a raised CK is suggestive of an inflammatory myopathy such as polymyositis.

3. A The previous episode of optic neuritis and currently the brainstem and cerebellum are affected making MS most probable.

4. C She has a thoracic myelopathy probably secondary to metastatic breast disease. The reduced tone and sometimes loss of reflexes in her legs is common initially in acute myelopathy.

5. G The early loss of postural reflexes, the supranuclear gaze palsy and the frontal signs (grasp reflexes and emotional lability) is characteristic of progressive supranuclear palsy.

6. 1. H This story is typical of a Pancoast tumour, which is usually caused by squamous cell carcinoma of the lung invading the lower brachial plexus and roots.

2. D Young patients may have pain throughout the arm and no neurological signs whereas older patients may have severe signs of median nerve damage with relatively few symptoms.

3. E There is often little sensory involvement and recovery occurs over months and may not be complete.

4. C   A mixture of upper and lower motor neuron signs above and below the neck is highly suggestive of motor neuron disease.

5. J   She has signs and symptoms consistent with a right C6 radiculopathy as well as a cervical myelopathy.

7.
1. A   Pure motor loss is usually due to a lacunar infarct.

2. J   Complete carotid occlusion can be fatal due to post-infarction oedema. In this example, it is probably due to left carotid artery dissection following a deceleration car accident and the sympathetic fibres are involved.

3. G   His symptoms have not fully resolved after 24 hours, therefore he has not had a TIA. His stroke did not involve all the territory supplied by the middle cerebral artery.

4. E   The posterior inferior cerebellar artery is usually involved but patients often make a good recovery.

5. F   This woman is starting to develop 'transtentorial herniation' with a false localizing early third nerve palsy and tonsillar herniation causing drowsiness. She needs an urgent CT head and referral to neurosurgery.

8.
1. A   Diabetic patients are at risk of acute mononeuropathies.

2. C   A sixth nerve palsy is a common finding in idiopathic intracranial hypertension and can be bilateral.

3. D   Ocular symptoms are very common in myasthenia gravis and are often fatigable.

4. G   This is a classic presentation of a cavernous sinus syndrome and is probably due to a benign tumour such as a meningioma, but because of their location they are very difficult to treat.

5. I   This woman has had a large right middle cerebral stroke and it involves the frontal gaze centre causing weakness of gaze to the left and hence deviation of her eyes to the right.

9.
1. C   A quadrantanopia usually occurs when one half of the optic radiation is affected – in this case the upper half in the parietal lobe.

2. A   Pain on moving the eye is typical of optic neuritis.

3. E   A pituitary macroadenoma is often associated with a bitemporal hemianopia that starts from the upper quadrants and progresses down.

4. B   The new onset of severe headache should be taken seriously in the elderly and giant cell arteritis can cause infarction of the optic nerve which may cause an altitudinal defect or complete visual loss.

5. J   Episodes of visual loss and constriction of the visual fields or 'tunnel vision' are concerning signs of impending further visual loss in patients with chronic progressive intracranial hypertension.

10.
1. J   A waddling gait can occur with orthopaedic problems, but when it is symmetrical and associated with muscle weakness and wasting it is usually caused by a long-standing myopathy.

2. E   This is the history of someone with a spastic paraparesis often associated with cerebral palsy.

3. D   Cerebellar disease causes a broad-based gait and it may be the only feature, especially with lesions of the cerebellar vermis.

4. G   Small, slow, shuffling steps in the context of frontal lobe disease is sometimes called 'marche à petit pas'. In contrast to Parkinson's disease, there is no festination and patients have no problem stopping, having started to walk.

5. H   The inconsistency of his disorder and the normal bedside examination are suggestive of an underlying functional disorder.

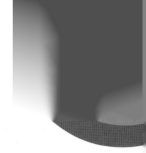

1. a. Polymyalgia rheumatica.
   b. Temporal arteritis.
   c. Occlusion of the ophthalmic artery or its ciliary branches and infarction of the optic nerve head and retina secondary to the arteritis.
   d. ESR (erythrocyte sedimentation rate) and a temporal artery biopsy.
   e. Corticosteroids, e.g. prednisolone 40–60 mg, must be started immediately. Treatment is often required for months and sometimes years. The dose of steroids is tailed down after a few months to the minimum required, to reduce the side effects.
   f. Once vision has been lost the prognosis for recovery is poor. Steroid treatment will reduce the risk of visual loss in the other eye.

2. a. • Peripheral vascular disease causing 'intermittent claudication'. The pain in this condition is usually in the calf muscles and is relieved by rest. The peripheral pulses in the leg are usually absent or reduced.
      • Cauda equina compression causing 'neurogenic claudication': results from mechanical compression of the lumbosacral roots within the cauda equina. The most common reason for this condition is congenital lumbar canal stenosis.
      • Atherosclerotic occlusive disease of the spinal arteries.
      • Intraspinal structural lesion.
      • Central lumbar disc prolapse.
      • Metabolic myopathy.
   b. For this man, a number of points make peripheral vascular disease unlikely:
      • Proximal distribution.
      • Improvement with bending forwards and ability to ride a bicycle without pain-flexing the body, the position used for riding a bicycle, opens up the lumbosacral canal, providing more room for the cauda equina and its blood flow.
      • Incontinence should always alert one to a neurogenic problem.
   c. Exercising the patient, especially if the 'claudication distance' is short, and re-examining when symptomatic may provide additional signs, e.g. weakness, sensory loss, and loss of previously present reflexes.
   d. Magnetic resonance imaging (MRI) of the lumbosacral spine is the investigation of choice.
      • If the patient presents early, without clear-cut neurological symptoms, then peripheral vascular investigations may be indicated.

3. a. The most likely diagnosis is Bell's palsy. Other conditions can cause an isolated lower motor neuron seventh nerve lesion. They include:
      • Ramsay Hunt syndrome – varicella zoster infection (shingles) of the seventh nerve (always look in the ear for vesicles).
      • Multiple sclerosis – a plaque involving the seventh nerve or its nucleus in the pons.
      • Sarcoidosis.
      • Lymphoma or leukaemia.
      • Lyme disease – *Borrelia* infection.
      • Carcinomatous meningitis.
      • Chronic meningitis – especially tuberculous and cryptococcal.
      • Mononeuritis multiplex – an unusual nerve to be involved, but rule out diabetes, connective tissue disease, and vasculitis.

      A lower motor neuron seventh nerve palsy may be the presenting feature of a cerebellopontine angle tumour, e.g. acoustic neuroma, therefore careful testing of facial sensation, including corneal reflexes, hearing, and cerebellar function, is mandatory.
   b. The facial nerve, in addition to supplying the muscles of facial expression, carries out the following:
      • Parasympathetic supply to the lacrimal gland with associated loss of tearing.
      • Taste from the anterior two-thirds of the tongue.
      • Supplies stapedius muscle – the nerve to stapedius exits from the seventh nerve proximal to the foramen spinosum. Damage causes hyperacusis.
      • Loss of taste and hyperacusis imply a lesion proximal to the foramen spinosum in the intracanalicular portion of the nerve.
   c. Usually, no investigations are carried out unless there are suspicions with the history or examination. Fine-cut MR images through the internal auditory canal may show thickening and enhancement of the seventh nerve. Further investigations would be aimed at ruling out the conditions listed in the differential diagnosis, especially diabetes.
   d. High-dose prednisolone, given within the first week, speeds up the recovery of idiopathic Bell's palsy. Oral aciclovir may also improve prognosis but this has not been fully verified by trial evidence.
   e. The prognosis is usually good. There is usually complete resolution within 3–6 months.

Occasionally, synkinesis due to aberrant reinnervation can occur. Examples of synkinesis include:

- 'Crocodile tears', when eating causes tearing.
- Eye closure causing the corner of the mouth to elevate.
- Pursing the lips causing contraction of the periorbital muscles, resulting in eye closure. For prolonged failure of eye closure, it is sometimes necessary to consider tarsorrhaphy.

4. a. Nocturnal epilepsy.
    b. A previous head injury may be relevant. In this patient, the neurological signs, even though subtle, should alert one to the possibility of a right hemispheric lesion.
    c. Imaging (either CT or MR) is important in this case.
       An electroencephalogram may help localize any pathology and provide evidence for epileptiform activity, although may be normal. Other important things to rule out are metabolic causes for seizures, e.g. hypoglycaemia, hypocalcaemia, renal failure. The commonest intracranial tumours are secondaries and therefore, if indicated, a chest X-ray may be helpful.

5. a. This is most likely to be transient global amnesia (TGA). The mechanism is poorly understood. The syndrome may be associated with migraine.
       Transient ischaemia of both temporal lobes has been postulated but there is little evidence for this. Patients often continue with complex activities, but at the end of an attack will be amnesic for the events that occurred during the period of apparent confusion. The differential diagnosis includes complex partial status epilepticus, hypoglycaemia (secondary to excess insulin – either exogenous or an insulinoma), and hysterical fugue.
    b. Screening tests for vascular disease; electroencephalography; and a 48-hour fast, if hypoglycaemia in a non-diabetic is seriously considered. Cranial MRI is indicated for short-lived attacks of possible epileptic origin.
    c. No specific treatment is required; however, one must modify risk factors for vascular disease. No strict policy with respect to driving is outlined.
    d. The prognosis is usually good. Most patients rarely have more than one TGA attack. When multiple attacks occur, it is usually due to a seizure disorder.

6. a. Tingling in both feet with reduced reflexes and an abnormal gait suggest a peripheral sensory neuropathy.
    b. The examination may reveal symmetrical sensory impairment of all modalities, which occurs in a distal pattern involving the feet, lower legs, and hands (less common), a 'glove-and-sock' sensory loss. Therefore, there will be impairment of light touch, vibration, joint position, pin-prick (pain), and temperature in the described distribution. In a sensorimotor neuropathy, there may be accompanying muscle weakness; in this situation there may be muscle wasting and fasciculations.
       The reflexes are diminished or lost and the plantar responses are flexor. A sensory neuropathy may give rise to a 'stamping' gait. The diagnosis may be established by nerve conduction studies.
    c. The most important issue for a patient who has a peripheral neuropathy is to determine whether there is a treatable cause. If this is not the case, the condition needs to be monitored and the management is then supportive.
       The approach to the history should be to first consider the most likely causes in a man of this age and then to consider the less likely possibilities.
- Diabetes – is there a history of diabetes?
- Alcohol/vitamin B_{12} – what is the patient's alcohol consumption? In this context does the patient eat regularly and well (B_{12}/B_1 deficiency); does he eat meat?
- Drugs – what medication is he taking and what has he taken in the past? Certain drugs can cause a peripheral neuropathy, in particular antiobiotics such as metronidazole, penicillin, chloramphenicol, nitrofurantoin. Is there a history of treatment for tuberculosis with the use of isoniazid? Although concomitant pyridoxine is used to prevent this from occurring, pyridoxine itself in rare situations can cause a peripheral neuropathy. Is the patient on treatment for a cardiac arrhythmia with amiodarone?
- Malignancy – is there evidence of malignant disease? Is the patient a longstanding smoker? Is there evidence of cachexia, finger clubbing, a history of haemoptysis? Primary small cell carcinoma of the lung may present with a peripheral neuropathy as a paraneoplastic manifestation of the disease. Peripheral neuropathy may occur in patients who have multiple myeloma, other monoclonal gammopathies, lymphoma, and amyloidosis. Has the patient been previously treated for a malignancy with chemotherapy; cisplatin and vincristine may cause a peripheral neuropathy.
- Chronic inflammatory demyelinating polyradiculopthy – this is a milder syndrome related to Guillain–Barré syndrome with a more protracted course; it is rarely preceded by an infection.
- Renal failure – does the patient have longstanding renal failure? Patients who have had a kidney transplant may also be taking ciclosporin.
- Heavy metals and toxins – what is the patient's occupation? Has there been any exposure to heavy metals or toxins, e.g. lead, arsenic, thallium, tri-ortho-cresyl phosphate?
- Hereditary – although the first presentation of a peripheral neuropathy at a later age is less likely to be hereditary, a family history should be obtained with regard to the hereditary motor sensory neuropathies. Acute intermittent porphyria is another uncommon hereditary

condition that has an autosomal dominant pattern of inheritance; however, this usually produces a predominantly motor neuropathy, abdominal pain, psychosis, and seizures, which may occur after the ingestion of certain drugs.

---

7. **Transient visual loss may arise as a result of:**

   a. Stenosis of the ipsilateral carotid artery with embolism into the retinal arterioles may give rise to amaurosis fugax. The patient complains of sudden unilateral altitudinal visual loss, often described as a shutter coming down from the superior to inferior part of the visual field. This lasts several seconds followed by complete recovery. The patient may give a history of transient ischaemic attacks involving the cerebral hemisphere – contralateral numbness or weakness of the face/arm/leg.

   Clinical examination may be entirely normal. Vascular risk factors may further support the diagnosis, e.g. hypertension, diabetes, smoking.

   b. Transient visual disturbance may occur in giant-cell arteritis. This is more common in women and usually occurs in patients over 60 years. If untreated permanent visual loss occurs from occlusion of the branches of the ophthalmic artery.

   Head pain is the primary complaint. There may be aching and stiffness of the proximal limb muscles; the patient may complain of jaw claudication and systemic manifestations of fever, anorexia, weight loss. The ESR is elevated although not invariably. Treatment is urgent with systemic steroids.

   c. Raised intracranial pressure within the optic nerve sheath impedes venous drainage and restricts axoplasmic flow in the nerve. In severe cases, fleeting bilateral loss of vision of a few seconds duration may be experienced. On examination, visual acuity is normal, but the blind spot is enlarged with restriction of the peripheral field of vision. The disc is swollen with blurring of the disc margin, engorgement of the retinal veins, and flame-shaped haemorrhages on or adjacent to the disc, features characteristic of papilloedema.

   Information from the history and additional clinical signs should be obtained to elicit the possible cause of the papilloedema:

   - Intracranial space-occupying lesion (tumour/abscess/haemorrhage) – focal neurological signs and symptoms including seizures; primary malignant neoplasia, e.g. lung, systemic ill health with a focus of infection, e.g. lung abscess/sinusitis/cutaneous abscess, head injury.
   - Central retinal vein thrombosis – isolated usually unilateral ophthalmological abnormality.
   - Malignant hypertension.
   - Venous sinus thrombosis – headache, focal neurological symtoms and signs; predisposing conditions – dehydration, a prothrombotic predisposition.
   - Hypercapnoea.
   - Idiopathic intracranial hypertension.
   - Malignant thyrotoxic exophthalmos.
   - Severe anaemia.

   d. The visual symptoms that accompany migraine headache can consist of unformed flashes of white or less commonly coloured lights (photopsia) or formations of dazzling zig-zag lines (fortification spectra). This visual aura can move across the visual field over 2–3 minutes leaving scotomatous defects, which are usually binocular and may be homonymous. However, transient monocular visual loss may also occur ('retinal migraine'). Aura symptoms generally precede the headache and last less than 60 minutes. The diagnosis is obtained by a history of recurrent paroxysmal attacks with headache.

---

8. a. Rapid development of limb weakness with pain and accompanying sensory symptoms in a previously well individual following an infective episode should suggest a diagnosis of Guillain–Barré syndrome, an inflammatory demyelinating polyradiculopathy.

   b. The clinical findings are:
   - Hypotonia in the limbs.
   - An ascending symmetrical paralysis usually involving the lower limbs before the upper limbs. The trunk, neck, cranial, and intercostal muscles may be affected later. There may be bilateral facial weakness of the upper and lower face; a bulbar palsy may develop later. The weakness can progress rapidly within a few days resulting in death from respiratory failure.
   - Paraesthesia in the extremities – an early feature; there may be mild variable objective sensory loss.
   - Areflexia and flexor plantar responses.
   - Autonomic dysfunction – sinus tachycardia/bradycardia, transient arrhythmias, fluctuating hypertension and hypotension.

   c. The diagnosis is supported by CSF examination and neurophysiological findings. The CSF is under normal pressure, with a raised protein content and normal cell content and glucose. There is a reduction in conduction velocities or conduction block on nerve conduction studies. The natural history of the condition is of recovery, which is complete in most patients. Significant beneficial effects of intravenous immunoglobulin therapy and in more severe cases plasma exchange have been established in the treatment of this syndrome.

   Supportive measures include the following:
   - Bed rest with careful nursing.
   - Physiotherapy to prevent the development of contractures.
   - Assisted ventilation in the event of respiratory failure.
   - Nasogastric feeding if the patient develops bulbar paralysis and is therefore likely to aspirate.
   - Treatment of haemodynamic compromise and prolonged arrhythmias.
   - Stool softeners for constipation; urinary retention is uncommon, but in this event catheterization may be needed for a short time.
   - Subcutaneous heparin while immobile; analgesia for muscle and back pain.

9. a. This patient presents with a history and examination consistent with acute meningitis, raised intracranial pressure, and a generalized seizure on the background of probable ongoing immunosuppression following treatment for leukaemia and his graft versus host disease. Patients are not immunologically fully competent for at least 1 year after treatment and are predisposed to atypical opportunistic organisms such as viruses, TB, fungi, and protozoa. He is also at risk from more conventional organisms that cause infective meningitis such as bacteria. Although an infective aetiology is most likely, neoplastic infiltration of the CSF is also a common complication of acute lymphatic leukaemia. Occasionally, patients who have received chemotherapy and radiotherapy can develop delayed neurological disease including vasculitis and demyelination but not meningitis. Acute meningitis can occur following the administration of intrathecal chemotherapy such as methotrexate.

b. The most important aspect of management is the speed at which it is recognized that he has an acute meningitis and that he is given broad-spectrum parenteral antibiotics even before any investigations are undertaken. If he is maintaining his airway, breathing normally and has a good blood pressure then the next step would be to perform a CT head prior to a lumbar puncture (LP).

If he had not had a fit and his GCS was 15 with no focal neurological signs, then an LP could be performed straight away without a CT scan. The CT scan looks for evidence of raised intracranial pressure and any gross lesions, such as abscesses or haemorrhages, within the brain.

The next most important point to note is that the patient is immunocompromised and will be susceptible to atypical infections. The CSF needs to be examined for cells, bacteria with a Gram stain, for acid-fast bacilli (TB) and India ink for *Cryptococcus neoformans*. The glucose in the CSF and serum, and the protein in the CSF also need to checked. A fresh sample of at least 30 mL CSF needs to be taken immediately to cytology to look for neoplastic cells. The CSF would be set up for culture for TB, bacteria, and fungus. Some hospitals have access to viral PCR tests for the herpes, JC and enterococcal viruses, although viral meningoencephalitis is less likely. Blood cultures should be taken before antibiotics are given, because they are often positive in bacterial meningitis and can be taken quickly. Blood cultures are sometimes better at culturing certain organisms than CSF, such as *Listeria monocytogenes*.

Serology should be taken for *Toxoplasma gondii*.

Finally, if the patient has had one seizure and is likely to have an underlying infective or neoplastic cause, an anticonvulsant should be started.

c. If the patient is managing to maintain his airway and his consciousness returns then he can be managed on a general ward. If his GCS remains low and/or he has difficulty maintaining his airway then he would best be managed in a high-dependency or intensive-care setting. This usually requires anaesthetic input. The haematologists should be informed especially with regard to the cytology on the CSF and examination of a blood film for recurrence of the laukaemia.

The microbiologists should be involved with regard to the special investigations outlined above for atypical organisms and advice regarding local antibiotic sensitivity.

10. a. Acute type II respiratory failure on the background of generalized myasthenia gravis.

b. The measurement of the vital capacity is essential not only to guide further management, but also to confirm the severity of his neuromuscular respiratory difficulties. The presence of muscle fatigability can be helpful in confirming the diagnosis.

c. The investigations should include an anti-acetylcholine receptor antibody titre, anti-striated muscle antibody, a CT chest to look for a thymoma, nerve conduction studies with repetitive stimulation to look for a decremental response, and 'jitter' on EMG. A Tensilon test may be performed if there is any doubt about the diagnosis.

d. His immediate management should be to monitor his vital capacity (VC) and arterial blood gases (ABG) carefully and if there are any signs of deterioration such as a VC less than 1 L or a rising carbon dioxide on the ABG, then anaesthetic review should be undertaken with a view to intubation and ventilation. If the patient is stable, then pyridostigmine can be slowly commenced with a cautious introduction of oral steroids in conjunction with gastric protection, e.g. ranitidine, and osteoporotic bone protection, e.g. a mixture of a bisphosphonate, calcium and vitamin D. Some patients may deteriorate, usually 7–10 days after commencement of steroids, before they improve. If the patient has a thymoma, then a thymectomy needs to be considered.

Index

Page numbers in **bold** refer to figures or tables.

305